Clinical Nursing Practices

SIXTH EDITION

Clinical Nursing Practices

SIXTH EDITION

Edited by

Sarah Renton MSc, PGCE, BScSpQ (Ortho), DipN, RN (Adult), FHEA
Assistant Head of Department, Nursing and Community Health
Lecturer in Nursing Studies
Deputy Director WHO Collaborating Centre
Department of Nursing and Community Health
School of Health and Life Sciences
Glasgow Caledonian University
Glasgow, UK

Claire McGuinness PhD, MSc, BSc, RLPE, FHEA, RN (Child)
Senior Lecturer and Programme Lead BSc/BSc Hons Professional Studies in Nursing
Department Learning and Teaching Lead
Department of Nursing and Community Health
School of Health and Life Sciences
Glasgow Caledonian University
Glasgow, UK

Evelyn Strachan MSc, PgCert TLHE, PgCert HEHP, BA, BA, DipPSN, RN, RNT, CCN, FHEA
Lead for Practice Learning
Department of Nursing and Community Health
School of Health and Life Sciences
Glasgow Caledonian University
Glasgow, UK

ELSEVIER   Edinburgh   London   New York   Oxford   Philadelphia   St Louis   Sydney   2020

First edition 1988
Second edition 1992
Third edition 1997
Fourth edition 2002
Fifth edition 2007
Sixth edition 2020

Notices

Practitioners and researchers must always rely on their own experience and knowledge in evaluating and using any information, methods, compounds or experiments described herein. Because of rapid advances in the medical sciences, in particular, independent verification of diagnoses and drug dosages should be made. To the fullest extent of the law, no responsibility is assumed by Elsevier, authors, editors or contributors for any injury and/or damage to persons or property as a matter of products liability, negligence or otherwise, or from any use or operation of any methods, products, instructions, or ideas contained in the material herein.

ISBN: 978-0-7020-7839-2

Content Strategist: Robert Edwards
Content Development Specialist: Carole McMurray
Project Manager: Anne Collett
Design: Brian Salisbury
Illustration Manager: Narayanan Ramakrishnan
Marketing Manager: Kristen Oyirifi

Printed in China

Last digit is the print number: 9   8   7   6   5   4   3   2   1

Working together
to grow libraries in
developing countries

www.elsevier.com • www.bookaid.org

CONTENTS

We are very pleased to have been asked to write the Foreword for this updated fifth edition of the classic textbook *Clinical Nursing Practices.* We are enjoying retirement from our various roles in nurse education but still have a keen interest in the role nursing has in the healthcare system.

When the first edition of the textbook appeared in 1988 we were lecturers in the Department of Nursing & Community Health at Glasgow Polytechnic (now Glasgow Caledonian University). Only a few institutions of higher education offered nursing degree programmes at that time and student numbers were small. This allowed us to be innovative in the programmes we offered and we were encouraged to try different approaches to teaching and learning. For example, our department was among the first to develop Clinical Simulation Laboratories and to investigate any benefits to students of skills analysis. At that time we felt there was a need for a nursing practice textbook that was research based and encouraged a holistic and individualized approach to care.

We have been involved with each edition since then - as authors and then as editors. Despite all the technology available, we are certain there is still a need for high quality research based nursing textbooks, so we are delighted that three current members of the Nursing Department at the School of Health & Life Sciences have taken on the role of editors for this updated edition. Sarah, Evelyn and Claire are well respected academics with vast and varied experience of nursing and nurse education. They have commissioned a team of contributors who are experts in their clinical areas and who have updated all the relevant practices and associated research while keeping the focus on patient centred, individualized care. The editors are very aware that the role of the nurse is developing at a rapid rate and are excited to be at the forefront of producing an appropriate textbook for current and future students.

We have been acting as consultants to help ease Sarah, Evelyn and Claire into their role as editors and are very happy to hand over the future development of our textbook to them and to recommend the benefit of *Clinical Nursing Practices* to you, the reader.

Liz Jamieson, Janice McCall and Lesley Whyte

PREFACE TO THE SIXTH EDITION

The first edition of this book was published in 1988, subsequent editions having evolved in response to the many changes that have taken and are taking place in nurse education and practice. The core philosophy of this book is still to encourage readers to deliver the highest-quality care to each individual patient, safely and effectively.

For this edition, we have taken on the role of editors, as we are now based in the university setting delivering the theory of nurse education and practice, rather than practising clinically. A team of clinical and education experts has therefore been commissioned to update the core practices contained within this text. They have also advised us on which practices are now obsolete and should be removed. To ensure continuity, the previous editors have acted as consultants in the development of this edition.

To reflect the continuing evolution of nursing and nursing practice, we have emphasized the importance of evidence-based practice, values-based care, person-centred care, health and social care integration and interprofessional education. We hope this will make the text more contemporary and address the wider issues that impact everyday nursing and healthcare practice.

To encourage reflective practice, the self-assessment questions remain at the end of each chapter for some disciplines. Where appropriate, certain practices are evidenced, mainly by National Guidelines and Standards such as Cardiopulmonary Resuscitation, Infection Control and Blood Transfusion; consequently, the presentation of the skill or procedure reflects this. Nursing research and practice evolve and new evidence is continually emerging; therefore we would encourage those who read this text to explore other sources of literature and evidence to supplement the knowledge gleaned here. As editors, we also acknowledge that these particular nursing practices are likely to continue to evolve within the lifetime of this edition, emphasizing the importance of continuing to seek current evidence to support nursing practice.

We really appreciate the enthusiasm, suggestions and material from our contributing team and we hope this edition will continue to be useful to our readers, irrespective of healthcare setting. Furthermore, we would like to take this opportunity to thank the previous editors, Elizabeth M. Jamieson, Janice M. McCall and Lesley A. Whyte, for their ongoing support and encouragement in developing this new edition.

Sarah J Renton
Claire McGuinness
Evelyn Strachan
Glasgow, 2018

The editors would like to acknowledge and offer grateful thanks for the input of all previous editions' contributors, without whom this new edition would not have been possible.

Mary T Ballentyne MSc, BSc, PGCE, RN, LPE, FHEA
Lecturer in Adult Nursing
Department of Nursing and
    Community Health
School of Health and Life Sciences
Glasgow Caledonian University
Glasgow, UK

Samantha Bannerman BSc, TQFE, Med
Lecturer in Adult Nursing
Department of Nursing and
    Community Health
School of Health and Life Sciences
Glasgow Caledonian University
Glasgow, UK

David Barber PgCert HSCE, MSc, BA (Hons)
Lecturer in Adult Nursing
Department of Nursing and
    Community Health
School of Health and Life Sciences
Glasgow Caledonian University
Glasgow, UK

Pamela Joannidis BSc (Hons), RGN, RSCN, MSc Infection Control
Nurse Consultant Infection Prevention
    and Control
West Glasgow Ambulatory Care
    Hospital
Glasgow, UK

Alexandra (Sandra) Johnston EdD, MSc, BN, RGN, RNT
Lecturer in Nursing
Programme Lead MSc Nursing Studies
    (Pre-registration) Programme
Department of Nursing and
    Community Health
School of Health and Life Sciences
Glasgow Caledonian University
Glasgow, UK

Helena Kelly MSc, PGCE (HPE), BSc, DipHE Nursing
Registered Nurse Teacher, Teaching
    Fellow, Programme Leader
Advanced Practice in District Nursing
Lecturer Nursing and Community
    Health
School of Health and Life Sciences
Glasgow Caledonian University
Glasgow, UK

Agnes Lafferty MN, PGCert Ed., RNT, fHEA, BA, RN
Lecturer in Nursing
Department of Nursing and
    Community Health
School of Health and Life Sciences
Glasgow Caledonian University
Glasgow, UK

Claire Lewsey MSc, PGCert Ed., RNT, SfHEA, BN, RN
Lecturer in Nursing
Department of Nursing and
    Community Health
School of Health and Life Sciences
Glasgow Caledonian University
Glasgow, UK

Louise McCallum MSc, BN, PGCert T&LHE, FHEA ENB 100, RN
Lecturer in Adult Nursing
Department of Nursing and
    Community Health
School of Health and Life Sciences
Glasgow Caledonian University
Glasgow, UK

Margaret McGarvey RGN
Transfusion Practitioner
Queen Elizabeth University Hospital
Glasgow, UK

Claire McGuinness PhD, MSc, BSc, RLPE, FHEA, RN (Child)
Senior Lecturer and Programme Lead
    BSc/BSc Hons Professional Studies
    in Nursing
Department Learning and Teaching
    Lead
Department of Nursing and
    Community Health
School of Health and Life Sciences
Glasgow Caledonian University
Glasgow, UK

Alison J McHarg BSc, Advanced Practice in Stoma Care, Cert. Counselling
Stoma Clinical Nurse Specialist
University Hospital Ayr
Ayrshire, UK

Laura Millar MSc, BSc, PGCert, TLHE, RN, RT, FHEA
Lecturer in Adult Field Nursing
Department of Nursing and
    Community Health
School of Health and Life Sciences
Glasgow Caledonian University
Glasgow, UK

Ben Parkinson MSc, BN, RNMH
Lecturer in Nursing
Department of Nursing and
    Community Health
School of Health and Life Sciences
Glasgow Caledonian University
Glasgow, UK

**Roland Preston MSc, PgCert TLHE,
BA, Dip Prof Studies, RN (Adult)**
Independent Prescriber, Nightingale
    Scholar
Lecturer Practitioner NHS Ayrshire
    and Arran University of the West
    of Scotland
University of the West of Scotland
Ayr, UK

**Sarah Renton MSc, PGCE, BScSpQ
(Ortho), DipN, RN (Adult), FHEA**
Assistant Head of Department,
    Nursing and Community Health
Lecturer in Nursing Studies
Deputy Director WHO Collaborating
    Centre
Department of Nursing and
    Community Health
School of Health and Life Sciences
Glasgow Caledonian University
Glasgow, UK

**Karen Robertson-Skene BSc, RGN,
MSc**
Lecturer in Adult Nursing
Department of Nursing and
    Community Health
School of Health and Life Sciences
Glasgow Caledonian University
Glasgow, UK

**Elizabeth Simpson MSc, BSc, RN,
LPE, SFHEA**
Lecturer, Simulation Centre
    Coordinator
Department of Nursing and
    Community Health
School of Health and Life Sciences
Glasgow Caledonian University
Glasgow, UK

**Elaine Steele BSc, PgCert Advanced
Practice**
Senior Charge Nurse
NHS Ayrshire and Arran
Crosshouse Hospital
Kilmarnock, UK

**Evelyn Strachan MSc, PgCert
TLHE, PgCert HEHP, BA, BA,
DipPSN, RN, RNT, CCN, FHEA**
Lead for Practice Learning
Department of Nursing and
    Community Health
School of Health and Life Sciences
Glasgow Caledonian University
Glasgow, UK

Morag Vickers RN
Nutrition Nurse Practitioner
Queen Elizabeth University Hospital
Glasgow, UK

**Craig M Walsh BN, RN, MSc
Advanced Nursing**
Lecturer in Adult Nursing
Department of Nursing and
    Community Health
School of Health and Life Sciences
Glasgow Caledonian University
Glasgow, UK

**Fiona Wilson BSc, PgCert
Advanced Practice**
Senior ENT Nurse Practitioner
NHS Ayrshire and Arran
Crosshouse Hospital
Kilmarnock, UK

ACKNOWLEDGEMENTS

We would like to thank our families for their ongoing support, patience and love whilst contributing to this edition of the book.

Sarah, Claire and Evelyn

Introduction to Contemporary Nursing Practice

Over the last decade the profession of nursing has evolved significantly in response to globalization and associated political, social, cultural, technological and economic factors (Ergin & Akin 2017). These changes are highlighted as part of the public's perception of the nursing profession and their experiences of healthcare, and contribute to several contemporary healthcare developments, including those outlined here. This chapter will therefore highlight the importance of contemporary nursing practice by offering an overview of:

- evidence-based practice
- values-based care
- person-centred care
- health and social care integration
- interprofessional education.

EVIDENCE-BASED PRACTICE

The evolution of healthcare and healthcare practice has led to an increasing demand for the delivery of safe, effective, person-centred care (Scottish Government 2010). Furthermore, increasing financial constraints nationally means that there is a demand for care that is also cost-effective at the point of delivery. The Kings Fund (2015, p. 3) articulates this when stating that the National Health Service (NHS) must *'focus on improving value and engaging clinicians at all levels in delivering better outcomes at lower cost'*. It is, however, an ongoing challenge to achieve these contemporary healthcare demands, emphasizing the importance of founding practice on the best possible evidence, rather than, as was often the case historically, custom and practice, and doing what was has always been done (Royal College of Nursing 2017).

Many definitions have been attributed to evidence-based practice over the years; *The Information Standard* perhaps provides a useful version when stating that

evidence based practice is the integration of best research evidence with clinical expertise and patients' values. This means that when health professionals make a treatment decision with their patient, they base it on

clinical expertise, the preferences of the patient and the best available evidence. (NHS England 2013, p. 3)

It is interesting to note that DiCenso & Cullum (1998), in earlier literature, allude to resources as a fourth component in terms of influencing the implementation of evidence-based practice. It is therefore clear that evidence-based practice is multifaceted (Fig. 1.1) and relies on integration of a variety of different components to achieve the desired outcome of cost-smart, safe, effective and person-centred care (Mackey & Bassendowski 2017).

In this context, it is appropriate to consider what constitutes best available evidence, mainly as there are, potentially, multiple sources that could be drawn on to inform care. It is as a consequence of this that a 'hierarchy of evidence' now exists to guide healthcare professionals in identifying this evidence (Beecroft et al. 2015). This hierarchy is instrumental not only in supporting the identification of different types of evidence, but also in assessing the credibility and quality of each source when considered within these parameters (Fig. 1.2). This is very important, as practitioners are increasingly expected to justify and/or provide a rationale for the care they deliver and the decisions they make (Royal College of Nursing 2017).

Positioning within this hierarchy is largely determined by research design. That is, studies that incorporate measures to minimize both researcher influence and potential errors in the research process are ranked top (Evans 2003). Such is the importance attributed to the types of evidence accessed by those providing care that the highest level is considered as the gold standard, elevating the status of this evidence in terms of care provision (Ingham-Broomfield 2016). Taking account of this, it is therefore important that those practising the skills and procedures contained within this text continue to review contemporary evidence, reflective of this hierarchy, as part of their ongoing professional development.

In addition to this hierarchy, it is becoming more apparent that care delivery is often underpinned by local and national protocols, standards, policies or guidelines; indeed, this is at times reflected in the literature cited as underpinning the practices advocated as part of this text. These documents are not developed in isolation, however, and are, again, usually underpinned by the evidence alluded to within the hierarchy, effectively demonstrating once more the importance of accessing best possible evidence to underpin care

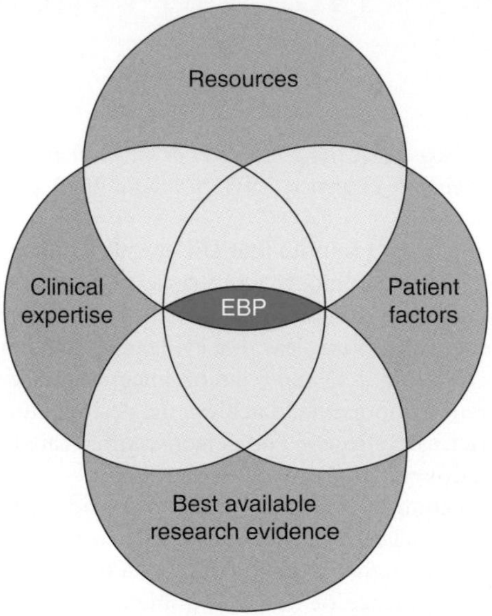

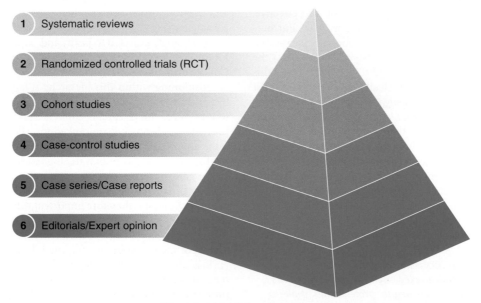

Fig. 1.1 The components of evidence-based practice (EBP).

(Nursing and Midwifery Council 2018a; Nursing and Midwifery Council 2018b).

Although dating from 2006, the definitions for each of these sources of evidence, provided by NHS Wales and shown in Table 1.1, remain clear and practical. These definitions also align with the expectations of contemporary nursing practice, in that there is a recognition that these sources will also inform care delivery in each local area.

In summary, it is imperative that those who are responsible for protecting the public act in the best interests of those in their care. To achieve this, the care delivered must be evidence-based, taking account of best available evidence, patient values and preferences, and clinical expertise. Recognition and acceptance of these components as central to practice in a contemporary healthcare setting will help to ensure that care is safe, effective, person-centred and cost-effective.

VALUES-BASED AND PERSON-CENTRED CARE

Values are important for professional nursing practice, as they influence and are reflective of professional nursing attitudes and behaviour. Rassin (2008, p. 614) considers that values represent the *'basic convictions of what is right, good or desirable, and motivates both social and professional behaviour'*. Baillie & Black (2015) further suggest that values and attitudes influence the prioritization of care and the

Fig. 1.2 A hierarchy of evidence.

TABLE 1.1	Definitions for Sources of Evidence
Document/Term	Definition
Protocol	An agreed framework outlining the care that will be provided to patients in a designated area of practice. It does not describe how a procedure is performed, but rather why, where, when and by who the care is given
Standard	A statement, reached through consensus, that clearly identifies the desired outcome. It is usually used within audit as a measure of success
Policy	A formal written statement detailing the particular action to be taken in a particular situation that is contractually binding
Guideline	A systematically derived statement that helps practitioners to make decisions about care in specific clinical circumstances. It should be research- or evidence-based

Modified from NHS Wales: Using Protocols, Standards, Policies and Guidelines to Enhance Confidence and Career Development, 2006. http://www.wales.nhs.uk/sitesplus/documents/861/Wipp%20Using%20Protocols%2Cstandards%2C%20 policies%20and%20guidelines.pdf.

quality of care provided. A consultation exercise by the Department of Health (2012) aimed to explore values for nursing, the results of which were published in *Compassion in Practice: Nursing, Midwifery and Care Staff: Our Vision and Strategy*. This vision identified nursing values, termed the 'Six Cs of Caring', to improve the quality of care for patients; these are care, compassion, competence, communication, courage and commitment (Department of Health 2012).

From a professional and regulatory perspective, the Nursing and Midwifery Council (NMC) (2018a) published *The Code: Professional Standards of Practice and Behaviour for Nurses, Midwives and Nursing Associates*. This grouped all professional standards into four themes: prioritizing people; practising effectively; preserving safety; and promoting professionalism and trust. The values and principles set out in *The Code* can be applied in any care setting, the key underpinning principle being 'to work within the limits of one's competence' in order to protect the public (Nursing and Midwifery Council 2018a, p. 4).

The NMC highlights the importance of values for professional nursing practice thus:

Platform 1: Being an accountable professional, proficiency 1.14

at the point of registration the registered nurse will be able to: provide and promote non-discriminatory, person-centred and sensitive care at all times, reflecting on people's values and beliefs, diverse backgrounds, cultural characteristics, language requirements, needs and preferences, taking account of any need for adjustments. (2018b, p. 9)

Nursing is therefore a dynamic and skilled profession that has public protection at its core. Registered nurses play a pivotal role in delivering, coordinating and leading compassionate, evidence-based, safe, effective and person-centred care (Nursing and Midwifery Council 2018b). The NMC's *Future Nurse: Standards of Proficiency for Registered Nurses* details the requirements for registration as a nurse from 2020 onwards (Nursing and Midwifery Council 2018b). These are split into two main sections: namely, the knowledge proficiencies – clustered into seven platforms – and the annexes. The two annexes are communication and relationship management skills (Annexe A), and nursing procedures that registered nurses must be able to demonstrate that they can perform safely by the end of their programme (Annexe B) (Nursing and Midwifery Council 2018b). The NMC suggests that, taken together, these will assure the public that nurses have the knowledge and skills to care for people safely and effectively across all care settings.

A number of policy documents exist, including *Vision 2030* (Scottish Government 2017); *Leading Change, Adding Value* (NHS England 2016); *The 2016 Challenge: A Vision for NHS Wales* (The Welsh NHS Confederation 2016); and *Health and Wellbeing 2026: Delivering Together* (Northern Ireland Department of Health 2017). These have underlined the value of preparing a workforce that is ready to meet people's needs, addressing unwarranted variations in care and delivering integrated, personalized care closer to people's homes or communities. It is therefore clear that being a nurse in the 21st century is founded on putting the patient firmly at the centre of their care. This includes viewing patients as equal partners in decisions about their care, and

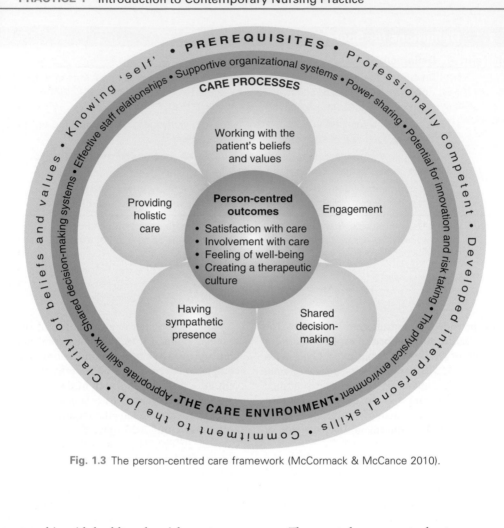

Fig. 1.3 The person-centred care framework (McCormack & McCance 2010).

working in partnership with health and social care teams to deliver care in a variety of settings.

Person-centred care can be viewed as an approach to care and is concerned with *'treating people as individuals; respecting their rights as a person; building mutual trust and understanding, and developing therapeutic relationships'* (McCormack & McCance 2010, p. 1). The person-centred care framework created by McCormack & McCance (2010) (Fig. 1.3) consists of four constructs: prerequisites; the care environment; person-centred processes; and expected outcomes. The prerequisites represent the attributes of the nurse, which include demonstrating competence, interpersonal skills and appropriate values for the role. The care environment focuses on where care is delivered, ensuring the right skills mix and organizational systems to facilitate shared decision-making. Person-centred processes include engaging with the patient and taking account of that person's values and beliefs; sharing decision-making; and holistic

care. The expected person-centred outcomes are at the centre of the person-centred care framework and include patient satisfaction and involvement with care, as well as a feeling of being valued and a sense of well-being (McCormack & McCance 2010, pp. 36–37).

Delivering safe and effective person-centred care within a health and social care system is the remit of integrated health and social care teams (see next section). Many healthcare practitioners now work at an advanced level, managing the complete clinical care of their patients (Scottish Government 2017). Within the UK, the integration of health and social care has created opportunities to review and redesign models of care to be delivered by multidisciplinary, integrated teams. The office of the Chief Nursing Officer for Scotland, for example, is committed to pushing the boundaries of traditional professional roles. The overall aims are to maximize the contribution of nursing, midwifery and allied health professionals and to improve the health of the people in Scotland. The series of papers outlining the *Transforming Roles* programme shows how nurses can develop the skills and expertise to work at an advanced level in each of the four pillars: clinical practice; facilitation of learning; leadership; and research, evidence and development (Scottish Government 2017).

In summary, drawing on the best available evidence suggests that a values-based approach is essential to ensure that the care delivered is person-centred, safe and effective, regardless of the health and social care setting. A number of policies and guidelines have outlined the importance of this approach and offer a framework for practitioners at all levels, thus ensuring best practice.

HEALTH AND SOCIAL CARE INTEGRATION AND INTERPROFESSIONAL EDUCATION

The number of people who have health problems that require both health and social care is increasing, and by 2035 the percentage of the population aged over 85 is expected to double (Department of Health and Social Care 2015; Scottish Government 2016). There are likely to be more people with 'complex health needs', described as more than one health problem, who require a combination of health and social care services (Department of Health and Social Care 2015). These services sometimes do not work well together, as it may be that people are sent to hospital, or stay in hospital too long, when it would have been better for them to have care at home. Also, individuals sometimes may access the same service twice, via the NHS and social care organizations, or an important part of their care is potentially missing (Goodwin et al. 2012). People may therefore not receive the joined-up services they need, leaving them vulnerable and at increased risk of harm. Crucial to the delivery of health and social care is the need for healthcare professionals, including nurses, to draw on each other's expertise to deliver collaborative and effective care (Annear et al. 2016). This is known as interdisciplinary working, and key to this approach to care are new ways of working and the integration of health and social care services.

Integration of health and social care services has been a goal of successive governments over the last 40 years (Humphries 2015). The bringing together of these two systems, health and social care, will allow for better integration built around people's needs. The key aim of the integration agenda is to improve care, and to do so, five factors must be considered: the quality of care; new models of care delivery; older people's needs; complex conditions; and workforce development (Department of Health and Social Care 2015). All four governments within the UK have a similar policy, based on the aforementioned areas, for achieving the integration of health and social care by 2020 (Kaehne et al. 2017).

To ensure that the integration of health and social care is effective, the use of evaluation and assessment will be essential in areas such as inspection of services; performance management; the meeting of set targets, such as length of hospital stay; clinical performance indicators; and the impact of user satisfaction or quality of life (Department of Health Northern Ireland 2011; Audit Scotland 2015; Department of Health and Social Care 2015; Care Quality Commission 2016; Welsh Government 2018).

Through developing the future health and social care workforce, interprofessional education (IPE) is key to ensuring interdisciplinary working between health and social care professions and to meeting the health and social care integration agenda (Centre for Workforce Intelligence 2013). Additionally, there is an increasing political and academic interest in improving coordination among health professionals through promoting co-responsibility for patients' needs and health outcomes (Silva et al. 2015).

The World Health Organization (2010, p. 13) defines IPE as 'the occurrence when students or members of two or more professions learn with, from and about each other, to improve collaboration and the quality of care, with the aim of generating effective interprofessional teams to lead to enhanced clinical outcomes'. Health and social care cannot be delivered exclusively by one service alone, but require the input of many services and a wide range of health and social care professionals. However, for this to work efficiently and effectively, the integration of services and teams is vital (Ketcherside et al. 2017). IPE has been recognized as important over the last few decades, and experts, as well as service users, have endorsed recommendations that IPE should be included in both nursing and healthcare education at pre-registration level (Armitage et al. 2009). Olson & Bialocerkowski (2014) suggest that university-based IPE in pre-registration nursing and allied health curricula is both feasible and effective.

Furthermore, in *Future Nurse: Standards of Proficiency for Registered Nurses* (2018b), the NMC recognizes that increasing integration of health and social care services requires registered nurses to negotiate boundaries and play a proactive role in interdisciplinary teams. Having the confidence and ability to think critically, apply knowledge and skills, and provide expert, evidence-based, direct nursing care therefore lies at the centre of all registered nursing care practice (Nursing and Midwifery Council 2018b). The standards set out the following proficiencies that directly link to interdisciplinary education and working:

By being an accountable professional, registered nurses will be able to demonstrate the knowledge and confidence to contribute effectively and proactively in an interdisciplinary team. Through assessing needs and planning care, registered nurses will be able demonstrate knowledge of when and how to refer people safely to other professionals or services for clinical intervention or support. By leading and managing nursing care and working in teams, registered nurses will be able to demonstrate an understanding of the roles, responsibilities and scope of practice of all members of the nursing and interdisciplinary team and how to make best use of the contributions of others involved in providing care. (Nursing and Midwifery Council 2018b, p. 3)

SUMMARY

This introductory chapter has highlighted contemporary aspects of nursing that will be useful to consider when delivering all of the clinical nursing practices within this textbook. The use of evidence-based practice is fundamental to ensuring that the most up-to-date and reliable evidence is utilized when delivering all clinical nursing practice. Having the right values and adopting a person-centred approach will allow clinical nursing practices to be delivered with care, compassion, competence, communication, courage and commitment. Finally, as the redesign of the health and social care system continues, the necessity for interprofessional education within nursing curricula will prepare the future nursing workforce for working in integrated teams.

REFERENCES

Annear, M., Walker, K., Lucas, P., et al., 2016. Interprofessional education in aged-care facilities: tensions and opportunities among undergraduate health student cohorts. Journal of Interprofessional Care 30 (5), 627–635.

Armitage, H., Pitt, R., Jinks, A., 2009. Initial findings from the TULIP (Trent Universities Interprofessional Learning In Practice) project. Journal of Interprofessional Care 23 (1), 101–103.

Audit Scotland, 2015. Health and Social Care Integration, Edinburgh: Audit Scotland.

Baillie, L., Black, S., 2015. Professional Values in Nursing. CRC Press, London.

Beecroft, C., Booth, A., Rees, A., 2015. Critical Appraisal of the Evidence. In: Gerrish, K., Lacey, A. (Eds.), The Research Process in Nursing, seventh ed. Wiley-Blackwell, Oxford, pp. 89–104.

Care Quality Commission, 2016. Building Bridges, Breaking Barriers. Care Quality Commission, Newcastle Upon Tyne.

Centre for Workforce Intelligence, 2013. Think Integration, Think Workforce, Department of Health and Social Care, London.

Department of Health, 2012. Compassion in Practice: Nursing, Midwifery and Care Staff: Our Vision and Strategy. Available

from: https://www.england.nhs.uk/wp-content/uploads/2012/12/compassion-in-practice.pdf.

Department of Health and Social Care, 2015. 2010 to 2015 government policy: health and social care integration, Department of Health and Social Care, London.

Department of Health Northern Ireland, 2011. Transforming your care: a review of health and social care in Northern Ireland, Department of Health and Social Care, Belfast.

DiCenso, A., Cullum, N., 1998. Implementation Forum - Implementing evidence-based nursing: some misconceptions. Evidence-Based Nursing 1 (2), 38–40.

Ergin, E., Akin, B., 2017. Globalisation and its Reflections for Health and Nursing. International Journal of Caring Sciences 10 (1), 607.

Evans, D., 2003. Hierarchy of evidence: a framework for ranking evidence and evaluating healthcare interventions. Journal of Clinical Nursing 12, 77–84.

Goodwin, N., Perry, C., Dixon, A., et al., 2012. Integrated care for patients and populations: improving outcomes by working together. A report to the Department of Health and the NHS. Future Forum, The King's Fund, London (2012).

Humphries, R., 2015. Integrated health and social care in England – progress and prospects. Health Policy 119, 856–859.

Ingham-Broomfield, R., 2016. A nurses' guide to the hierarchy of research designs and evidence. Australian Journal of Advanced Nursing 33 (3), 38–43.

Kaehne, A., Birrell, D., Miller, R., Petch, A., 2017. Bringing integration home – Policy on health and social care integration in the four nations of the UK. Journal of Interprofessional Care 25 (2), 84–98.

Ketcherside, M., Rhodes, D., Powelson, S., et al., 2017. Translating interprofessional theory to interprofessional practice. Journal of Professional Nursing 33 (5), 370–377.

McCormack, B., McCance, T., 2010. Person-Centred Nursing: Theory and Practice. Wiley-Blackwell, Chichester.

Mackey, A., Bassendowski, S., 2017. The history of evidence-based practice in nursing education and practice. Journal of Professional Nursing 33 (1), 51–55.

NHS England, 2016. Leading Change, Adding Value. Available from: https://www.england.nhs.uk/leadingchange.

NHS England (The Information Standard), 2013. Finding the Evidence: A Key Step in the Information Production Process. Available at: https://www.england.nhs.uk/wp-content/uploads/2017/02/tis-guide-finding-the-evidence-07nov.pdf.

NHS Wales, 2006. Using Protocols, Standards, Policies and Guidelines to Enhance Confidence and Career Development. Available at: http://www.wales.nhs.uk/sitesplus/documents/861/Wipp%20Using%20Protocols%2Cstandards%2C%20policies%20and%20guidelines.pdf.

Northern Ireland Department of Health, 2017. Health and Wellbeing 2026: Delivering Together. Available from: https://www.health-ni.gov.uk/sites/default/files/publications/health/health-and-wellbeing-2026-delivering-together.pdf.

Nursing and Midwifery Council, 2018a. The Code: Professional Standards of Practice and Behaviour for Nurses, Midwives and Nursing Associates. London: NMC. Available at:

https://www.nmc.org.uk/globalassets/sitedocuments/nmc-publications/nmc-code.pdf.

Nursing and Midwifery Council, 2018b. Future Nurse: Standards of Proficiency for Registered Nurses. London: NMC. Available at: https://www.nmc.org.uk/globalassets/sitedocuments/education-standards/future-nurse-proficiencies.pdf.

Olson, R., Bialocerkowski, A., 2014. Interprofessional education in allied health: a systematic review. Medical Education 48 (3), 236–246.

Rassin, M., 2008. Nurses' professional and personal values. Nursing Ethics 15 (5), 616–622.

Royal College of Nursing, 2017. Three Steps to Positive Practice – a Rights Based Approach to Reviewing the Use of Restrictive Interventions. Royal College of Nursing, London.

Scottish Government, 2010. The Healthcare Quality Strategy for NHS Scotland. Scottish Government: Edinburgh. Available at: https://www.gov.scot/publications/healthcare-quality-strategy-nhsscotland/.

Scottish Government, 2016. Health and Social Care Delivery Plan, APS Group Scotland. Available at: https://www.gov.scot/publications/health-social-care-delivery-plan/.

Scottish Government, 2017. Chief Nursing Officer's Directorate (CNOD) Transforming Nursing, Midwifery and Health Professions' (NMaHP) Roles. Paper 2: Advanced nursing practice. Available from: https://www.nes.scot.nhs.uk/media/4031450/cno_paper_2_transforming_nmahp_roles.pdf.

Scottish Government, 2017. Vision 2030. Available from: https://www.gov.scot/publications/nursing-2030-vision-9781788511001/.

Silva, J.A., Peduzzi, M., Orchard, C., Leonello, V.M., 2015. Interprofessional education and collaborative practice in primary health care. Univ. Sao Paulo Nurs. Sch. J. 49, 16–24.

The Kings Fund, 2015. Better Value in the NHS: The Role of Changes in Clinical Practice. London: The Kings Fund. Available at: https://www.kingsfund.org.uk/sites/default/files/field/field_publication_file/better-value-nhs-Kings-Fund-July%202015.pdf.

The Welsh NHS Confederation, 2016. The 2016 Challenge: A Vision for NHS Wales. Available from: https://www.nhsconfed.org/resources/2015/10/the-2016-challenge-a-vision-for-nhs-wales.

Welsh Government, 2018. A Healthier Wales: Our Plan for Health and Social Care. Available at: https://gov.wales/topics/health/publications/healthier-wales/?lang=en.

World Health Organization, 2010. Framework for Action on Interprofessional Education & Collaborative Practice. WHO Press, Geneva.

WEBSITES

https://www.gov.uk/health-and-social-care/health-and-social-care-integration *UK Government health and social care*

https://www.health-ni.gov.uk/topics/health-policy/transforming-your-care *Northern Ireland Department of Health: Transforming your Care*

https://www.kingsfund.org.uk/publications/integrated-care-patients-and-populations-improving-outcomes-working-together *The King's Fund*

https://www.nmc.org.uk *Nursing and Midwifery Council*

Administration of Medicines

There are six parts to this chapter:
1. Principles of medicine administration
2. Routes of medicine administration
3. Immunization
4. Syringe driver
5. Patient-controlled analgesic devices
6. Patient compliance devices.

LEARNING OUTCOMES

By the end of this chapter, you should be able to:
- support and prepare the patient for this practice
- collect and prepare the equipment
- carry out the administration of medicines safely and accurately
- educate the patient on follow-up care.

BACKGROUND KNOWLEDGE REQUIRED

- Revision of the pharmacology of the medicine to be administered (Downie et al. 2007; McGavock 2015)
- Revision of the metric system of volume and weight used in the dose calculation of a medicine (Boyd 2013a; Tyreman 2013)
- Review of the Medicines Act 1968
- Review of the Misuse of Drugs Act 1971, including all its amendments
- Review of *The Human Medicines Regulations* 2012
- Review of *The Code* (Nursing and Midwifery Council 2018a)
- Review of *Future Nurse: Standards of Proficiency for Registered Nurses* (Nursing and Midwifery Council 2018b)
- Review of the Medicinal Products: Prescription by Nurses Act 1992
- Review of the *Immunisation Against Infectious Disease* document (Department of Health 2018)
- Review of local health policy regarding the patient's medicine prescription and recording documents, the administration of drugs, the disposal of equipment and the management of anaphylaxis

INDICATIONS AND RATIONALE FOR THE ADMINISTRATION OF MEDICINES

A medicine can be administered by a variety of routes and for many different reasons:
- to prevent disease
- to cure disease
- to alleviate pain or other symptoms caused by disease, injury or surgery
- to alleviate a manifestation of disease.

PROFESSIONAL ISSUES TO CONSIDER PRIOR TO THE PROCEDURE

The role of the nurse involved in medicine administration is multifaceted. Therefore prior to commencing this procedure, it is important to be aware of the following issues:
- The nurse in charge of the ward, department, and unit or treatment room at any time of the day or night is responsible for maintaining the safe and correct storage of all medicines, these storage requirements being enforced by law through the Medicines Act 1968, Misuse of Drugs Act 1971 and *The Human Medicines Regulations 2012* (Nursing and Midwifery Council 2018b). *The Human Medicines Regulations 2012* is a consolidation of medicines law, which will influence the practice of non-medical prescribers and those working with medicines (Griffith 2012). Medicines kept in patients' own homes are their responsibility but the community nurse has an important role in educating patients on all aspects of their regime. The manufacturer's recommendations for safe storage and expiry date should be adhered to or the composition of the medicine may be altered. This is particularly relevant to vaccines, which, if not stored in accordance with the manufacturer's instruction, can lose their effectiveness (Health Protection Scotland 2017; Driver 2018).
- A nurse can administer a medicine only on the written instruction of a medical practitioner, dentist or nurse. Changes to regulations in May 2006 enable nurses who

are trained as independent prescribers to prescribe licensed medicines that they are professionally competent to work with. District nurses and health visitors continue to be entitled to prescribe from a limited formulary known as the 'Nurse Prescribers' Formulary for Community Practitioners', which can be accessed in the *British National Formulary* (2018a).

- The medicine prescription should be written legibly in ink, making it indelible (British National Formulary 2018b). Information given in the prescription should include the date, the patient's full name, age and date of birth, the name (not abbreviated) of the medicine, the dosage to be given and the time or interval of administration (British National Formulary 2018b). *The Code* (Nursing and Midwifery Council 2018a) details that all records are to be completed accurately at the time of, or as soon as possible after, the event. In relation to the name of the medicine, the drug name should be written, not the brand name, i.e. paracetamol as opposed to Calpol; omeprazole rather than Losec; peptac liquid and not Gaviscon.

- A nurse administering medicine is responsible for the correct administration and documentation of a prescribed medicine (Nursing and Midwifery Council 2018a; Nursing and Midwifery Council 2018b). The nurse has a responsibility to ensure that documentation related to the administered medicine is accurate (Nursing and Midwifery Council 2018a).

- A student nurse is supervised by a Nursing and Midwifery Council (NMC) registrant if working with medicines; this includes medicines management and the administration of medicines (Nursing and Midwifery Council 2018c).

- Should any error during administration or an adverse reaction to the medicine occur, this must be reported using the local health policy to allow the appropriate action to be implemented (Nursing and Midwifery Council 2018a; Nursing and Midwifery Council 2018b).

- Nurses must understand the importance of practising with and administering medicine safely. The Five Rights of Medicine Administration should be adhered to by every nurse before and during administration. The Five Rights are: right patient, right drug, right dosage, right time and right route (Edwards & Axe 2015). Utilizing the Five Rights, when handling or administering medicines, can reduce the risk of a medicine error occurring (Edwards & Axe 2015).

- Nurses must have knowledge and an understanding of the therapeutic action of the medicines being administered. This includes being able to recognize the impact of the medicine and monitor for possible side-effects (Nursing and Midwifery Council 2018b).

OUTLINE OF THE PROCEDURE

The administration of medicine encompasses many different procedures, depending on the needs of the patient. The NMC (2018b) lays great emphasis on issues of accountability for all nurses undertaking this practice. It is vital that nurses follow guidelines and local health policy when handling, checking or administering medicine (Nursing and Midwifery Council 2018b). The majority of hospital settings require two nurses or two registered professionals to administer controlled medicines (Taylor et al. 2015), with appropriate documentation and signatories to record such administration.

◎ EQUIPMENT

- Means of identifying the patient (local health policy should be followed)
- Patient's medicine prescription and recording documents
- Trolley, tray or suitable work surface for equipment
- Medicine to be administered
- Equipment for use during medicine administration, e.g.:
  - oral administration: medicine cup, oral syringe, glass of water
  - injection: appropriately sized sterile needles and syringe, disposable gloves, alcohol-impregnated cleansing swab, gauze swab and adhesive plaster
- Sharps box
- Receptacle for soiled material
- Emergency equipment/medicine for the treatment of anaphylaxis (as per local health policy; *see* 'Anaphylaxis', Ch. 8)

1. PRINCIPLES OF MEDICINE ADMINISTRATION

GUIDELINES AND RATIONALE FOR THIS NURSING PRACTICE

All Forms of Medicine Administration

- Discuss the procedure with the patient, asking whether they have any known allergy to this medicine, other medicines and/or any other substances (e.g. eggs, which are used as a carrier substance in some medicine), and obtain consent (this may not always be possible, e.g. if the patient is unconscious). Observe this practice *to inform the patient about the procedure, discuss any concerns or queries, identify any known allergies and ensure that the patient is aware of their rights as a patient.*

- Wash the hands *to reduce the risk of cross-infection.*
- Select a suitable clean surface and lay out the equipment *to provide a suitable protected work surface.*
- Identify the medicine to be administered on the prescription document. The prescription should be complete and legible *to ensure that all details about the medicine can be clearly identified on the prescription documentation.*
- Check that the medicine has not already been administered *to ensure that only one dose of the medicine is given.*
- Select the appropriate medicine, checking against the prescription documentation *to ensure that the right medicine is administered.*
- Check the medicine's name, dosage, timing and expiry date. If the medicine has been dispensed to a specific patient, check the right name is on the container *to ensure that all the relevant details are listed on the medicine container.*
- Remove the prescribed dosage from the container *to ensure that the right amount of medicine is ready for administration to the patient.*
- Check the prescription and dosage against the medicine container *to ensure that the prescription matches the medicine.*
- Identify the patient to whom the medicine is to be administered. In an institution, this will normally be achieved by checking the details on the patient's identification bracelet. In a community setting, verbal verification should be obtained from either the patient or the carer *to ensure that the medicine is administered to the right patient.*
- Administer the medicine by the right route as prescribed.
- Observe the patient throughout this procedure *to identify any adverse effects or response to the medicine.*
- Ensure that the patient is comfortable following administration of the medicine.
- Follow local health policy regarding the time that a nurse must remain with a patient following the administration of certain medicines. This is particularly relevant when the medicine is being administered in the patient's own home or in a treatment room *to ensure prompt recognition and treatment of any reaction to the drug* (see 'Anaphylaxis', Ch. 8).
- Record the medicine details on the patient documentation, monitor any after-effects and report abnormal findings immediately *to ensure that there is a permanent record of the medicine administration and that any side-effects are appropriately treated and documented.*
- Dispose of contaminated equipment according to local health *policy to prevent the transmission of infection or the poisoning of other persons.*
- If the patient has difficulty swallowing an oral preparation, the nurse may request that the medicine be supplied in another form. The pharmacist should be consulted and permission sought and documented before any tablet is crushed or halved (as this may affect the composition or absorption of the medicine). Pills, capsules and sachets should be supplied in the dosage stated on the prescription sheet.
- In undertaking this practice, nurses are accountable for their actions, the quality of care delivered and record-keeping (Nursing and Midwifery Council 2018a; Nursing and Midwifery Council 2018b).

Controlled Medicines (Often Referred to as Controlled Drugs)

Institutional Setting

The administration of a controlled drug within an institutional setting must involve two nurses, or a nurse and another registered professional such as a medical practitioner or operating department practitioner. A controlled drug register is kept on each ward or department, giving details of the stock and administration of controlled drugs. Controlled drugs should be checked (stock count) as per local health policy; this could be once a day or, most frequently, at each shift change.

- As for all forms of medicine administration, check that the controlled drug has not already been administered, both on the patient's prescription chart and in the controlled drug register.

In the presence of another registered practitioner, perform the following checks and procedures:

- Remove the appropriate controlled drug from the controlled drug store, and check the stock number against the number detailed in the controlled drug register, *to ensure that the number of controlled drugs in the container matches the number recorded in the register.*
- Check the date of the prescription *to ensure that the controlled drug is administered on the right date.*
- Check the time of administration *to ensure that the controlled drug is given at the right time.*
- Check the method of administration *to ensure that the right route of administration is used.*
- Remove the appropriate dose from the stock of controlled drugs, checking the name and dosage with the second nurse or registered practitioner. Check and record the stock number of the remaining controlled drug *to ensure that the right dose is withdrawn from the container and the remaining balance recorded.*
- Enter the following in the controlled drug register, on the appropriate page, *to ensure that there is a permanent record of the administration details:* date, time, patient's name, drug dosage and initials of the staff administering the controlled drug on this occasion.
- Continue as for 'All forms of medicine administration'.

Community Setting

The administration of a controlled drug within the patient's own home may be carried out by the patient or carer (this being the normal practice for medicines in tablet or liquid form). When medicines/drugs are given by injection, as a suppository or via a syringe driver, this is normally carried out by the community nurse(s). The number and grade of staff depend on local health policy.

Controlled drugs belong to the patient and remain within their home. Advice should be given to the patient/carer on the safe storage of these drugs. A controlled drug record sheet giving details of any drug administered by the nurse and a balance of stock should be placed in the patient's home, along with a specific prescription sheet for controlled drugs (completed and signed by the general practitioner or hospital consultant in charge of the patient's care). Nurses should familiarize themselves with local or national policy and best practice guidelines for controlled drug management in primary care (Griffith 2015).

- Proceed as for 'All forms of medicine administration' up to the guideline 'Check that the drug has not already been administered'.
- Check the stock number of drugs against the number detailed in the controlled drug record sheet *to ensure that the number of drugs in the container matches the number recorded in the controlled drug register.*
- Check the date of the prescription *to ensure that the controlled drug is administered on the right date.*
- Check the time of administration *to ensure that the controlled drug is given at the correct time.*
- Check the method of administration *to ensure the correct route of administration.*
- Remove the appropriate dose from the stock of controlled drugs, checking the name and dosage. Check and record the stock number of the remaining controlled drugs *to ensure that the correct dose is withdrawn from the container and the remaining balance recorded.*
- Enter the appropriate information in the controlled drug register *to ensure that there is a permanent record of the administration details:* date, time, medicine dosage and signature of staff.
- Continue as for 'All forms of medicine administration'.

2. ROUTES OF MEDICINE ADMINISTRATION

ORAL PREPARATIONS

- As for all forms of medicine administration, check the prescription *to identify the medicine, route of administration and prescribed dose.*

- Remove the required number of tablets or capsules from the medicine container without contaminating the preparation. Place into the medicine cup *to ensure that the correct drug dosage is dispensed.*
- Alternatively, for liquid medicine:
  - Check the medicine and dosage prescribed.
  - Identify the correct medicine in liquid form.
  - Check the dose of medicine in liquid (e.g. 250 mg/5 mL) and calculate the required number of millilitres (mL) for the prescribed dose.
  - Shake the liquid medicine preparation well *to ensure that it is mixed and the medicine is evenly dispersed throughout the liquid.*
  - Pour it into the appropriate container at eye level and on a solid flat surface, pouring away from the label. Wipe the bottle after pouring the liquid *to prevent contamination.*
  - If the medicine is a powder that needs to be mixed with water, follow the instructions on the container.
  - Draw it up into an oral *syringe to ensure accurate medicine dose measurement.*
- Identify the right patient, according to local health policy, *to ensure that the medicine is administered to the correct person.*
- Administer the medicine and offer the patient water (if allowed) *to aid the swallowing of an oral preparation.*
- Continue as for 'All forms of medicine administration'.

INJECTION PREPARATIONS: INTRAMUSCULAR AND SUBCUTANEOUS ROUTES

◎ EQUIPMENT

- Appropriately sized needles (21G, 23G and 25G) and syringes
- Alcohol-impregnated swab
- Drug ampoule or vial
- Diluent, if required
- Prescription
- Personal protective equipment: gloves and apron
- Gauze swab
- Sterile adhesive plaster, if required

GUIDELINES AND RATIONALE FOR THIS NURSING PRACTICE

- As for 'All forms of medicine administration', follow the guideline that begins 'Check the medicine's name, dosage, timing and expiry date'.

- Personal protective equipment should be worn as appropriate *to prevent medicine contact or contamination and to protect against infection transmission.*

Ampoule

- Snap the neck of the ampoule using a gauze swab *to protect from laceration by glass splinters,* should the medicine be stored in a glass ampoule.
- If any glass enters the ampoule, discard the ampoule and start the process with a new one, as glass particles may have contaminated the medicine. It is becoming more commonplace for clinical areas, i.e. some ward areas, to have filter needles to draw up medicine, which prevent glass splinters entering the syringe.
- If the solution is already present in the ampoule, draw up the required amount of medicine into the syringe.
- If the medicine is in powder form, draw up the required amount of diluent and inject it slowly into the powder within the ampoule *to enable the medicine to be dissolved.*
- Gently rotate the ampoule and inspect it for any visible particles of undissolved powder *to ensure that the powder is fully dissolved.*
- Withdraw the required amount of drug solution into the syringe *to ensure that the correct amount of medicine is dispensed.*
- Gently tap the side of the syringe barrel with finger *to move any air bubbles to the neck of the syringe to enable them to be expelled prior to injecting the patient with the solution.*

Vial

- Remove the protective cap and cleanse the rubber top with an alcohol-impregnated swab *to cleanse the entry point.*
- Insert the first needle, ensuring that the tip is above the fluid level *to release the vacuum within the vial.*
- Draw air into the syringe attached to the second needle to equal the amount of medicine solution to be withdrawn from the vial *to enable the easier withdrawal of solution from the vial.*
- Insert the second needle attached to the syringe, and expel the air into the vial. Draw up the required amount of medicine, expelling any air bubbles prior to removing the needle from the vial *to prevent spray of the medicine solution into the atmosphere on withdrawal of the needle.*
- If the medicine is in powder form, draw up the required amount of diluent and inject it slowly into the powder within the vial *to enable the medicine to be dissolved in diluent.*

- Gently rotate the ampoule and inspect for any visible particles of undissolved powder *to ensure that the powder is fully dissolved.*

Ampoule and Vial

- Change the needle to the required size for the route of administration; if an intramuscular injection is to be given, a clean needle prevents irritation of the subcutaneous tissue as the needle is being inserted into the muscle (Ogston-Tuck 2014b).
- Place the prepared syringe and the empty ampoule or vial on a foil tray *to retain the original medicine container so that a final check can be made prior to administering the medicine.*
- Identify the patient to whom the medicine is to be administered and recheck the prescription details with the medicine, container and dosage drawn up in the syringe *to ensure that the correct medicine is administered to the correct patient.*
- Ensure the patient's privacy.
- Cleanse the skin surface (if required); the policy on skin cleansing prior to and following injection may vary according to local health policy; therefore it is important to check this as appropriate. Patients receiving insulin injections should not have the area cleansed with an alcohol-impregnated swab, as this will toughen the skin over time.
- Expose the chosen site and inject the medicine.

Intramuscular Injection

Sites for intramuscular (IM) injection are shown in Fig. 2.1. Ogston-Tuck (2014b) and Mraz et al. (2018) suggest four injection sites, including the ventrogluteal region; despite its advantages, however, use of the latter is still limited. Using the Z-track method with IM injection (Fig. 2.2) will prevent leakage of liquid after injection, which may discolour and irritate the skin and surrounding tissues (Ogston-Tuck 2014b).

- Using the non-dominant hand, stretch the skin over the site; with the dominant hand, insert the needle two-thirds of the way in, at an angle of 90 degrees, *to ensure that the needle is inserted into the muscle.*
- Withdraw the piston of the syringe. If blood is drawn up into the syringe, withdraw the needle and syringe from the patient's tissue. Replace the needle and start the procedure again *to prevent the medicine being injected into a blood vessel.*
- If no blood is withdrawn into the syringe, inject the medicine solution slowly at a rate of 1 mL per 10 seconds (Ogston-Tuck 2014b) *to reduce patient discomfort and/or tissue damage.*

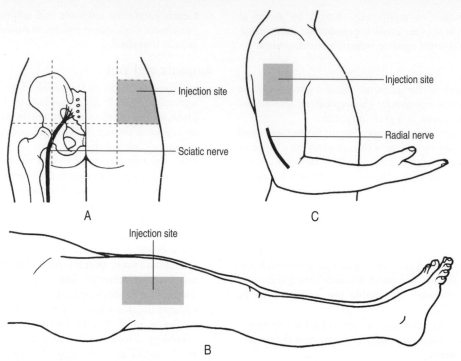

Fig. 2.1 Administration of medicines: sites used for intramuscular injection. (A) Upper outer quadrant of the buttock. (B) Anterior lateral aspect of the thigh. (C) Deltoid region of the arm.

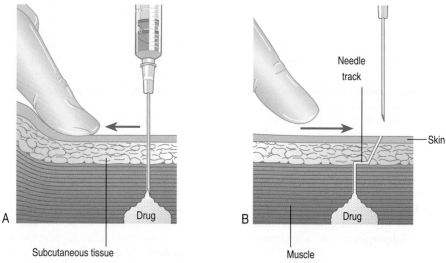

Fig. 2.2 Z-track technique. (A) The practitioner pulls back the skin, then proceeds to insert the needle at a 90-degree angle, administering the injection. (B)Once the needle is removed, the practitioner immediately lets go of the skin. The skin returns to its normal position but creates the Z track, preventing injected liquid from escaping.

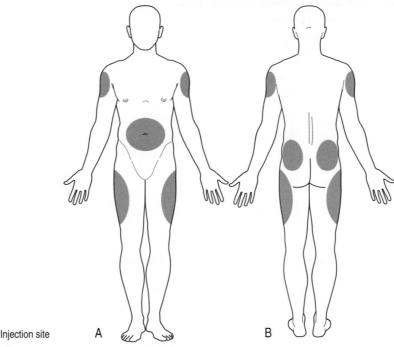

Injection site   A   B

Fig. 2.3 Administration of medicines: sites used for subcutaneous injection. (A) Anterior aspect. (B) Posterior aspect.

Subcutaneous Injection

Sites for subcutaneous (SC) injection are shown in Fig. 2.3. Use a pinch-skin technique (Fig. 2.4):

- Introduce the needle at a 90-degree angle (Ogston-Tuck 2014a; Diggle 2018) *to ensure that the medicine is delivered into the subcutaneous tissue.*
- For subcutaneous injections there is no need to draw back, as the needle size and the pinch-skin technique will ensure that a blood vessel is not targeted.
- If a patient is receiving SC injections over a period of time, the site of injection should be rotated *to reduce subcutaneous tissue irritation and maintain the medicine's absorption rate* (Diggle 2018).
- For more information on insulin therapy, *see* 'Administration of Insulin' later in this chapter.

All Injections

- Hold the needle in situ for 10 seconds *to allow the diffusion of the medicine into the tissues* (Ogston-Tuck 2014b).
- Withdraw the needle smoothly *to prevent the occurrence of a needle-stick injury;* **never** resheath the needle.

- Apply pressure to the site of the injection using a gauze swab. If bleeding occurs, apply a small adhesive plaster to prevent blood leakage.
- Always follow the specialized administration instructions provided by the manufacturer.

The nurse should always be aware of the possibility of anaphylaxis following the administration of medicines. Local health policy should be followed regarding the length of time for which the patient should be monitored following the administration of the medicine. This is particularly important for patients receiving medicines in the community. (For further information, *see* 'Anaphylaxis', Ch. 8.)

Administration of Insulin

Insulin may be given via special insulin syringes or by an insulin pen device, and is delivered subcutaneously. For patients who are self administering insulin, the pen system is often more practical, as the vial in the pen holds enough insulin for several doses. Some pen systems have a needle that is shorter than the standard one used for subcutaneous injections. A number of manufacturers advise that insulin pens be introduced at a 90-degree angle, but there has been

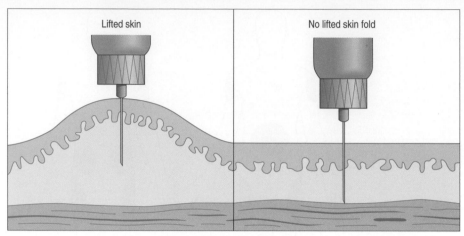

Fig. 2.4 Pinch-skin technique.

some debate over whether this technique causes insulin to be injected into the muscle rather than the subcutaneous tissue. The nurse should therefore adopt an injection technique that ensures the muscle is not injected. Patients injecting insulin should be taught the technique advised by the diabetic specialist of the particular local health authority, and local health policy should be reviewed as appropriate prior to administration of this injection (Diggle 2018).

Intradermal Route

According to Prausnitz et al. (2004), transdermal medicine delivery has been one of the most important innovations that offers a number of advantages over the oral route. However, Van Damme et al. (2009) communicate that although intradermal medicine delivery is promising, adoption of an intradermal injection technique remains challenging. This is because intradermal injection requires a trained practitioner and is difficult to perform with standard injection needles; the injection of a medicine into the dermis remains a skilled injection technique (Van Damme et al. 2009). When it is used for immunizations such as bacillus Calmette–Guérin (BCG), the nurse must meet the criteria for immunization prior to administering this or any other vaccine via this injection route. The sites where the injections can be given may vary according to the type of vaccination being administered; local health policy should therefore be followed.

TOPICAL APPLICATION

Topical application is another common method of medicine administration; this is because the medicine can be applied to a specific site requiring treatment (Boyd 2013b). The topical medicine route is used when administering eye drops and applying a nicotine patch or a cream/ointment to the skin (Boyd 2013b).

A patch is an adhesive material impregnated with a medicine, which is applied to the patient's skin. Patches should normally be applied to clean, dry skin. The length of time for which they should be worn depends on the medicine involved and the prescription. The site of the patch should be rotated to reduce the risk of a skin reaction, and care should be taken to ensure that only one patch is in place at a time, thus ensuring that the correct dose of medicine is administered. Further information on medicines delivered via this route is available from the manufacturers of these patches and should be read as appropriate prior to siting of the patch.

3. IMMUNIZATION

Immunization and vaccination are public health interventions aimed at saving lives and preventing disease (Kraszewski 2017).

Nurses working in both community and institutional settings are increasingly undertaking immunization. This may include child immunization regimes, vaccinations for travel abroad, the administration of influenza vaccines and the giving of antitetanus or hepatitis B vaccinations within accident and emergency units or treatment rooms. Driver (2018) comments that health professionals should check to make sure they are qualified and authorized to administer vaccinations.

The Department of Health has issued guidance for immunization by nurses; this information can be found in *The Green Book* (Department of Health 2013).

For immunization to take place (particularly for large groups), knowledge of patient group directions (PGDs) is essential (Driver 2018). A PGD is a written instruction used by a nurse or other registered professional, to supply and administer medicine to a patient group previously identified before presenting for treatment (Department of Health 2013).

To be considered qualified and authorized to administer a PGD, the nurse or healthcare practitioner must:

- undertake additional training in immunization
- undertake training in the management of anaphylaxis and basic life support
- be competent in the practice of immunization and be able to recognize contraindications to vaccination
- be accountable for their practice (Nursing and Midwifery Council 2018a).

Student nurses **cannot** administer PGD medicines; these must only be given by a registered nurse or medical professional, primarily because of the risk of anaphylaxis (*see* 'Anaphylaxis', Ch. 8 for more information).

4. SYRINGE DRIVER

INDICATIONS AND RATIONALE FOR USE OF A SYRINGE DRIVER

A patient who requires a continuous dose of medicine may have this administered via a syringe driver. Some manufacturers of syringe drivers also refer to theses as 'pumps'; however, for the purposes of this chapter, the term 'syringe driver' will be used. Syringe drivers permit the steady infusion of medicine, contributing to the maximization of a desired medicine effect. More information can be obtained by accessing the *British National Formulary*, available at https://www.bnf.org.

A syringe driver may be used when:

- the patient is unable to tolerate oral medicine (e.g. because of a pathological lesion, unresolved nausea or vomiting, or a reduced level of consciousness)
- adequate pain control cannot be achieved by oral medicine
- the patient's symptoms or presenting condition require that the medicine be administered via the SC route over a period of time.

OUTLINE OF THE PROCEDURE

A syringe driver administers a continuous amount of a prescribed medicine via the SC route over a set period of time (e.g. 24 hours). It may be used when a continuous infusion of a medicine is required, such as to manage postoperative pain or to control symptoms during the terminal stage of an illness (Thomas & Barclay 2015). More than one medicine may be administered at a time via this route. The use of a syringe driver to deliver medicine to patients needing palliative care is considered best practice, mainly due to improved symptom control (Cruickshank et al. 2010).

In many settings, this practice has to be undertaken by two people, although local health policy may vary, particularly in the community setting. Within an institutional setting, the medicine is often prepared beforehand by the pharmacist or doctor and delivered to the area. In this situation, the syringe should be sealed and clearly labelled with details of the syringe contents (including the medicine and diluent, medicine dose, expiry date and the initials of those who prepared the syringe). In a community setting, the medicine is likely to be made up by the district nurse in the patient's own home. Nurses must have an understanding of local health policy and know their own professional accountability and their limitations before undertaking this practice.

Different models of syringe drivers with differing operating instructions are available; consequently, it is essential for all who work with this equipment to have a clear understanding of the particular manufacturer's instructions (Lee 2014). As a consequence of the variation in terms of local health policy and manufacturer's equipment, it is possible to provide only general guidelines for this skill. These guidelines should be followed, but must be read in conjunction with the appropriate local health policy guidance and the relevant manufacturer's instructions.

◎ **EQUIPMENT**

- Syringe driver and battery (if required) and/or connection for mains power
- Manufacturer's instructions for the syringe driver
- Local guidelines for the administration of medicines via a syringe driver
- Giving set: sterile tubing that links the syringe driver to the cannula in the patient
- Patient's medicine prescription and recording documentation
- Trolley, tray or suitable work surface for equipment
- Medicine to be administered (including diluents)
- 22G butterfly cannula and giving set
- Syringes (type and size as instructed by the manufacturer of the syringe driver)
- Sterile needles: must have a glass filter if medicine is being drawn up from a glass ampoule
- Disposable gloves
- Sterile gauze
- Semi-permeable adhesive film dressing
- Sharps container
- Receptacle for soiled material
- Adhesive label

GUIDELINES AND RATIONALE FOR THIS NURSING PRACTICE

The following steps should be undertaken in conjunction with local health policy and the instructions of the manufacturer of the syringe driver. These guidelines also briefly consider the insertion of an appropriate subcutaneous cannula. Furthermore, it is imperative for student nurses to ensure that they are appropriately supported and supervised when undertaking this skill:

- Select the site for infusion (the same as for 'Subcutaneous Injection'; *see* earlier for further details); however, when inserting the cannula, do so at a 45-degree angle.
- Once the cannula is inserted, secure it with a semi-permanent transparent adhesive dressing *to prevent it from becoming dislodged and to ensure that the cannula entry site is clearly visible while the infusion is taking place.*
- Proceed as for 'All forms of medicine administration' (*see* earlier), up to the guideline 'Check that the medicine has not already been administered' before preparing the infusion. If a controlled medicine is to be administered, the guidelines provided under 'Controlled medicines' (*see* earlier) should be followed.
- Ensure that the syringe driver is functioning by following the checking procedure advised by the manufacturer and local health authority. This normally involves inserting the battery or attaching the pump to the mains supply and ensuring that the indicator light is on. As applicable, a check of the inbuilt alarm system should also be carried out *as part of any recommended safety checks.*
- In an institutional setting: collect the prepared syringe containing the prescribed medicine and check the details on the syringe (patient's name and hospital number, date, medicine name(s) and diluent, dosage, total volume of fluid in the syringe, starting time of administration, expiry date, and signature of the person preparing the medicine). This information should be checked against the details given on the patient's prescription sheet *to ensure that the medicine details on the syringe match those on the prescription sheet.*
- In a community setting: prepare the medicine for administration as per the patient's prescription sheet (note that although a prescription may state how much of a medicine or medicines should be in the syringe, a suitable diluent will need to be added; this should have also been prescribed). A label should be attached to the barrel of the syringe giving information on the contents of the syringe (date, name and dosage of the medicine, volume of drug and diluent, starting time of administration, and signature of the nurse) *to identify the contents clearly.*

- Attach the giving set to the syringe and prime the tubing with the medicine solution to ensure that all air is expelled from the tubing. This can be confirmed by checking along the length of the tubing for any air bubbles and flushing the medicine solution through until these are ejected from the end of the giving set. Attach the giving set to the patient's cannula only once all air bubbles have been removed from the giving set.
- Following the manufacturer's instructions, set the prescribed rate on the syringe driver *to ensure the correct infusion rate.*
- Secure the syringe in the driver, ensuring that the plunger mechanism is correctly positioned and that any securing straps are in place to enable the administration of the medicine and *to ensure that the syringe does not become dislodged from the pump.* **The giving set should be in the closed position when the syringe is attached to the syringe driver pump to prevent the administration of an inadvertent bolus of the medicine to the patient in error at this stage.**
- Start the syringe driver at the set rate as per the prescription and observe it for the time specified by the local health authority *to ensure that the syringe driver is functioning.*
- Place the syringe driver in a safe position (a carrying case is normally available for patients who are mobile or the driver may be attached to a pole with other infusions in an institutional setting) and ensure that it is kept away from water *to prevent the infusion set being dislodged from the syringe driver and to avoid damage to equipment.*
- The syringe driver should be checked regularly and recordings such as fluid volume length (the amount of fluid in the syringe barrel, normally measured in millilitres) documented (remembering that the checks to be carried out, and their frequency, may vary according to local health policy) *to ensure that the device is continuing to function correctly.*
- Check the infusion site regularly and report any signs of localized pain, inflammation or swelling; in the community setting the patient or carer may be taught how to check the site. If any problems occur at the infusion site, then a new cannula may have to be inserted at an alternative site for infusion to continue; this should be documented in the patient's notes.
- Observe the patient's symptoms *to monitor the effectiveness of the medicine being administered.*
- In undertaking this practice, nurses are accountable for their actions, the quality of care delivered and record-keeping in accordance with *The Code* (Nursing and

Midwifery Council 2018a) and *Future Nurse: Standards of Proficiency for Registered Nurses* (Nursing and Midwifery Council 2018b).

- Regular maintenance and calibration of the pump by the local health authority or manufacturer is essential. As part of this maintenance, syringe pump drivers should have a label in situ on the equipment, stating the due date of the next maintenance/calibration check.

5. PATIENT-CONTROLLED ANALGESIC DEVICES

Patient-controlled analgesia (PCA) is a method of medicine administration for patients experiencing postoperative pain (Alawy et al. 2018). Analgesic medicine is usually administered via a locked and programmed device, enabling the patient to administer small, controlled doses of prescribed analgesic by pressing a button (McNicol et al. 2015). An inbuilt safety and timeout mechanism helps control the frequency of medicine administration. The main administration route is intravenous (Alawy et al. 2018). The benefits of this system are that the patient is more empowered and less anxious about effective pain control. The patient is also not heavily reliant on the nurse managing their pain, which can result in greater patient satisfaction (Alawy et al. 2018).

Patient-controlled analgesia may be prescribed for patients following surgical procedures. It allows the patient to administer frequent small boluses of analgesia for pain relief without becoming over-sedated. Good pain control enables the patient to mobilize earlier and enhances postoperative recovery in many situations.

Patients who have access to a PCA device must be monitored regularly to prevent medicine overdose and to detect signs of medicine toxicity; local health policy should be used to guide this practice. Note, however, that hourly checks of both patient and syringe pump driver are often viewed as best practice, helping the nurse to identify any adverse effects as part of these checks.

Venous Access: Specialized PCA Devices

These devices consist of a syringe that is prepared with the prescribed analgesic medicine by the nursing staff. The fluid from the syringe flows through a filter and associated tubing to the patient when the demand button is pressed (Fig. 2.5). Many devices are available and the individual manufacturer's instructions must always be followed.

Patients administer their own dose of analgesia by pressing the demand button, which may take the form of a wrist button or a small, hand-held demand set. When further analgesic is required, the demand button is again

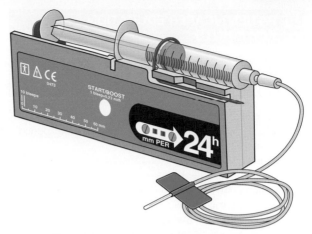

Fig. 2.5 Patient-controlled analgesia device.

pressed and a small amount of medicine is administered. The equipment has an inbuilt safety mechanism that allows only a certain amount of medicine to be administered over a set period of time, so there is less chance of a medicine overdose. The strength of the individual bolus will be prescribed by the medical or nurse practitioner after assessing the patient's pain. The amount transfused each hour should be recorded, monitored and documented, along with the patient's conscious level and respiratory rate.

6. PATIENT COMPLIANCE DEVICES

There are many types of device available to assist the patient to administer their medicines. All patients should be fully assessed before a device is given, and checks made that the medicines can be stored in the device safely. Interactions between medicines should also be checked; it is therefore essential for a pharmacist to be involved at all stages. The medicine device may consist of individual trays for every day of the week, each with different compartments for the different times of day when the patient must take the medicine; this is often referred to as a blister pack (Payne 2018). The trays are usually filled and sealed by the pharmacist, with all the patient's medicines for up to 1 week in advance. There are several advantages to using blister packs: they can aid the patient in self-management of medicine, and carers can use blister packs to administer medicines to patients (Payne 2018). However, nurses should be aware of the different patient compliance devices available. Local health policy will dictate if these devices can be used in other care settings.

PATIENT/CARER EDUCATION: KEY POINTS

Nurses also have a responsibility to provide education to patients and families if administering a medicine as part of the patient's treatment plan. This education should include:

- the risks of non-compliance if medicines are prescribed for a particular time of day and/or over a set period of time
- the action of the prescribed medicine
- the potential side-effects
- if appropriate, any potential interaction with other prescribed medicines.

It is therefore vital that nurses can provide appropriate and informed education when administering medicines (Nursing and Midwifery Council 2018b).

Nurses must also ensure that they seek the expertise of others as appropriate in each situation, in particular the pharmacists involved in the dispensing of the medicines.

REFERENCES

Alawy, H., Paxton, R., Giuliano, C., 2018. Patient controlled analgesic: the impact of an 8 versus 10-minute lockout interval in postoperative patients. Journal of Perioperative Practice 28 (7&8), 177–183.

Boyd, C., 2013a. Calculation Skills for Nurses. Wiley-Blackwell, Oxford.

Boyd, C., 2013b. Medicine Management Skills for Nurses. Wiley-Blackwell, Oxford.

British National Formulary, 2018a. Nurse Prescribers' Formulary, National Institute for Health and Care Excellence. Available from: https://bnf.nice.org.uk/nurse-prescribers-formulary/.

British National Formulary, 2018b. Prescription Writing, National Institute for Health and Care Excellence. Available from: https://bnf.nice.org.uk/guidance/prescription-writing.html.

Cruickshank, S., Adamson, E., Logan, J., Brackenridge, K., 2010. Using syringe drivers in palliative care within a rural, community setting: capturing the whole experience. International Journal of Palliative Nursing 16 (3), 126–132.

Department of Health, 2013. The Green Book, DOH, London. Available from: https://www.gov.uk/government/collections/immunisation-against-infectious-disease-the-green-book.

Department of Health, 2018. Immunisations, DOH, London. Available from: https://www.gov.uk/government/collections/immunisation.

Diggle, J., 2018. Injecting insulin safely and effectively. Practice Nursing 29 (3), S13–S16.

Downie, G., MacKenzie, J., Williams, A., 2007. Pharmacology and Medicines Management for Nurses, fourth ed. Churchill Livingstone, Edinburgh.

Driver, C., 2018. Vaccine storage and administration. Nurse Prescribing 16 (5), 218–222.

Edwards, S., Axe, S., 2015. The 10 'R's of safe multidisciplinary drug administration. Nurse Prescribing 13 (8), 399–406.

Griffith, R., 2012. Medicines law overhaul with Human Medicines Regulations 2012. British Journal of Community Nursing 17 (9), 445–447.

Griffith, R., 2015. Understanding the Code: use of medicines. British Journal of Community Nursing 20 (12), 616–618.

Health Protection Scotland, 2017. Guidance on Vaccine Storage and Handling, Version 3, Health Protection Scotland, Glasgow.

Kraszewski, S., 2017. Childhood immunisation. Nurse Prescribing 15 (2), 66–70.

Lee, P., 2014. Syringe driver safety issues: an update. International Journal of Palliative Nursing 20 (3), 115–119.

McGavock, H., 2015. How Drugs Work: Basic Pharmacology for Healthcare Professionals, fourth ed. CRC Press, Florida.

McNicol, E., Ferguson, M., Hudcova, J., 2015. Patient controlled opioid analgesia versus non-patient controlled opioid analgesia for postoperative pain (Review). The Cochrane Database of Systematic Reviews (6), CD003348.

Medicinal Products: Prescription by Nurses Act 1992, C.28. Available from: https://www.legislation.gov.uk/ukpga/1992/28/contents.

Medicines Act 1968, c.67. Available from: https://www.legislation.gov.uk/ukpga/1968/67/introduction.

Misuse of Drugs Act 1971, c.38. Available from: https://www.legislation.gov.uk/ukpga/1971/38/contents.

Mraz, M., Thomsas, C., Rajcan, L., 2018. Intramuscular injection CLIMAT pathway: a clinical practice guideline. British Journal of Nursing 27 (13), 752–756.

Nursing and Midwifery Council, 2018a. The Code: Professional Standards of Practice and Behaviour for Nurses, Midwives and Nursing Associates. London: NMC. Available from: https://www.nmc.org.uk/globalassets/sitedocuments/nmc-publications/nmc-code.pdf.

Nursing and Midwifery Council, 2018b. Future Nurse: Standards of Proficiency for Registered Nurses. London: NMC. Available from: https://www.nmc.org.uk/globalassets/sitedocuments/education-standards/future-nurse-proficiencies.pdf.

Nursing and Midwifery Council, 2018c. Part 2: Standards for Student Supervision and Assessment. London: NMC. Available from: https://www.nmc.org.uk/globalassets/sitedocuments/education-standards/student-supervision-assessment.pdf.

Ogston-Tuck, S., 2014a. Subcutaneous injection technique: an evidence-based approach. Nursing Standard 29 (3), 53–58.

Ogston-Tuck, S., 2014b. Intramuscular injection technique: an evidence-based approach. Nursing Standard 29 (4), 52–59.

Payne, D., 2018. Medicine at home. British Journal of Community Nursing 23 (6), 292–295.

Prausnitz, M.R., Mitragotri, S., Langer, R., 2004. Current status and future potential of transdermal drug delivery. Nature Reviews Drug Discovery 3 (2), 115–124.

Taylor, V., Middleton-Green, M., Carding, S., Perkins, P., 2015. Hospice Nurses' views on single nurse administration of controlled drugs. International Journal of Palliative Nursing 21 (7), 319–327.

The Human Medicines Regulations 2012. Available from: http://www.legislation.gov.uk/uksi/2012/1916/made.

Thomas, T., Barclay, S., 2015. Continuous subcutaneous infusion in palliative care: a review of current practice. International Journal of Palliative Nursing 21 (2), 60–64.

Tyreman, C., 2013. How to Master Nursing Calculations, second ed. Kogan Page, London.

Van Damme, P., Oosterhuis-Kafeja, F., Van der Wielen, M., et al., 2009. Safety and efficacy of a novel microneedle device for dose sparing intradermal influenza vaccination in healthy adults. Vaccine 27 (3), 454–459.

SELF-ASSESSMENT

1. Make a note of all the acceptable methods that may be used to identify patients prior to administering any prescribed medicine in your work area.
2. What advice would you give to a patient who was self-administering insulin?
3. What legislation, guidelines and policy govern the administration of medicines and what area of practice does each relate to?
4. What is the nurse's role in relation to patient education with regard to medicine administration?
5. In what situation would a patient compliance device be used in the community?
6. In what situation would a patient group directive be used?

Blood Gases and Profiles

Traditionally, it was only medical staff who performed this procedure, but with changes in practice, nurses and clinical support workers may also carry it out. **Practitioners should undertake this procedure only after theoretical instruction and supervision from a properly trained, experienced and competent person** (World Health Organization 2010). Nurses may be asked to assist, however, so this chapter will describe the procedure for sampling arterial blood from the radial artery.

INDICATIONS AND RATIONALE FOR ARTERIAL BLOOD SAMPLING

Arterial blood gases (ABGs) are collected from an artery and the results provide information about the patient's oxygenation, ventilation and metabolic status. The results obtained include information on:
- the partial pressure of arterial oxygen (PaO_2)
- the partial pressure of arterial carbon dioxide ($PaCO_2$)
- the saturation of oxyhaemoglobin (SaO_2)
- the acidity/alkalinity (pH) of the blood
- the bicarbonate (HCO_3^-) level (World Health Organization 2010).

Some blood gas analysers also measure levels of haemoglobin, blood glucose, electrolytes and lactate, which are important when caring for patients with critical illness.

The British Thoracic Society (2017) advocates that ABGs should be checked in:
- all critically ill patients
- patients whose oxygen saturations drop below 94%
- patients with increasing breathlessness
- patients on oxygen therapy who are at risk of carbon dioxide (CO_2) retention
- breathless patients who are at risk of metabolic conditions such as diabetic ketoacidosis
- patients in renal failure
- patients whose condition unexpectedly deteriorates with an increase in National Early Warning Score (NEWS).

Function

The function of an arterial blood gas sample is to allow for the assessment of:
- oxygenation levels
- respiratory/metabolic derangements
- acid–base status
- lactate levels
- electrolyte and haemoglobin levels
- response to treatments and interventions.

Choice of Site

The ideal site for ABG sampling is the radial artery, which is located on the thumb side of the wrist, but because this is a small artery, skill is required to access it. Alternative sites for arterial sampling are both the brachial and the femoral arteries but these too have inherent disadvantages, such as:
- being harder to locate because they lie deeper than the radial artery
- having poor collateral circulation

- presenting an increased chance of damage to surrounding structures if there is poor technique (World Health Organization 2010).

Contraindications

- Absent ulnar circulation (*see* 'Performing a modified Allen test' later)
- Impaired circulation, e.g. Raynaud's disease
- Distorted anatomy or trauma to the limb proximal to the proposed site of sampling
- Anticoagulation therapy or a history of clotting disorders
- Coagulopathy
- History of arterial spasms
- Infection at or near the proposed site of sampling

Complications and Hazards

ABG sampling is associated with several complications:
- spasm of the artery
- haematoma formation
- nerve damage causing paraesthesia and numbness
- distal ischaemia
- infection
- fainting or a vasovagal response (World Health Organization 2010; Danckers & Fried 2013).

◎ EQUIPMENT

Obtaining an ABG sample should be done under aseptic technique (The Royal Marsden NHS Trust 2015) and the following equipment is required:
- Trolley
- Sterile dressing pack
- Apron
- Sterile gloves
- Clean tray or receiver
- Sharps container
- Sterile gauze and tape
- 2% chlorhexidine in 70% alcohol wipe
- ABG sampling kit: contains a pre-heparinized arterial blood gas syringe (Fig. 3.1), a small-gauge safety needle and a syringe cap, although the contents of the kit vary, depending on the manufacturer. Some syringes are vented or self-filling while others require the user to draw back to fill
- Local anaesthetic and an additional single-use sterile syringe and safety needle, where applicable
- Container with crushed ice for transportation, if the ABG sample is going to be sent to the laboratory for analysis.

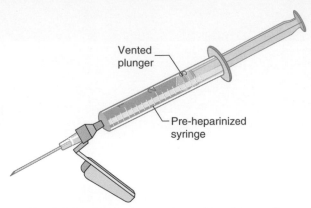

Fig. 3.1 Arterial blood gas syringe with safety needle.

GUIDELINES AND RATIONALE FOR THIS NURSING PRACTICE

Preparing for Radial Artery Puncture

The radial artery is the vessel most often used in practice because of the fact that it is superficial and easily palpated. Prior to any attempt at arterial puncture of the radial artery, the practitioner **must** perform the modified Allen test (World Health Organization 2010).

- Explain the procedure to the patient *to obtain their consent;* in certain situations, consent may not be possible due to a diminished conscious level and/or critical illness.
- The amount of oxygen being delivered to the patient should be recorded (as a percentage), as well as the patient's temperature, as both these parameters must be known in order *to interpret the blood gas result accurately.*
- The patient's coagulation screen results should be checked (if this test has been carried out) and any prescribed anticoagulation therapy noted, as this helps *to ascertain the possible risk of bleeding and haematoma formation post procedure* (Danckers & Fried 2013).
- Put on the apron and gather all necessary equipment and prepare the trolley *to ensure all the equipment is available and ready for use.*
- Ensure that the patient is in a comfortable position *to maintain the quality of this nursing practice.*
- The skin of the proposed site chosen for sampling should be inspected for bruising, broken skin or signs of infection, as this will help *to decide the best site to use.*
- The practitioner will locate and palpate the radial artery and perform a modified Allen test *to ensure there is sufficient collateral circulation* (*see* below).

Performing a Modified Allen Test

This test is performed *to ascertain that there is sufficient collateral circulation* from the ulnar artery in

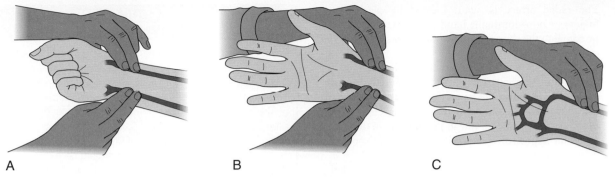

A   B   C

Fig. 3.2 The Modified Allen test. (A) Occlusion of both the radial and ulnar arteries with a clenched fist. (B) A blanched palm; when the ulnar artery is released, the palm should become pink. (C) Ulnar circulation is sufficient to provide circulation to the hand.

the event that a thrombosis of the radial artery occurs (Fig. 3.2).

- Position the patient's arm on a firm, flat surface with the wrist slightly extended *to maintain the quality of this practice.*
- With the middle and index finger of both hands, the radial and ulnar arteries are compressed and the patient is asked to clench and unclench the fist until blanching of the skin of the hand occurs.
- The practitioner then releases the pressure from the ulnar artery and assesses how quickly the skin colour returns to normal; approximately 5 seconds after release of the artery, the extended hand should blush, owing to capillary refilling.
- If blanching is prolonged, i.e. for more than 5 seconds, then this is an indication that the collateral circulation to the hand is poor with insufficient palmar arch circulation. Sampling from this site could lead to ischaemia of the hand.
- Poor collateral circulation must be documented in the patient's notes and arterial sampling from this hand **should NOT be performed** (World Health Organization 2010).

Collecting the Arterial Sample (if there is sufficient collateral circulation)

- Perform hand hygiene (World Health Organization 2018): open the dressing pack and place all the sterile equipment required for the procedure on to it *to reduce the risk of cross-infection.*
- The practitioner will place a sterile field under the patient's wrist and maintain an aseptic technique throughout the procedure.
- If local anaesthetic is going to be used, then the practitioner will inject 1 mL of 1% lidocaine close to the identified sample site (British Thoracic Society 2017).

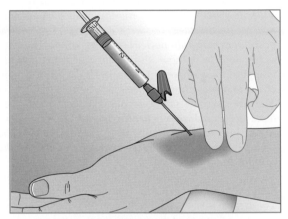

Fig. 3.3 Collecting the arterial sample.

- The practitioner will then decontaminate their hands, apply gloves (following hospital policy as regards whether the gloves should be sterile or non-sterile), and then disinfect the sample site with 2% chlorhexidine in 70% alcohol wipe rub for 30 seconds; this is allowed to dry for 30 seconds.
- The ABG sampling kit should be prepared following the manufacturer's instructions.
- The procedure will be performed by a suitably qualified practitioner.
- Place the patient in the supine position; with the patient's forearm facing upwards, the practitioner will gently extend the wrist but avoid over-extension (assistance may be required), which brings the radial artery to a more superficial plane (Danckers & Fried 2013) (Fig. 3.3).
- The ABG syringe and needle are held with two fingers of the dominant hand like a dart, angling the needle at a 30-degree to 45-degree angle away from the patient's hand towards the upper arm, and keeping the bevel of the needle facing upwards *to ensure correct technique.*

- The radial artery is again located by placing two fingers of non-dominant hand on to the radial artery proximal to the chosen puncture site *to ensure use of the correct site.*
- The needle is slowly advanced in the direction of the artery until bright red arterial blood fills the syringe, *thus indicating that the correct vessel has been entered.* The practitioner should not need to pull back the plunger, as the syringe should fill due to the pressure in the artery, but in the hypotensive patient a gentle pull of the plunger may be required.
- A minimum of 1 mL of blood is required but check the recommended amount of blood as directed by the manufacturer's guidelines or hospital laboratory.
- Once the ABG sample has been obtained, the needle is withdrawn and firm pressure applied immediately using a sterile gauze swab for a minimum of 5 minutes *to achieve haemostasis;* the wrist is returned to a neutral position *to maintain patient comfort*. For patients with a coagulopathy or those who are anticoagulated, pressure is applied for a longer time (World Health Organization 2010) *to achieve haemostasis.*
- The ABG syringe safety needle is activated and then discarded *to reduce any health hazard.*
- All air bubbles are expelled from the syringe, and the syringe is then capped *to preserve the quality of the sample.*
- The syringe is gently rolled for a few seconds to mix the blood with the heparin **but it must not be shaken.**
- The sample is labelled with the patient's details and sent immediately to the laboratory or ABG analyser, where it will be processed. Note that a delay of more than 10 minutes from sampling to analysis requires the sample to be stored in ice *to prevent the sample from deteriorating* (World Health Organization 2010).

After-Care

- After 5 minutes of firm pressure, check the puncture site and apply a new sterile gauze dressing, taping it in place. Assess the patient for any altered sensation or changes in temperature of the hand, as well as pain, *to ensure there are no complications*.
- Dispose of all equipment according to hospital policy *to reduce any health hazard.*
- Accurately and clearly document the procedure in the patient's notes, along with the results of the analysis, and inform the appropriate staff *to maintain the quality of this practice.*
- In undertaking this practice, nurses are accountable for their actions, the quality of care delivered and record-keeping in accordance with the NMC's *The Code* (Nursing and Midwifery Council 2018).

 PATIENT/CARER EDUCATION: KEY POINTS

In partnership with the patient/carer, the nurse should ensure that the patient understands the reason for this procedure, as they may be anxious about the test results. The patient and/or carer should be given an explanation of the procedure and the information should then be repeated if necessary.

The patient and/or carer should be told of the results and any implications for treatment should be explained. It is beneficial for the nurse to have an awareness of services available to support the patient, should the test findings indicate potentially life-changing treatment, e.g. long-term home oxygen therapy.

REFERENCES

British Thoracic Society, 2017. Guideline for emergency oxygen use in adults in healthcare and emergency settings. Available from: https://www.brit-thoracic.org.uk/standards-of-care/guidelines/bts-guideline-for-emergency-oxygen-use-in-adult-patients.

Danckers, M., Fried, E.D., 2013. Arterial blood gas sampling. Available from: http://emedicine.medscape.com/article/1902703-overview.

Nursing and Midwifery Council, 2018. The Code: professional standards of practice and behaviour for nurses, midwives and nursing associates. NMC, London. Available from: https://www.nmc.org.uk/globalassets/sitedocuments/nmc-publications/nmc-code.pdf.

The Royal Marsden NHS Trust, 2015. The Royal Marsden Manual of Clinical Nursing Procedures, ninth ed. Available from: http://www.rmmonline.co.uk/manual/c10-fea-0054.

World Health Organization, 2010. WHO Guidelines on Drawing Blood: Best Practices in Phlebotomy. WHO Document Production Services, Geneva.

World Health Organization, 2018. Five moments for hand hygiene. Available from: https://www.who.int/gpsc/5may/background/5moments/en/.

SELF-ASSESSMENT

1. What are the indications for obtaining an ABG?
2. Which sites may be used for ABG sampling?
3. What are the potential complications of arterial sampling?
4. Once they are analysed, what basic information do the results show?
5. What is the modified Allen test and why is it required?

Blood Glucose Monitoring

4

LEARNING OUTCOMES

By the end of this chapter, you should be able to:
- collect and prepare the equipment required for blood glucose monitoring
- prepare the patient for this nursing practice
- carry out blood glucose measurement.

BACKGROUND KNOWLEDGE REQUIRED

- Anatomy and physiology of the endocrine system, with special reference to the regulation of blood glucose
- Clinical knowledge of type 1 and type 2 diabetes
- Target range of individual patient blood glucose level
- Knowledge of the normal range of blood glucose concentration
- Manufacturer's information on the selected test strip
- Knowledge of blood glucose meters and lancing devices
- Revision of local policy on blood glucose monitoring
- Principles of infection control with respect to blood-borne infection

INDICATIONS AND RATIONALE FOR BLOOD GLUCOSE MEASUREMENT

Blood glucose measurement is the measurement of the level of blood glucose using a chemical test strip inserted into a blood glucose meter. This investigation may be carried out to:
- assist in the preliminary diagnosis of diabetes mellitus caused by pancreatic disease or other hormonal disorders *through the measurement of the level of glucose in the blood*

- monitor the blood glucose level in patients with established diabetes *to facilitate an acceptable blood glucose level and to detect abnormal levels* (Diabetes UK website)
- monitor patients receiving parenteral nutrition (*see* Ch. 26) *to ensure that the blood glucose level is kept within an acceptable range.*

OUTLINE OF THE PROCEDURE

The nurse must be aware of the theory underpinning glucose monitoring practice and have a knowledge of the normal range for blood glucose level in order for any abnormal readings to be immediately recognized and treatment initiated according to local policy. Blood glucose levels are measured in mmol/L. Diabetes UK currently recommends that people with diabetes should aim to keep their blood glucose levels between 4 and 6 mmol/L before meals (preprandial) and at no higher than 10 mmol/L 2 hours after meals (postprandial) (Diabetes UK website). The acceptable range for each individual patient (particularly those with longstanding diabetes) may vary slightly but should be identified by the medical practitioner and recorded in all patient documentation. Health promotion may be carried out in relation to an underlying disease, e.g. in a diabetic patient attending for blood glucose monitoring.

EQUIPMENT

- Lancing device
- Cotton wool balls
- Blood glucose testing strip and blood glucose meter
- Disposable gloves
- Tray for equipment
- Sharps box
- Receptacle for soiled material
- Patient documentation and personal diabetic diary (if appropriate)

27

GUIDELINES AND RATIONALE FOR THIS NURSING PRACTICE

There are several different lancing devices and blood glucose meters available in the UK (Fig. 4.1) and so the manufacturer's instructions for use must always be followed. Diabetes UK provides up-to-date information on a wide range of devices and meters on their website.

The frequency of blood glucose monitoring will usually be advised by the medical practitioner.

- Familiarize yourself with the instructions for the device you are using *to ensure correct, safe practice.*
- Check the expiry date of the test strip *to ensure that the strips are within the 'use by' date.*
- Confirm that the device is calibrated to the test strip *to reduce the risk of an erroneous result being recorded.*
- Discuss the practice with the patient *to inform the patient about the practice, gain consent and encourage participation in care.*
- Select a suitable clean surface and lay out the equipment *to provide an appropriate work surface.*
- Wash and dry your hands *to reduce the risk of cross-infection.*
- Ask or assist the patient to wash their hands with soap and warm water, ensuring that all traces of soap have been rinsed off and that the hands are dried thoroughly *to ensure that the skin surface is clean and free of any sugars that may be present on the patient's fingers and that there is no residual soap, which may affect the accuracy of the reading.* Using warm water will also help to dilate the small blood vessels in the fingertips, making it easier to obtain blood.
- The patient's finger should not be cleansed with an alcohol-saturated wipe *to prevent the alcohol from contaminating the specimen. The use of alcohol wipes can cause the skin to harden with constant use.*
- Any test strip accidentally contaminated by the nurse or patient must be discarded, as *contamination of the test pad or the patient's blood could lead to inaccurate results.*

- Help the patient into a comfortable position (either sitting or lying supine) *to ensure patient comfort and prevent injury in the event that the patient feels faint during the procedure.*
- Select an appropriate puncture site (normally the soft flesh at either side of the top of the finger). If blood glucose monitoring is a regular practice, the site should be rotated *to avoid overuse of any one site and thus reduce discomfort for the patient.* The World Health Organization (2010) recommends the use of the middle or ring finger for glucose monitoring (Diabetes UK website). Where frequent blood glucose monitoring is required in an acutely ill patient, the earlobe may be a viable alternative site (Anzalone 2008).
- Put on gloves *to protect the patient and yourself from potential blood-borne infection.*
- Using the lancing device, prick the patient's finger *to pierce the skin with minimal discomfort.*
- Gently squeeze the finger to obtain an adequate amount of blood. *Obtain a suitable amount of blood to cover the test strip. Squeezing the finger tightly should be avoided, as it may dilute the specimen with plasma from the tissue and is likely to cause haemolysis* (World Health Organization 2010). If the finger needs to be squeezed hard, consider lancing the finger again.
- Allow the drop of blood to come into contact with the test strip as per the manufacturer's instructions, without smearing and spreading the blood, *to ensure even coverage of the strip.*
- Continue as per the manufacturer's instructions for the specific device in use.
- Apply a clean cotton wool ball with firm pressure to the skin site for approximately 30–60 seconds or until bleeding has stopped (the patient may be able to undertake this activity) *to prevent any further bleeding after the sample has been obtained and prevent haematoma formation.*
- Read the result on the glucose meter device *to obtain the blood glucose level.*

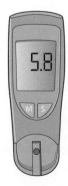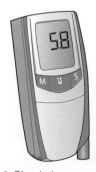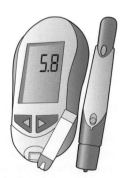

Fig. 4.1 Blood glucose monitoring devices.

- Dispose of contaminated equipment according to local policy *to prevent cross-infection.*
- Remove and dispose of the gloves and wash your hands *to prevent cross-infection.*
- Note and document the results in both the nursing/medical notes and the patient's personal diabetic diary (where applicable). Some meters can store results in the memory. The patient is normally informed of the result *to ensure that they are aware of their condition and to encourage participation in care.*
- The result must also be communicated to the medical practitioner who requested the test *to inform subsequent treatment.*
- Any abnormal results must be reported to a medical practitioner immediately. If the practice is being carried out in the patient's own home, the nurse may be required to remain with the patient until the blood glucose level has stabilized *to ensure that prompt and appropriate treatment is initiated. There may be a local protocol to be followed when abnormal glucose readings are detected by nursing staff.*
- Ensure that the patient is feeling comfortable and well after the practice (especially if the practice has been carried out in the patient's own home) *to ensure that any potential complications of the procedure are addressed promptly.*
- Discuss the points raised under 'Patient/carer education: key points' later. If the patient is unable to participate in follow-up self-care, this should be undertaken by the nurse or an appropriate adult carer *to ensure that the patient, carer and/or nurse are aware of, and understand, follow-up self-care.*
- In undertaking this practice, nurses are personally and professionally accountable for their actions, and for the safety, quality, assessment, evaluation and documentation of care delivered (Nursing and Midwifery Council 2018a; Nursing and Midwifery Council 2018b).

ADDITIONAL INFORMATION

- All test strips should be stored in a locked cupboard or drawer when not in use, in order to comply with health and safety at work regulations. The nurse in the community should encourage patients to keep all equipment in a safe place away from children. The manufacturer's recommendations for the conditions of storage and blood glucose monitoring technique must be observed; otherwise, inaccurate results may be obtained from the glucose meters.
- It is advisable to record the date when the strips were opened, as these may need to be used within a given timeframe. Regular checking of the glucose meter device

with the control solution provided by the manufacturer is recommended (Diabetes UK website).
- The nurse should assess the blood glucose level at the specific time requested by the medical practitioner. This is dependent on the type of diabetes, the treatment regime and the patient's experience. The use of blood glucose diaries can be useful to help the nurse, medical staff, patient and carers spot trends and build up a profile over time.

 PATIENT/CARER EDUCATION: KEY POINTS

In partnership with the patient and/or carer, ensure that they are competent to carry out any practices required. Information should be given on an appropriate point of contact for any concerns that may arise.

Diabetes UK has a wide range of educational materials on its website.

If the blood glucose results are not disclosed to the patient immediately after undertaking the practice, the patient should be informed of when they will be available and of the process for obtaining them.

For newly diagnosed diabetic patients, the teaching of blood glucose estimation should be part of an individual education package on disease and symptom management. Teaching the patient about blood glucose estimation should incorporate the following main stages:

- education on the practice (including the rationale and the treatment of any abnormal readings) using verbal and written information
- demonstration of the blood glucose monitoring technique
- supervision of the patient carrying out blood glucose estimation
- regular monitoring of the technique as part of the ongoing management programme of care for the patient with diabetes.

Patient education is likely to be shared between hospital, clinic and community staff.

Patient education material is available from many of the manufacturers who produce test strips and glucose meters, and from the Diabetes UK website.

Hospitalized insulin-dependent diabetics who are self-caring in this practice should be encouraged to continue self-testing, as this provides an opportunity to assess their technique and reinforce good practice.

An opportunity should be given for the patient and/or carer to discuss anxieties or issues concerning any newly diagnosed disease.

REFERENCES

Anzalone, P., 2008. Equivalence of earlobe site blood glucose testing with finger stick. Clinical Nursing Research 17 (4), 251–261.

Nursing and Midwifery Council, 2018a. The Code: Professional Standards of Practice and Behaviour for Nurses, Midwives and Nursing Associates. London: NMC. Available at: https://www.nmc.org.uk/globalassets/sitedocuments/nmc-publications/nmc-code.pdf.

Nursing and Midwifery Council, 2018b. Future Nurse: Standards of Proficiency for Registered Nurses. London: NMC. Available at: https://www.nmc.org.uk/globalassets/sitedocuments/education-standards/future-nurse-proficiencies.pdf.

World Health Organization, 2010. WHO Guidelines on Drawing Blood. WHO, Geneva.

WEBSITES

https://www.diabetes.co.uk/ *Diabetes UK*

https://www.diabetes.co.uk/blood-glucose/how-to-test-blood-glucose-levels.html *Diabetes UK How to test your blood glucose*

https://www.diabetes.co.uk/diabetes_care/blood_glucose_monitor_guide.html *Diabetes UK Blood glucose meter guide*

https://www.diabetes.org.uk/guide-to-diabetes/managing-your-diabetes/testing *Diabetes UK Diabetes and checking your blood sugars*

? SELF-ASSESSMENT

1. What are the recommended ranges for normal blood glucose in healthy adults?
2. What part of the finger should you use for obtaining a sample of blood?
3. What action should you take if an abnormal blood glucose result is returned?
4. What patient education should you give a diabetic patient when teaching them to monitor their blood glucose level independently?

5

Pulse and Blood Pressure

There are two parts to this chapter:
1. Pulse
2. Blood pressure.

1. PULSE

INDICATIONS AND RATIONALE FOR ASSESSING THE PULSE

The pulse is described as the alternating expansion and recoil of the arteries following each contraction of the left ventricle (systole) as part of the cardiac cycle (Tortora & Derrickson 2017). The contraction of the heart creates a pressure wave that may be detected by manual palpation where the artery passes over a bony prominence and is close to the skin surface, known as a pulse point. There are a number of pulse points throughout the body; however, as the radial artery at the wrist is easily accessible, this is the most frequently checked in clinical practice (Marieb & Hoehn 2010). Fig. 5.1 shows some of the most commonly used pulse points.

Three important aspects are considered when assessing a patient's pulse: rate, rhythm and quality (also known as strength/amplitude).

Automated machines, such as blood pressure monitors and pulse oximeters, are able to give the pulse rate but often do not provide other important information, such as the rhythm and quality of the pulse. Alexis (2010) highlights that nurses should not always rely on automated machines to provide an accurate recording of vital patient observations and that they must have the required skills and knowledge to assess, measure and record the pulse correctly by manual means. This is further supported by the Nursing and Midwifery Council (NMC) (2018a), which requires all nurses to be competent in measuring, recording and interpreting vital signs both manually and through the use of technological devices.

The pulse may be assessed for a number of reasons, including:

- On admission to hospital or on enrolment to a service, *to establish a baseline and to ascertain if this falls within the normal range for the person's age.*
- Preoperatively or prior to an invasive procedure, *to ascertain the patient's baseline heart rate, rhythm and quality so that comparisons can be made postoperatively or post procedure.*
- Postoperatively or post procedure, *to monitor the rate, rhythm and quality as vital indicators of the patient's cardiovascular and general clinical stability.*
- *To help estimate, in general terms, the degree of fluid loss when circulating blood volume is reduced,* e.g. in excessive vomiting, diarrhoea, dehydration or haemorrhage. With severe fluid loss the pulse is thready and rapid.
- *To obtain information about the overall health and well-being of the individual,* as part of a holistic assessment, which should also consider the general appearance

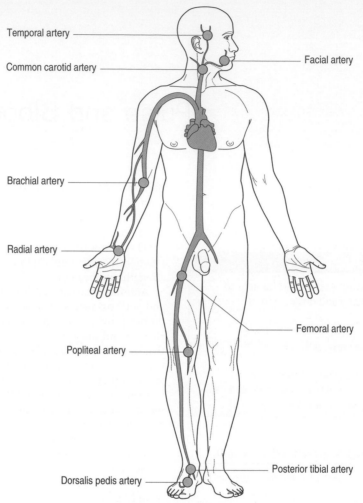

Fig. 5.1 Locating the pulse. From Trim J: 2005 Monitoring pulse. Nursing Times 101(21):30–31. Copyright Emap Public Sector Ltd 2005. Reproduced with the permission of Nursing Times.

of the patient, along with the feel and colour of their skin.

- As part of the cardiovascular assessment, *to obtain an overview of cardiovascular status and detect abnormalities*.
- *To assess the response to an intervention or medication* (e.g. to assess a patient's response to being given a beta-blocker).
- To monitor a patient during the administration of a treatment, e.g. during a blood transfusion, *to detect and respond to any signs of deterioration or adverse reaction promptly.*
- *To assess blood supply to specific areas of the body where there is evidence of peripheral vascular disease or risk*

of comprised circulation, e.g. checking pedal pulses in a patient who has a femoral line in situ.

CHARACTERISTICS OF THE PULSE

All three characteristics of the pulse – rate, rhythm and quality – should be assessed when taking a patient's pulse. Any changes in these should be compared to the patient's baseline or expected observations. Taking the patient's pulse is a fundamental observation, which should be part of a structured and holistic patient assessment. Any concerns in relation to the pulse rate, rhythm or quality should be recorded and reported to senior nursing or medical staff.

Rate

The heart rate should be obtained by counting the pulse over a timed 60-second period. The nurse should have knowledge of the normal ranges and be able to act accordingly if any results are a cause for concern.

The resting pulse varies, depending on a number of factors, including age, level of cardiovascular fitness and emotions. Despite variations in normal pulse rate, it is generally accepted that the average resting pulse rate is between 60 and 80 beats per minute (bpm) in a healthy adult or adolescent (Donaldson & Ness 2009).

Individuals with a pulse rate below 60 bpm are considered to be bradycardic (slow pulse), while those with a pulse rate above 100 bpm are considered to be tachycardic (fast pulse).

Tachycardia can be the result of pain, anger, fear or anxiety, all of which stimulate the sympathetic nervous system and cause the release of adrenaline (epinephrine). Additionally, a number of cardiac conditions, raised body temperature and certain drugs can all elevate the pulse (Marieb & Hoehn 2010). Furthermore, the pulse will be elevated during exercise, as part of the physiological response to the increased oxygen demands of the body (Tortora & Derrickson 2017).

Bradycardia (a slow pulse rate) occurs in any condition that stimulates the parasympathetic nervous system, such as raised intracranial pressure. Specific heart conditions, such as damage to the conducting mechanism after a myocardial infarction, can also cause bradycardia. It also occurs in athletes, who develop a very efficient heart muscle action. Bradycardia can also occur as a result of taking certain medications, such as digoxin and beta-blockers.

The National Early Warning Score (NEWS) (Royal College of Physicians 2017) identifies a pulse rate of 50 bpm and below, or above 91 bpm, as being outside the normal range and these are therefore considered to be 'trigger points' for increased monitoring or action, as appropriate, to maintain patient safety.

Rhythm

When the pulse is manually checked, the heart rhythm is assessed through the sequence of beats detected by the fingers and the regularity, or pattern, of these. There are a range of different cardiac conduction defects that give rise to cardiac arrhythmias and an irregular pulse. It is important to recognize that an abnormality in a patient's heart rhythm should be investigated to establish if this is new or is a cause for concern. Normally an electrocardiogram should be performed and this should be discussed with medical staff. When assessing a patient's heart rhythm through taking the manual pulse, the nurse should first establish if this is regular or irregular. If irregular, then consider whether the irregularities are occurring at regular intervals or irregular intervals.

It is important to acknowledge that in younger patients (under 40 years), irregularity is often linked to the respiratory pattern, with heart rate increasing on inspiration and decreasing on expiration; this is considered to be normal and is known as 'sinus arrhythmia' (Woods et al. 2009).

Quality

This refers to the strength (or amplitude) of each detected pulse and the elasticity of the arterial wall as the contraction travels through it. There can be fluctuations in these factors, reflecting alternating 'weak' and 'strong' contractions of the heart (Bickley et al. 2017). It is important to be able to recognize significant changes in the quality of the pulse; for example, a faint, thready pulse may be present in a profoundly hypovolaemic patient (shock), while a strong, bounding, irregular pulse may be present in an individual experiencing palpitations (Dougherty & Lister 2015).

OUTLINE OF THE PROCEDURE

The pulse can be felt by placing one, two or three fingers over any artery lying close to the skin surface; suitable arteries are easier to detect over underlying firm tissue or bony prominences (pulse points). Nurses should be aware that the thumb has a pulse, which can be misinterpreted as the patient's own pulse, leading to inaccuracy, and should therefore not be used (Dougherty & Lister 2015).

 EQUIPMENT

- Watch or digital counter that can count seconds
- NEWS observation chart
- Black pen

GUIDELINES AND RATIONALE FOR THIS NURSING PRACTICE

- Explain the nursing practice to the patient **to obtain informed consent and cooperation** (Nursing and Midwifery Council 2018b).
- Wash your hands with suitable liquid soap and warm water, and dry thoroughly; alternatively, decontaminate with alcohol gel **to reduce the risk of cross-infection** (National Institute for Health and Care Excellence 2014).
- Ensure that the patient is in a comfortable and relaxed position. Ideally the patient should refrain from physical activity for 20 minutes before the pulse is assessed (Dougherty & Lister 2015), **to help the nurse to gain a true baseline measurement.**

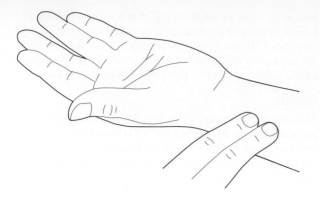

Fig. 5.2 Taking a radial pulse. From Trim J: 2005 Monitoring pulse. Nursing Times 101(21):30–31. Copyright Emap Public Sector Ltd 2005. Reproduced with the permission of Nursing Times.

- Observe the patient throughout this activity *to note any signs of distress.*
- Locate one of the pulse points (identified in Fig. 5.1); most commonly the radial pulse is used. The radial artery runs along the lateral (outer) aspect of the anterior forearm and can be felt most clearly just at the wrist crease (Fig. 5.2).
- Place the first and second (and, if preferred, third) fingers along the artery and apply sufficient pressure *to allow the pulse of blood passing through the artery to be detected by your fingers* without fully occluding the artery (Fig. 5.2).
- Once a pulse has been detected, begin counting each pulse felt for a total of 60 seconds; a watch or digital timer should be used to establish a 60-second period accurately. *Recording the pulse for a full minute allows sufficient time to detect any irregularities or other defects.*
- If you are unable to locate the radial pulse, then an alternative pulse point, such as the brachial or carotid pulse, can be checked.
- Document the findings carefully, as set out by local protocol and in accordance with your responsibilities for accurate record-keeping as a nurse (Nursing and Midwifery Council 2018b). This may be in the NEWS chart. Seek advice on any findings that are outside the patient's normal or expected parameters *to ensure patient safety in line with your NMC requirements* (Nursing and Midwifery Council 2018b).
- Ensure the patient is left feeling comfortable and wash your hands in line with local policy *to reduce the risk of cross-infection.*

2. BLOOD PRESSURE

INDICATIONS AND RATIONALE FOR MEASURING BLOOD PRESSURE

Blood pressure is the hydrostatic pressure exerted on the inner walls of blood vessels and is generated by the contraction of the ventricles of the heart (Tortora & Derrickson 2017). The systolic blood pressure occurs during ventricular systole (contraction of the ventricles) and is represented by the top figure in a standard blood pressure recording; the diastolic blood pressure relates to pressure at the end of diastole (relaxation of the ventricles) and is represented by the bottom figure in the blood pressure reading.

The measurement of blood pressure is essential to monitor a patient's cardiovascular status and haemodynamic stability, and is recognized as being a key component in identifying the deteriorating patient (Unsworth et al. 2015). Furthermore, it is argued that all nurses, across all fields, should be able to measure and record blood pressure accurately and to respond appropriately. This is endorsed by the NMC (Nursing and Midwifery Council 2018a), which requires all nurses to be competent in measuring, recording and interpreting vital signs both manually and through the use of technological devices.

Reasons for measuring blood pressure may include:
- to aid in the diagnosis of disease
- to aid in the assessment of the cardiovascular system during and after illness
- to assess the efficacy of antihypertensive (blood pressure–lowering) medication
- preoperatively, to assess the patient's usual range of blood pressure (as a baseline)
- to aid in the assessment of the cardiovascular system and haemodynamic stability following medication, surgery or trauma, or during pregnancy.

◎ EQUIPMENT

- Sphygmomanometer: manual aneroid auscultatory device (Fig. 5.3A) or electronic oscillometric device (Fig. 5.3B)
- Blood pressure cuff: different-sized cuffs are available for use on a baby, a child or an obese person
- Stethoscope: for use with a manual device only
- Alcohol-impregnated swabs to clean stethoscope ear-pieces and diaphragm
- NEWS observation chart
- Black pen

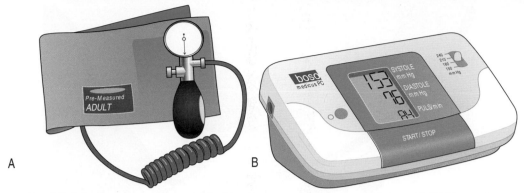

Fig. 5.3 Sphygmomanometers used for blood pressure measurement. (A) Aneroid. (B) Electronic.

GUIDELINES AND RATIONALE FOR THIS NURSING PRACTICE

- Explain the nursing practice to the patient *to gain consent and cooperation.*
- Wash your hands *to reduce the risk of cross-infection.*
- Ensure the patient's privacy *to reduce anxiety and/or embarrassment.*
- Select the most appropriately sized blood pressure cuff available *to ensure accuracy in the measurement* (consult the manufacturer's guidelines for a sizing chart).
- Collect the equipment, ensuring that this is cleaned both before and after the procedure (as per local policy), *to assist in the planning and implementation of the practice and to reduce the risk of cross-infection.*
- Observe the patient throughout the nursing practice *to note any signs of distress.*
- Help the patient into a suitable position, either sitting or lying; the legs should be uncrossed with both feet on the ground if sitting, and any restrictive clothing should be removed from the arm. The patient's arm should be supported *to ensure accuracy in the measurement and to maintain patient comfort.*
- Ensure that the patient is reassured, comfortable and rested prior to beginning the procedure, *as factors such as anxiety and recent exertion (e.g. rushing to a clinic appointment) can increase blood pressure.* The patient should be allowed to rest for at least 5 minutes in the above position before the procedure is begun (British and Irish Hypertension Society 2017).
- A quiet, relaxed location at normal room temperature should be provided, *as these factors can affect the accuracy of the blood pressure recording* (National Institute for Health and Care Excellence 2011).
- Ideally the patient should have refrained from smoking, eating or taking caffeine for 30 minutes prior to the procedure (National Institute for Health and Care Excellence 2011). Ask the patient to remain quiet when the measurement is taken, as talking can also influence the blood pressure. *These factors can affect the accuracy of the blood pressure recording.*
- In most circumstances, blood pressure can be checked on either arm, although on occasion there may be significant differences recorded between the patient's left and right arms. When a diagnosis of hypertension (high blood pressure) is being considered, the National Institute for Health and Care Excellence (2011) advises that blood pressure is measured in both arms. There are, however, some important reasons why blood pressure should be checked only in either the right arm or the left arm for some patients. For example, the Royal College of Nursing (2011) warns that, unless it is a medical emergency, blood pressure checks (and venepuncture) should be avoided in the 'at risk' arm of a patient following mastectomy, on the affected side of their body, due to the risk of lymphoedema. This should be taken into consideration as part of a person-centred approach to patient assessment. Record blood pressure as clinically appropriate *to assess the patient's individual needs and to identify anyone who may need further investigation or referral.*
- Apply the correctly sized cuff 2 cm above the point at which the brachial artery can be palpated (located in the antecubital fossa area) (British and Irish Hypertension Society 2017) (Fig. 5.4). If preferred, the cuff can be positioned so that the tubes are at the top, as this can avoid them interfering with the placement of the stethoscope (for manual blood pressure measurements) (British and Irish Hypertension Society 2017). Avoid any venous or arterial access devices when locating the cuff *to make correct use of the equipment and obtain an accurate and reliable blood pressure reading.*

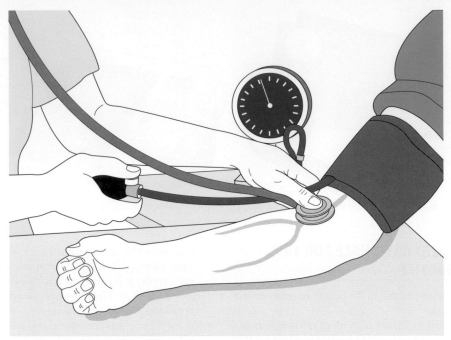

Fig. 5.4 Stethoscope over the brachial artery.

The cuff should be applied smoothly and firmly, covering 80% of the arm circumference but not more than 100% (British and Irish Hypertension Society 2017; Williams et al. 2004), with the middle of the rubber bladder lying directly over the brachial artery. Many blood pressure cuffs have an arrow to indicate the mid-point of the bladder; where one is present, align it with the brachial artery. Ensure that the cuff is level with the patient's heart. The cuff should be tight enough to allow you to insert one finger on the inside of it with only slight resistance. Follow these guidelines *to make correct use of the equipment and obtain an accurate and reliable blood pressure reading.*

Electronic Sphygmomanometers

- With the cuff now in situ, activate the device by switching it on and pressing 'go' or 'start'. The electronic device will automatically inflate the cuff to just above systolic blood pressure, before gradually reducing the pressure and recording the diastolic figure. These numbers are normally shown on a digital display; record the results as per local policy and take any actions necessary. Follow these guidelines *to make correct use of the equipment, obtain an accurate and reliable blood pressure reading,*

document blood pressure accurately and act on any concerns.

Manual Sphygmomanometers
Estimating Systolic Blood Pressure Using the Radial or Brachial Artery

- Ask the patient to rest the arm, with the forearm at heart level, on a suitable firm surface to ensure patient comfort and prevent movement of the limb, which may lead to inaccurate results.
- With the cuff now in place, palpate the radial or brachial pulse and inflate the cuff rapidly, while ensuring patient comfort, until the pulse has been obliterated. Inflate for a further 20 mmHg above this point. Release the valve slowly, taking note of the reading on the gauge when the radial/brachial pulse returns. Allow all the air to escape from the cuff via the control valve to provide an initial estimate of the systolic blood pressure.

Measuring Blood Pressure

- Palpate the brachial pulse, place the diaphragm of the stethoscope over the site, and inflate the cuff to 20–30 mmHg above the previously noted reading. Slowly release the valve to allow air to escape, at a rate of around 2 mmHg/second; deflating the cuff too quickly can lead to an underestimation of systolic and overestimation of diastolic blood pressures (National Institute for Health and Care Excellence 2011). When the first pulse is heard (first Korotkoff sound, K1), the reading on the gauge should be noted: this is the systolic pressure. Do this *to provide an accurate assessment of the systolic pressure without excessive discomfort to the patient through over-inflation of the cuff.*

- Continue to deflate the cuff slowly; the pulse sounds will change to muffled sounds until they finally disappear. Make a note of the point on the gauge at which you can no longer hear the sounds: this is considered to be the diastolic figure (British and Irish Hypertension Society 2017; National Institute for Health and Care Excellence 2011). *This provides an accurate assessment of the diastolic pressure.*
- Carefully record both the systolic and diastolic figures (document which arm was used), as set out by local protocol and in accordance with your responsibilities for accurate record-keeping as a nurse (Nursing and Midwifery Council 2018b). Seek advice on any findings that are outside the patient's normal or expected parameters *to ensure patient safety in line with your NMC requirements* (Nursing and Midwifery Council 2018b).
- If necessary, as indicated earlier, repeat the process on the other arm, carefully documenting the results.
- When the procedure has been completed, ensure that the patient is left feeling comfortable; dispose of any single-use equipment and sanitize any reusable equipment in line with local policy. Wash and dry your hands thoroughly in line with local policy *to reduce the risk of cross-infection.*

Recording Lying and Standing Blood Pressure

- Allow the patient to rest in either a supine or a seated position for at least 5 minutes before following the above procedure for checking blood pressure (using a manual or automated device); ideally, check both arms (one followed by the other). Use whichever arm gives the highest blood pressure reading for the remainder of the procedure (National Institute for Health and Care Excellence 2011) *to ensure accuracy and reliability in the blood pressure measurements.*
- Follow the procedure detailed earlier for providing the blood pressure as a routine observation; however, after recording these lying/seated values, record the blood pressure again with the patient standing. Allow the patient to stand for 1 minute before commencing the standing measurement.

PATIENT/CARER EDUCATION: KEY POINTS

It is important, where possible, to involve the patient and/or carer in any meaningful conversations about the pulse and blood pressure to encourage their participation in their own care and to help them to understand any treatment recommendations.

Some patients may be keen to learn how to check their own pulse, particularly those who are aware that they are prone to an irregular pulse, or those who are involved in cardiac rehabilitation programmes where they are increasing their physical activity levels.

Electronic sphygmomanometers are now available for patients to buy, and many people will be keen to use these themselves to check their own blood pressure in the home. The nurse should instruct the patient and/or carer in the appropriate use of these devices.

Information regarding the common lifestyle factors that are known to affect blood pressure should be discussed with patients and/or carers. This may allow the patient to make an informed choice about whether or not to continue such practices. Offer support and referral for patients who are keen to make positive health choices.

REFERENCES

Alexis, O., 2010. Providing best practice in manual pulse measurement. The British Journal of Nursing 19 (4), 228–234.

Bickley, L., Szilagyi, P., Hoffman, R., 2017. Bates' Guide to Physical Examination and History Taking, twelvth ed. Wolters Kluwer, Philadelphia.

British and Irish Hypertension Society, 2017. Blood Pressure Measurement Using Manual Blood Pressure Monitors. Poster. Available from: https://bihsoc.org/resources/bp-measurement/measure-blood-pressure/.

Donaldson, J., Ness, V., 2009. Maintaining a safe environment. In: Docherty, C., McCallum, J. (Eds.), Foundation Clinical Nursing Skills. Oxford University Press, Oxford.

Dougherty, L., Lister, S., 2015. The Royal Marsden Manual of Clinical Nursing Procedures. John Wiley & Sons, Chichester.

Marieb, E.N., Hoehn, K., 2010. Human Anatomy and Physiology, eighth ed. Pearson/Benjamin Cummings, San Francisco.

National Institute for Health and Care Excellence, 2011. Hypertension in Adults: Diagnosis and Management - Clinical Guideline [CG127]. NICE, London.

National Institute for Health and Care Excellence, 2014. Infection Prevention and Control – Quality Standard [QS61]. NICE, London.

Nursing and Midwifery Council, 2018a. Future Nurse: Standards of Proficiency for Registered Nurses. NMC, London. Available at: https://www.nmc.org.uk/standards/standards-for-nurses/standards-of-proficiency-for-registered-nurses.

Nursing and Midwifery Council, 2018b. The Code: Professional Standards of Practice and Behaviour for Nurses, Midwives and Nursing Associates. NMC, London. Available at: https://www.nmc.org.uk/globalassets/sitedocuments/nmc-publications/nmc-code.pdf.

Royal College of Nursing, 2011. Reducing the Risk of Upper Limb Lymphoedema: Guidance for Nurses in Acute and Community Settings. Royal College of Nursing, London.

Royal College of Physicians, 2017. National Early Warning Score (NEWS) 2: Standardising the Assessment of Acute-Illness Severity in the NHS. Updated report of a working party. London: Royal College of Physicians.

Tortora, G.J., Derrickson, B.H., 2017. Tortora's Principles of Anatomy and Physiology, Global Edition. Wiley, Singapore.

Unsworth, J., Tucker, G., Hindmarsh, Y., 2015. Man versus machine: the importance of manual blood pressure measurement skills amongst registered nurses. Journal of Hospital Administration 4 (6), 61.

Williams, B., Poulter, N.R., Brown, M.J., et al., 2004. British Hypertension Society Guidelines for Hypertension Management 2004 (BHS-IV): summary. British Medical Journal 328 (7440), 634–640.

Woods, S., Woods, S.L., Froelicher, E.S., et al., 2009. Cardiac Nursing, sixth ed. Lippincott Williams and Wilkins, Philadelphia.

SELF-ASSESSMENT

1. What do you understand by the terms rhythm and quality in relation to assessing a patient's pulse?
2. Name three sites, other than the radial artery, where a pulse measurement may be taken.
3. What do the terms bradycardia and tachycardia mean, and why might patients experience these?
4. Why is the measurement of a patient's blood pressure an important nursing observation?
5. What does the top figure in a blood pressure recording refer to?
6. Why might a patient have low blood pressure?

Blood Transfusion

INDICATIONS AND RATIONALE FOR A BLOOD TRANSFUSION

The term 'blood transfusion' is used to describe the transfusion of red cells. Whole blood is rarely transfused nowadays. Red cells are supplemented with other blood components, such as fresh frozen plasma or platelet concentrates, if required, as this is considered more effective treatment (McClelland 2013). This practice will refer to the transfusion of red cells; however, the same safety issues relate to the administration of all blood components.

A 'blood transfusion' is the introduction of compatible donor red cells into the circulation of a recipient. It may be indicated for the following reasons:
- to support a patient who has lost a large volume of blood
- to enable a patient to have surgery that may involve the loss of a large volume of blood
- to support a patient receiving treatment for leukaemia or cancer
- to maintain or improve the lives of patients with some chronic conditions (Murphy et al. 2017).

Several countries have established a haemovigilance programme to collect data on the serious adverse effects of transfusion. The UK Serious Hazards of Transfusion (SHOT) scheme was launched in 1996. It is a voluntary scheme covering both NHS and independent hospitals, and aims to use the information gathered to improve safety standards for blood transfusion. The scheme has consistently reported that human error contributes significantly to the morbidity and mortality of patients receiving blood transfusion (SHOT 1998–2016; *see* https://www.shotuk.org/). The majority of these occurred because of an error in patient identification, either at the time of blood component collection from the storage site, or at the patient's bedside. Correct identification of the patient is therefore the main focus of transfusion safety.

OUTLINE OF THE PROCEDURE

The decision to transfuse a patient is made by a medical practitioner.

It is not a legal requirement in the UK for consent to be obtained before a transfusion of blood components; however, it is considered a required standard of good transfusion practice to ensure that the patient/carer or parent receives adequate information regarding the transfusion. Guidance on obtaining consent for blood component transfusion is available from the Advisory Committee on the Safety of Blood Tissues and Organs (2011).

When a decision to transfuse the patient is made, a venous blood sample is taken and sent to the hospital transfusion laboratory, along with a request for the blood component

TABLE 6.1	Blood Component Storage Conditions	
Component	**Shelf Life**	**Storage Conditions**
Red blood cells Whole blood	35 days	+4°C (±2°C) in an authorized blood fridge
Platelets	7 days	+22°C (±2°C) on an agitation rack in the hospital transfusion laboratory
Fresh frozen plasma	3 years	−30°C in the hospital transfusion laboratory
Octaplas Solvent detergent plasma	4 years	−30°C in the hospital transfusion laboratory
Cryoprecipitate	2 years	−30°C in the hospital transfusion laboratory

required. Tests are undertaken on the sample to identify the patient's ABO and RhD group, and to establish whether there are any specific antibodies, before selecting a compatible donor unit for issue.

Each of the blood components has specific storage requirements (Table 6.1), and it is the responsibility of the hospital transfusion laboratory to ensure that blood components are stored appropriately (Guidelines for the Blood Transfusion Services in the UK 2013).

The final patient identification check can be undertaken by one or two people, depending on local policy. Some health boards have adopted a single-person check, as it has been suggested that it may be more appropriate for one registered practitioner to take full responsibility (British Society for Haematology 2017). It is important to check current policy regarding the checking procedure in place.

TRANSFUSION REACTIONS

A reaction can occur with all blood components; ensuring the patient's safety is therefore the most important aspect of caring for a patient during the transfusion (Table 6.2). Any adverse event experienced by a patient should be considered as a possible transfusion reaction. Immediate recognition and prompt nursing and medical action are required to prevent further complications and possible death. This is particularly important if the patient is unconscious or cannot report symptoms.

If any transfusion reaction is suspected, the transfusion must be **stopped** and urgent medical attention sought. Acute

reactions can occur during, or within the first 24 hours of, transfusion. Delayed transfusion reactions can occur days, weeks, months or even years later. These include delayed haemolytic reaction, and signs and symptoms of infectious disease such as hepatitis C or human immunodeficiency virus (HIV).

Treatment will depend on the cause and severity of the reaction, and is dictated by the patient's clinical condition. Close observation and monitoring of the patient should be maintained and should include temperature, pulse, respiratory rate, blood pressure, blood loss and urinary output. All serious transfusion reactions must be reported to the hospital transfusion laboratory and duty haematologist, to ensure appropriate investigation, further management and reporting of the reaction (The Blood Safety and Quality Regulations 2005). There will be a local policy for the method of reporting. The adverse event should also be documented in the patient's medical and nursing notes.

◎ EQUIPMENT

- As for 'Intravenous Therapy' (*see* Ch. 22)

Additional Equipment
- Sterile blood administration set
- Infusion device
- Non-sterile gloves and apron

In Emergency Situations
- Intravenous fluid pressure infusion bag
- Blood-warming equipment

GUIDELINES AND RATIONALE FOR THIS NURSING PRACTICE

You should refer to your local transfusion policy, as there may be some variations in practice.

Practical Aspects of Transfusion

- Blood components should be transfused via an intravenous route separate from all other infusions, *to prevent clotting of the transfused component in the infusion tubing.*
- Blood components must be administered through a blood administration set with an integral filter, *to filter macroaggregates (white cells, platelets and coagulum), which collect in stored blood.*
- No drugs should be added to any blood component, *as they may contain additives such as calcium that can cause the citrated blood to clot.*

TABLE 6.2	Acute Transfusion Reactions	
Type	**Cause**	**Symptoms**
Volume overload	Transfusion of too much fluid or transfusion of a component too rapidly	Dyspnoea, hypertension and tachycardia
Febrile	An immune response of the recipient to white cell antigens or white cell fragments in the blood component	Headache, mild fever (temperature rise of up to 2°C) and a moderate tachycardia without hypotension
Allergic Urticarial or Anaphylactic	An immune response of the recipient to plasma proteins in the blood component	Urticarial: headache, rash and pruritus without hypotension Anaphylaxis: nausea, vomiting, facial swelling, wheezing and laryngeal oedema
Haemolytic	Transfusion of an ABO-incompatible component in the majority	Rigors, loin pain, muscle aches, tachycardia, hypotension and haemoglobinuria
Septic shock	A bacterially contaminated component	Chills, high fever, vomiting, abdominal cramps, diarrhoea and signs of shock

- Infusion devices, which are certified as suitable for use with blood components, can be used *to assist with regulation of flow rate.*

Preparing the Patient for Transfusion

- Gloves and apron should be worn to prevent contamination with body fluids.
- Ensure that the blood component has been prescribed and check the prescription for the following information:
  - the name and date of birth of the patient
  - the patient identification number
  - the date and time of the transfusion
  - the type of blood component prescribed, e.g. red cells or platelets
  - the number of units prescribed
  - the rate of transfusion
  - the signature of the medical practitioner.
- Help to explain the nursing practice to the patient, *to gain their consent and cooperation, and to encourage their participation in their care.*
- Collect and prepare the equipment, *to make efficient use of time and resources.*
- Ensure that the patient is in a setting where they can be directly observed, *to ensure visual observation of the patient.*
- Assist the patient into a comfortable position and ensure the patient's privacy, *to respect and maintain self-esteem and promote acceptance of the transfusion.*
- Wash your hands, *to prevent cross-infection.*
- Prime the administration set with normal saline; *dextrose 5% or Ringer lactate solution should not be used, as this may lead to clotting of the blood component.*

- Assist the medical practitioner with the insertion of an intravenous cannula, if required.

Collecting Blood Components from the Hospital Transfusion Laboratory or Satellite Fridge

- Collect the blood component immediately before it is required, *so that the blood component is stored at the correct temperature until administered.*
- In a non-emergency situation, collect one blood component at a time, *to reduce the risk of a patient identification error.*
- Take written patient identification information when collecting blood components, *as failure of correct patient identification is a major source of incorrect blood component incidents.*
- Check the written patient identification details against the information on the blood component label, *to ensure that the patient identification details match.*
- Record the collection of the blood component on the blood fridge register, *to ensure traceability of the blood component* (The Blood Safety and Quality Regulations 2005).
- Deliver the blood component promptly to the clinical area, *to ensure that the transfusion is commenced without delay.*

Pre-Administration Checking Procedure

- Check the prescription for the blood component, *to identify if the patient has any special requirements, e.g. irradiated blood, or a concomitant drug is being given, e.g. a diuretic.*

Red Blood Cells

Compatibility/Traceability label

The compatibility/traceability label is generated in the hospital transfusion laboratory. It is attached to the blood component and contains the following patient information: *Surname, Forename(s), Date of birth, Gender, Hospital number/ CHI number, Hospital and Ward*

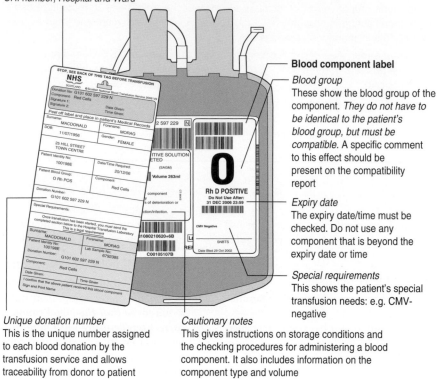

Blood component label

Blood group
These show the blood group of the component. *They do not have to be identical to the patient's blood group, but must be compatible.* A specific comment to this effect should be present on the compatibility report

Expiry date
The expiry date/time must be checked. Do not use any component that is beyond the expiry date or time

Special requirements
This shows the patient's special transfusion needs: e.g. CMV-negative

Unique donation number
This is the unique number assigned to each blood donation by the transfusion service and allows traceability from donor to patient

Cautionary notes
This gives instructions on storage conditions and the checking procedures for administering a blood component. It also includes information on the component type and volume

Fig. 6.1 Blood component label and compatibility/traceability label. *CHI,* Community Health Index number (Scotland only).

- Take a reading of the patient's temperature, pulse, respiration and blood pressure, ***to provide a set of baseline observations before the start of the blood transfusion.***
- Check the expiry date of the component and undertake a visual inspection of the component, ***to ensure that the component is safe to use*** (Fig. 6.1).
- If there are any discrepancies, do not proceed; ***contact the hospital transfusion laboratory for advice and inform the nurse in charge and medical staff.***

Final Patient Identification Checking Procedure

- Establish the patient's identity; wherever possible, ask the patient to tell you their first name, surname and date of birth.
  - Check this information against the patient's wristband for accuracy.
- Check that the patient's identification details on the wristband match the patient details on the compatibility/traceability label attached to the blood component.
- Check that the blood group and donation number on the compatibility/traceability label are identical to the information on the blood component label (Fig. 6.2).
- If there are any discrepancies, **do not proceed; contact the hospital transfusion laboratory for advice and inform the nurse in charge and medical staff.**
- Transfer the donation number to the patient's transfusion record/chart and complete all documentation, ***to ensure there is traceability of the transfused component and a record of professional responsibility.***

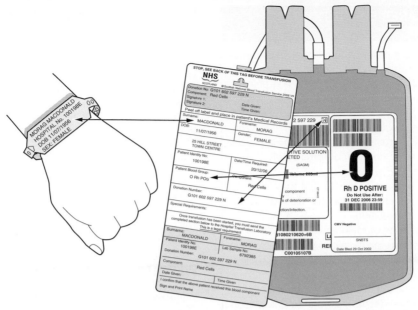

Fig. 6.2 Checking the information on the patient's wristband and the compatibility/traceability label attached to the blood component.

- Connect the blood component to the administration set and commence the transfusion at the prescribed rate.
- Each unit of red cells should be transfused within 4 hours of removal from controlled storage.

Monitoring the Patient During Blood Transfusion

- Ensure that the patient has access to the nurse call bell system, *to enable the patient to gain assistance immediately.*
- Observe the patient throughout the transfusion, paying particular attention to the first 15 minutes, *as the majority of major transfusion reactions occur within this time period.* Observations (pulse, blood pressure, temperature and respiratory rate) should be undertaken and documented for every unit transfused. Minimum monitoring of the patient should include the following:
  - pre-transfusion observations taken and recorded no more than 60 minutes before the start of the component transfusion
  - observations 15 minutes after the start of each unit
  - post-transfusion observations taken and recorded not more than 60 minutes after the end of the component transfusion (British Society for Haematology 2017), *to ensure early detection of an adverse reaction.* Some health boards may undertake observations more frequently; therefore you must check local policies.

- If a transfusion reaction is suspected, the transfusion must be stopped immediately and urgent medical advice sought, *to ensure prompt action in the event of an adverse reaction.*

On Completion of the Transfusion

- Record the volume of the blood component transfused, *to ensure accurate monitoring of patient's fluid balance status.* There are approximately 250–300 mL in a unit of red cells.
- If other intravenous fluids are to be administered, change the blood administration set when the transfusion is completed, *as there may be residue of the blood component in the infusing tubing.*
- Dispose of the equipment safely, *to prevent the risk of sharp injuries and the transmission of infection.*
- File all transfusion documentation in the patient's case notes, *to ensure compliance with traceability legislation* (The Blood Safety and Quality Regulations 2005).
- In undertaking this practice, nurses are accountable for their actions, the quality of care delivered and record-keeping, according to *The Code* (Nursing and Midwifery Council 2018) and *Standards for Medicines Management* (Nursing and Midwifery Council 2007).

PATIENT/CARER EDUCATION: KEY POINTS

In partnership with the patient and/or carer, ensure that they are competent to carry out any required practices. Information should be given on an appropriate point of contact for any concerns that might arise.

Explain the reason for the transfusion, and state the time expected for the completion of each unit. This makes it easier for the patient to tolerate the practice.

Advise the patient to notify you immediately if they become aware of any symptoms such as shivering, flushing, pain or shortness of breath or if they begin to feel anxious. This will enable early identification of any adverse effects of transfusion.

Explain the importance of maintaining the cannula by keeping the cannulated limb as still as possible. Emphasize the dangers of disconnection of the infusion lines.

Explain the importance of immediately reporting any soreness or redness at the site of the transfusion, which may be a sign of local infection, even after completion of the transfusion.

If the patient has had a specific antibody identified on pre-transfusion testing, this will be documented by the hospital transfusion laboratory for future reference. The patient should also be given written information on the details of the particular antibody. They should be advised to give this to the doctor or nurse the next time they need to be transfused.

REFERENCES

Advisory Committee on the Safety of Blood, Tissues and Organs, SaBTO, 2011. Patient consent for blood transfusion. https://www.gov.uk/government/publications/patient-consent-for-blood-transfusion.

British Society for Haematology, 2017. Administration of Blood Components guideline. Available at: https://b-s-h.org.uk/guidelines/guidelines/administration-of-blood-components/.

Guidelines for the Blood Transfusion Services in the UK, 2013, eighth ed. The Stationery Office, London.

McClelland, D.B.L. (Ed.), 2013. The Handbook of Transfusion Medicine, fifth ed. The Stationery Office, London.

Murphy, M.F., Pamphilon, D.H., Heddle, N.M., 2017. Practical Transfusion Medicine, fifth ed. Wiley, Oxford.

Nursing and Midwifery Council, 2007. Standards for Medicines Management. NMC, London.

Nursing and Midwifery Council, 2018. The Code: Professional Standards of Practice and Behaviour for Nurses, Midwives and Nursing Associates. NMC, London. Available at: https://www.nmc.org.uk/globalassets/sitedocuments/nmc-publications/nmc-code.pdf.

The Blood Safety and Quality Regulations, 2005. No. 50. Available at: www.legislation.gov.uk/uksi/2005/50.

WEBSITE

https://www.shotuk.org/ *Serious Hazards of Transfusion*

 SELF-ASSESSMENT

1. What is the most common cause of an incompatible transfusion?
2. What checks should be completed when collecting a red cell unit from the hospital blood bank or satellite fridge?
3. What vital signs should be recorded on a patient receiving a red cell transfusion?
4. What is the first step you should take if you suspect a transfusion reaction?

Body Temperature

INDICATIONS AND RATIONALE FOR TAKING A TEMPERATURE

Body temperature can be considered as the balance of heat lost from the body and heat gained. Both behavioural and physiological mechanisms maintain core body temperature at 37°C ± 1°C. Abnormal body temperature recordings can be an indication of a deterioration in patients' condition and vital signs. The normal range of body temperature is 36°C –37.5°C but this may vary, according to the site used for measurement and from individual to individual (Amoore 2010). Factors naturally influencing the patient's body temperature include: age, ingestion of fluids and food, hormonal changes, smoking and room temperature. The Nursing and Midwifery Council (2018b) states that nurses should demonstrate and apply a knowledge of body systems when undertaking patient assessment. For this to happen, it is vital for the nurse to be able to identify normal and abnormal values in temperature. Combining temperature readings with other observational values, patient history and presentation, the nurse should be able to make a nursing diagnosis and provide evidence-based interventions for the patient (Sund-Levander & Grodzinsky 2013).

Grant & Crimmons (2018) detail parameter values and scores as part of the National Early Warning Score (NEWS). The nurse should have an awareness of what the following temperature values may indicate:
- moderate/severe hypothermia (≤35°C)
- mild hypothermia (35.1°C–36°C)
- normal temperature (37.1°C–38°C)
- mild pyrexia (38.1°C–39°C)
- hyperthermia (≥39.1°C).

Although Grant & Crimmons (2018) consider a temperature between 37.1°C and 38°C as normal, Amoore (2010), as well as Garner & Fendius (2010), states that a temperature above 37.5°C is considered as pyrexia. When looking after patients with a temperature recording within these parameters, the nurse must be aware that although the patient may not score on a NEWS chart, the temperature may still be a sign of deterioration in the patient's condition.

Temperatures of more than 38°C are normally recognized as a sign of infection. Similarly, a patient with a temperature of less than 36°C would be classed as being potentially hypothermic. However, the patient could be showing signs of infection with pyrexia and hypothermia, and the healthcare professional should remember this when assessing the patient (Lat et al. 2018).

NEWS charts may vary slightly, depending on the health authority; therefore the healthcare professional should pay attention to the documentation being used to assess vital signs

The recording of body temperature may be required:
- *to establish a baseline temperature,* e.g. when patients are admitted to the hospital or clinic
- *to monitor fluctuations in temperature,* as may occur during the postoperative period, *because temperature*

fluctuations can indicate developing infection or the presence of a deep venous thrombosis

- *to monitor signs of incompatibility when patients are receiving a blood transfusion*
- *to monitor the temperature of patients being treated for an infection*
- *to monitor the temperature of patients recovering from hypothermia*
- *to monitor temperature during and following invasive diagnostic procedures.*

The frequency of measurement will be dependent on the patient's condition, recorded temperature and instructions provided as part of the NEWS tool.

◎ EQUIPMENT

- Tray
- Appropriate thermometer, e.g.:
  - disposable thermometer
  - electronic thermometer, probe and disposable cover
  - tympanic thermometer and disposable cover
- Watch with a second hand
- Black pen
- Observation or NEWS chart
- Tissues
- Receptacle for disposable items

TYPES OF THERMOMETER

The nature of this practice means that there is a risk of cross-infection if the nurse does not adequately clean the thermometers between each patient and dispose of any single-use equipment.

Disposable Thermometers

A variety of disposable thermometers are available, two of the more common types being the chemical dot thermometer and the liquid crystal heat-sensitive synthetic strip (Fig. 7.1). These are for single use only and the manufacturer's instructions for use must be followed to ensure an accurate recording. These thermometers tend to be used in a community or domestic setting.

Electronic Thermometers

Electronic thermometers (Fig. 7.2) have, for some time now, replaced traditional mercury glass thermometers as one of the most common methods of measuring body temperature in hospitals. The electronic thermometer can be used to measure both oral and axillary temperatures, and some may have a separate probe for rectal use; refer to the information given later regarding rectal temperature measurement prior to engaging in this skill. In addition, the electronic thermometer may require the correct mode of use, e.g. oral or rectal, to be selected prior to use. Regardless of which site

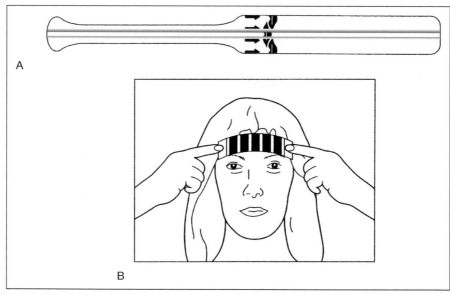

Fig. 7.1 (A) Disposable chemical dot thermometer. (B) Liquid crystal disposable synthetic strip.

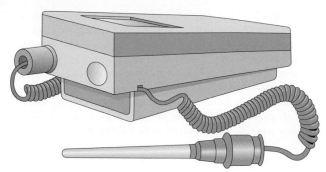

Fig. 7.2 Types of thermometer: electronic. From Torrance C, Semple M: Practical procedures for nurses No 6.1. Recording temperature 1. Nursing Times 94(2), 1998. Copyright Emap Public Sector Ltd 1998. Reproduced by permission of Nursing Times.

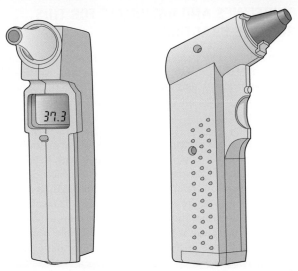

Fig. 7.3 Types of thermometer: tympanic. From Torrance C, Semple M: Practical procedures for nurses No 6.1. Recording temperature 1. Nursing Times 94(2), 1998. Copyright Emap Public Sector Ltd 1998. Reproduced by permission of Nursing Times.

is chosen, research indicates that the accuracy of the recording is dependent on correct probe placement and the skill of the healthcare professional using the equipment (Amoore 2010). The thermometer will automatically give out an audible signal when the temperature has been recorded. As an accountable nurse, it is your responsibility to know how to operate equipment, and reference to the manufacturer's instructions is essential.

Tympanic Thermometers

Used widely, tympanic thermometers (Figs 7.3 and 7.4) have a probe with a disposable cover that is inserted into the ear canal. They detect infrared energy that is emitted from the tympanic membrane at the end of the ear canal and surrounding tissue; this is then displayed digitally as a temperature reading. Literature suggests that tympanic thermometers represent a more accurate picture of actual body temperature due to the fact that the tympanic membrane shares the same arterial blood supply as the hypothalamus (the temperature-regulating centre within the brain) (El-Radhi 2013).

The thermometer must be covered by a disposable cover in order to function, and the detection window must be kept clean to obtain an accurate result. Grainger (2013) communicates that for patients who have been lying down on their side, tympanic measurement should not be conducted in the ear on which the patient was lying; this can give a false reading, as heat will have built up in and around the ear.

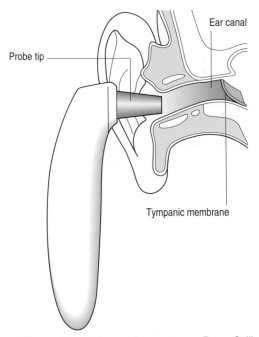

Fig. 7.4 Tympanic membrane thermometer. From Gallimore D: Reviewing the effectiveness of tympanic thermometers. Nursing Times 100(32):32–34, 2004. Copyright Emap Public Sector Ltd 2004. Reproduced by permission of Nursing Times.

GUIDELINES AND RATIONALE FOR THIS NURSING PRACTICE

The patient should be assessed carefully to identify the most appropriate site for temperature measurement, which will ensure an accurate and safe result. Once chosen, the same site should be used for consistent measurement.

Axilla

The axillary site is inappropriate when a patient's peripheral circulation is shut down, such as in people with hypothermia. In addition, the axillary site is the least accurate for reflecting core body temperature (El-Radhi 2013). In elderly patient groups who are emaciated, there may be insufficient body mass to ensure that the probe is surrounded by skin tissue. The presence of surgical wounds should also indicate the avoidance of this site as a means of temperature measurement.

- Wash your hands and clean the thermometer *to prevent cross-infection.*
- Explain the nursing practice *to gain consent and cooperation, and encourage participation in care.* Ensure that the patient has not recently had a hot bath, ingested fluid or food or engaged in strenuous exercise, *as these will cause a temporary rise in body temperature.*
- Ensure the patient's privacy *to respect their dignity.*
- Help the patient into a comfortable position, either sitting or lying, with the back and shoulders well supported, *so that the position can be maintained for a few minutes.*
- Help the patient to remove or adjust the clothing *to expose one axilla.*
- Observe the patient throughout this activity *to monitor any adverse effects.*
- Dry the skin of the axilla by wiping with a tissue; *a film of moisture between the skin and the thermometer probe can lead to an inaccurate reading.*
- Place the probe of the thermometer in the axilla where the skin surfaces will surround it *to gain an accurate temperature reading.*
- Help the patient to hold the arm across the chest *to retain the thermometer in the correct position.*
- Leave the thermometer in position as per the manufacturer's instructions *to ensure an accurate technique.*
- Remain with the patient, if required, *to reassure the patient and ensure that the thermometer remains in the correct position.*
- Remove the thermometer *when the optimum time for accurate recording has been reached.*
- Read the temperature measured by the thermometer *for an accurate recording to be monitored and documented.*

- Ensure that the patient is left feeling as comfortable as possible *to reassure the patient and reduce anxiety.*
- Clean/dispose of equipment safely *to prevent cross-infection.*
- Document the temperature reading in the patient's records, compare the reading with previous recordings, and report any abnormal findings immediately, *to ensure safe practice and enable prompt, appropriate medical and nursing intervention to be initiated.*
- In undertaking this practice, nurses are accountable for their actions, the quality of care delivered and record-keeping, as stated in *The Code* (Nursing and Midwifery Council 2018a).

Oral Cavity

Accuracy in measuring body temperature utilizing this site is often determined by thermometer placement. Accuracy of the reading will also be affected by mouth breathing, oxygen therapy, fluid or food ingestion and smoking. The oral cavity should be avoided in patients who are at risk of seizure or of biting down on the thermometer, people who are confused and perhaps non-compliant, and those who have undergone oral surgery. Oral measurement of body temperature should not take place routinely to measure the temperature of children under 5 years of age (Royal College of Nursing 2017). These factors should be considered prior to proceeding to use this site.

- Wash your hands and clean the thermometer *to prevent cross-infection.*
- Explain the nursing practice *to gain consent and cooperation.* Ensure that the patient has not recently had a hot or cold drink or a hot bath, or engaged in strenuous exercise, *as this may temporarily raise the body temperature.*
- Help the patient into a comfortable position *so that they will more readily tolerate the thermometer probe.*
- Prepare the thermometer as per the manufacturer's instructions.
- Apply a disposable sleeve, if required, *to prevent the transmission of infection.*
- Place the thermometer probe under the patient's tongue so that the probe lies adjacent to the frenulum at the junction of the floor of the mouth and the base of the tongue, on either the right or the left side. *A maximum temperature recording will be obtained from one of these two 'heat pockets' in the mouth* (Fig. 7.5). This is also the position for disposable oral thermometers.
- Explain to the patient the importance of only closing the lips round the thermometer and not biting it, *so that the oral temperature is maintained and not distorted by the inspiration of air through the mouth.*
- Leave the thermometer in position for the required time *to take an accurate recording.*

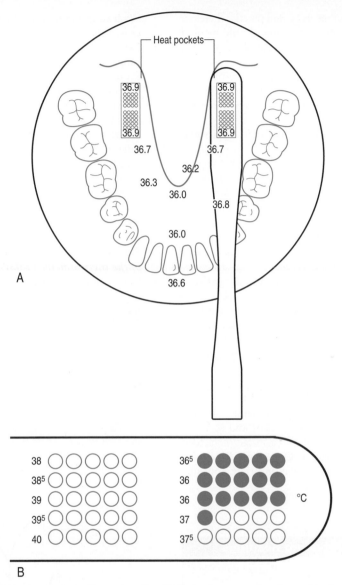

Fig. 7.5 (A) Heat pockets in the oral cavity. (B) Recording area of a disposable thermometer.

- Remove the thermometer probe and proceed as for an axillary temperature recording.

Rectum

The rectal site should not be used in patients with rectal trauma such as haemorrhoids, those who have had rectal surgery or those who have difficulty in lying on their left side. Rectal temperature recording should not be used in children under 5 years of age (Royal College of Nursing 2017) and is indicated only in very specific situations for use in those over 5 years; as such, it is imperative to review local health policy to ensure adherence.

Sund Levander & Grodzinsky (2013) describe a difference between rectal temperature readings and those taken at other sites. It can take approximately 20 minutes for temperatures in the rectum to adjust to core body temperature. It is therefore essential for nurses taking a rectal temperature to be aware of the potential for different temperature readings compared to those taken at other areas. Best practice therefore suggests that rectal temperature recording should be used only if clinically indicated (Royal College of Nursing 2017) and supported by local health policy.

- Wash your hands, apply gloves and clean the thermometer to *prevent cross-infection.*
- Explain the nursing practice to the patient *to gain consent and cooperation.*
- Ensure the patient's privacy *to respect their dignity and maintain self-esteem.*
- Help the patient into a comfortable position lying on their side with the knees bent, *so that access is easier and the patient is distressed as little as possible.*
- Prepare the thermometer probe as per the manufacturer's instructions.
- If suggested by the manufacturer, lubricate the end of the thermometer probe *to make insertion easier and prevent any damage to the mucosa.*
- Gently insert the thermometer probe into the patient's anus for 2–4 cm (depending on the patient; seek advice if unsure) and hold it in position for the required time *to take an accurate recording of the temperature.*
- Remove the thermometer probe, dispose of the probe and soiled glove, and proceed as for an axillary temperature recording.

Ear Canal: Tympanic Thermometer Only

A number of factors must be considered prior to using the tympanic route. The comfort of the patient and accuracy of the recording could be affected by a range of factors. These are summarized in Box 7.1. Once these have been considered, you can then, if safe and appropriate, continue with tympanic measurement.

- Wash your hands and clean the thermometer *to prevent cross-infection.*
- Explain the nursing practice *to gain consent and cooperation.*
- Ensure that the patient has not recently had a hot or cold drink or a hot bath, or engaged in strenuous exercise, *as this may temporarily raise the body temperature.*
- Help the patient into a comfortable position *to gain safe access to the ear canal and to enable the patient to tolerate the practice more readily.*
- Prepare the thermometer as per the manufacturer's instructions *to ensure an accurate measurement.*
- Apply a disposable sleeve *to prevent the transmission of infection and allow the device to function.*
- Switch the device on *to ensure that it is calibrated and ready to take an accurate measurement.*
- Stabilize the patient's head *to ensure the safe introduction of the thermometer probe.*
- Gently pull the ear lobe downwards and position the probe so that it occludes the canal; this will *straighten the ear canal and permit the probe to view the tympanic membrane without interference from ambient air temperature* (Fig. 7.6).
- Hold the thermometer steady and take the recording as per the manufacturer's instructions, *to take an accurate recording.*
- Remove the thermometer probe, dispose of the cover and return the equipment to its storage case *to prevent breakage and prolong usage.*
- Proceed as for an axillary temperature recording.

BOX 7.1   Factors Affecting Readings

Most studies acknowledge some of these factors but none considers them all:

- Wax in the ear
- Incorrect placement of the probe tip in the ear canal
- Inner ear infection
- Lying on the side of the head that will be measured before a temperature recording
- Hair in the ear
- The removal of a hearing aid up to 20 minutes before a reading is taken.

From Gallimore D: Reviewing the effectiveness of tympanic thermometers. Nursing Times 100(32):32–34, 2004. Copyright Emap Public Sector Ltd 2004. Reproduced by permission of Nursing Times.

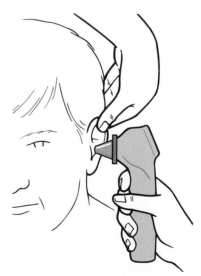

Fig. 7.6 Using a tympanic thermometer.

ADDITIONAL INFORMATION

The measurement of body temperature is an invaluable observation of the patient's condition and one that can inform the decisions made about treatment and care (Sund-Levander & Grodzinsky 2013). It is vital for the appropriate equipment to be selected for use, for the correct site to be chosen and for the temperature to be accurately recorded as part of the patient's nursing notes. Prompt recognition and reporting of temperature abnormalities and irregularities are also essential.

Body temperature measurement can be obtained from many different areas; however, healthcare professionals should be aware that temperature readings may vary across different sites. It is important to note that the core temperature can be more than 0.4°C higher than a peripherally measured temperature, and more than 0.2°C lower than a temperature recorded via the rectal route (Amoore 2010). Oral, rectal and axillary temperature can be taken using a digital electronic probe, and the tympanic route can be chosen for use with a special handheld device having a probe that is inserted into the patient's ear canal. For each patient, the preferred site should be used consistently so that any change in temperature can be accurately monitored (Grainger 2013). This should be based on an assessment of the most appropriate site for measurement to be recorded. The contraindications and aspects for consideration in relation to the use of rectal temperature measurement must also be borne in mind, and advice sought as appropriate, in advance of using this approach to temperature measurement.

It is important to note that the measurement of body temperature does not rely solely on the thermometer alone but should include a general observation of the patient. Particular observations should include whether the patient looks flushed, if the skin is hot or cold, if the patient sweating and clammy to the touch, if they are shivering or if they are showing any signs of confusion and disorientation.

PATIENT/CARER EDUCATION: KEY POINTS

In partnership with the patient and/or carer, ensure that they are competent to carry out the practice required when undertaking measurement of temperature. Information should be given to educate the patient and/or carer appropriately on the practice of this skill, and an appropriate point of contact should be provided, should they have any concerns.

Explain the importance of monitoring the body temperature for evaluating the progress and treatment of the patient's condition.

The patient should understand the importance of the thermometer remaining in position for the correct period of time.

Explain the importance of reporting headaches, excess sweating, shivering or general feelings of distress, which may indicate a change in body temperature.

Patients with pyrexia should understand the importance of drinking an adequate amount of fluid in order to prevent dehydration.

Elderly patients should be given advice on how to prevent heat loss at home and told of the dangers of hypothermia. This should be reinforced with written advice and specific information about the resources available, and should involve family and carers as applicable.

The procedure should be explained to the patient and instruction given on their role in achieving an accurate measurement, e.g. the need to restrain from speaking during oral recording.

REFERENCES

Amoore, D., David, A., 2010. Best practice in the measurement of body temperature. Nursing Standard 24 (42), 42–49.

El-Radhi, A., 2013. Temperature measurement: the right thermometer and site. The British Journal of Nursing 22 (4), 208–211.

Garner, A., Fendius, A., 2010. Temperature physiology assessment and control. British Journal of Neuroscience Nursing 6 (8), 397–400.

Grainger, A., 2013. Principles of temperature monitoring. Nursing Standard 27 (50), 48–55.

Grant, S., Crimmons, K., 2018. Limitations of track and trigger systems and the National Early Warning Score. Part 2:

sensitivity versus specificity. The British Journal of Nursing 27 (12), 705–710.

Lat, S., Mashlan, W., Heffey, S., Jones, B., 2018. Recognition and clinical management of sepsis in frail older people. Nursing Older People 30 (2), 35–38.

Nursing and Midwifery Council, 2018a. The Code: Professional Standards of Practice and Behaviour for Nurses, Midwives and Nursing Associates. NMC, London. Available at: https://www.nmc.org.uk/globalassets/sitedocuments/ nmc-publications/nmc-code.pdf.

Nursing and Midwifery Council, 2018b. Future Nurse: Standards of Proficiency for Registered Nurses. NMC, London. Available at: https://www.nmc.org.uk/globalassets/ sitedocuments/education-standards/future-nurse- proficiencies.pdf.

Royal College of Nursing, 2017. Standards for Assessing, Measuring and Monitoring Vital Signs in Infants, Children and Young People, second ed. Royal College of Nursing, London. Available from: https://www.rcn.org.uk/ professional-development/publications/pub- 005942.

Sund-Levander, M., Grodzinsky, E., 2013. Assessment of Body temperature measurement options. The British Journal of Nursing 22 (15), 880–888.

SELF-ASSESSMENT

1. What is the normal temperature range in a healthy adult?
2. What observations could you use to assess your patient's temperature apart from a thermometer?
3. Write down the numerical values of the following temperature ranges:
   hyperthermia
   mild hypothermia
   borderline pyrexia
   moderate hypothermia.
4. Identify the contraindications to the use of the following sites for recording temperature:
   tympanic
   oral
   axillary
   rectal.
5. Ray Martin is a 75-year-old gentleman who lives alone in sheltered accommodation. What advice would you give to Ray to prevent hypothermia?

Cardiopulmonary Resuscitation and Anaphylaxis

There are six parts to this chapter:

1. Identifying patients at risk of cardiorespiratory arrest
2. Using the ABCDE approach
3. Cardiac arrest and rationale for in-hospital cardiopulmonary resuscitation (CPR)
4. Healthcare provider CPR in the primary care environment
5. Respiratory arrest
6. Anaphylaxis

LEARNING OUTCOMES

By the end of this chapter, you should be able to:

- identify patients at risk of cardiorespiratory arrest
- apply the theory of altering physiology to the patient's clinical deterioration
- manage these patients using the structured ABCDE approach
- confirm and manage cardiac arrest, both in hospital and out of hospital
- identify essential equipment required in a clinical emergency.

BACKGROUND KNOWLEDGE REQUIRED

- Revision of the anatomy and physiology of the cardiovascular and respiratory systems
- Review of local health authority/board policy pertaining to the procedure of CPR and calling criteria for the emergency team

INTRODUCTION

Within the context of the in-hospital environment, adult resuscitation involves management of the critically ill patient with acutely altered physiology, in addition to CPR. This chapter will look briefly at a systematic approach to recognition and management of the 'at risk' patient; in-hospital CPR; out-of-hospital CPR for the healthcare provider; respiratory arrest; and anaphylaxis. The procedures involved in advanced life support (ALS) are beyond the remit of this chapter; the focus will therefore be on first-responder CPR and the use of automated external defibrillators (AEDs).

1. IDENTIFYING PATIENTS AT RISK OF CARDIORESPIRATORY ARREST

In simple terms, in order for the body to maintain function of the vital organs, these must be perfused with oxygen. This requires an open **A**irway; the ability to **B**reathe in oxygen and to obtain adequate gaseous exchange in the lungs; and a pump to **C**irculate this oxygen to the organs. Failure at any point in this process will result in reduced oxygen delivery to the tissues (hypoxia), organ failure and, ultimately, death.

Recognition of deteriorating physiology and prevention of cardiac arrest are the first components of the chain of survival, as outcomes from cardiac arrest are poor with only around 20% of these patients surviving to hospital discharge (Soar et al. 2015). Close monitoring of the patient may allow early recognition of deteriorating physiology, provide an opportunity for appropriate treatment, and in some cases may prevent cardiac arrest.

The majority of in-hospital cardiac arrests in non-monitored ward areas are predictable, and as many as 80% of patients will experience a slow, progressive physiological deterioration (Hodgetts et al. 2002; Smith & Pitcher 2015).

The clinical signs of acute illness are similar in all patients, regardless of the original cause, and are a consequence of failing respiratory, cardiovascular and neurological systems (Soar et al. 2015). The common clinical presentation of vital signs includes:

- tachypnoea in response to rising carbon dioxide levels and falling oxygen levels
- tachycardia as the body attempts to circulate oxygen to the vital organs

- hypotension, as when the cardiac output drops, the blood pressure will fall
- reduced conscious level as the perfusion of the brain is diminished.

RELATED PHYSIOLOGY

Respiratory rate is a very significant observation in the critically ill patient and the most sensitive of the vital signs to alterations in physiology (Cullinane & Findlay 2005). As blood oxygen levels fall and carbon dioxide levels rise, an increase in respiratory rate will be triggered by the respiratory centre in the brain. This increase may be subtle initially but should be closely monitored. These patients should be given high-flow oxygen as soon as possible (O'Driscoll et al. 2017) and help should be sought, according to local criteria (Soar et al. 2015). As the demand for oxygen increases, the heart rate will rise. From the equation:

$$\textit{Heart rate (HR)} \times \textit{Stroke volume (SV)} = \textit{Cardiac output (CO)}$$

(Waugh & Grant 2014), it is clear that as the heart rate increases, the cardiac output will increase. This will achieve compensation for a period of time. However, as the rate increases, the refilling time during the resting phase of the cardiac cycle (diastole) will be reduced; this will ultimately lead to a fall in stroke volume and a fall in cardiac output.

By applying the principles of the equation:

$$\textit{Blood pressure (BP)} = \textit{Cardiac output (CO)} \times \textit{Peripheral resistance (PR)}$$

(Waugh and Grant 2014), it can be demonstrated that as cardiac output falls, the body will respond by further increasing the peripheral resistance in an attempt to maintain an adequate blood pressure and organ perfusion. This will result in a weak, thready pulse. This compensation cannot be maintained in the long term; ultimately, perfusion of the organs will stop and, subsequently, they will fail. The organ that will be protected most is the brain. As the conscious level begins to deteriorate, the brain is no longer being adequately perfused and this patient could be considered to be in severe difficulty.

Nurses must work within their level of competence (Nursing and Midwifery Council 2018) and must summon help as early as possible, as soon as signs of deterioration are identified. Many hospitals have an early warning score system in place to help identify 'at risk' patients, and the calling criteria for emergency teams may vary from place to place. Regardless, care must be escalated to those with the skills and expertise to manage deteriorating physiology, and information should be communicated to them using a structured tool (e.g. Situation, Background, Assessment, Recommendation (SBAR); Marshall et al. 2009).

2. USING THE ABCDE APPROACH

GUIDELINES AND RATIONALE FOR THIS NURSING PRACTICE

A common method used to identify and treat problems is known as the ABCDE approach. This refers to **A**irway, **B**reathing, **C**irculation, **D**isability, **E**xposure (Simpson 2016). The ABCDE approach is a systematic framework that allows the healthcare professional to identify problems and to act on these without delay (Table 8.1). The process is continuous and staff should reassess the casualty at each point, where intervention takes place, for signs of improvement or deterioration. Nurses should only work to their own level of clinical expertise and should be aware of their limitations. It is essential to call for help as soon as it is required and to acknowledge your limitations.

Airway

- The airway should be assessed to determine whether it is patent, partially obstructed or completely obstructed. *If a patient can give a verbal response, then it is likely that the airway is patent* (Jevon 2010).
- If there is evidence of noise (e.g. stridor or wheeze), then the airway is partially obstructed. *Stridor often indicates an upper airway obstruction and wheeze usually indicates a lower airway obstruction.*
- Simple manoeuvres should be used to open the airway. If the patient is conscious, and assuming there is no neck injury, *the patient may attempt to optimize their own airway by sitting upright.* If this is clearly ineffective and the patient remains conscious, then lifting the chin forward may help. If the patient is unconscious, the head tilt–chin lift manoeuvre can be used (Jevon 2010). In situations where there is suspicion or risk of cervical spine injury, the head should not be tilted and a jaw thrust or chin lift manoeuvre should be used instead to open the airway (Soar et al. 2015). Nevertheless, the requirement to open and maintain an adequate airway is paramount, and attempts to protect the cervical spine must not compromise oxygenation and ventilation (Deakin et al. 2010).
- Therefore, if life-threatening airway obstruction persists despite use of a jaw thrust or chin lift manoeuvre, head tilt can be added in small increments until the airway is open (Soar et al. 2015).
- If these manoeuvres are ineffective, airway adjuncts may be considered (e.g. a nasopharyngeal airway in a conscious patient with a glossopharyngeal (gag) reflex or an oropharyngeal airway in an unconscious casualty

ABCDE	Assessment	Response
TABLE 8.1 Summary of Rapid Assessment of ABCDE*		
A	Checking of patency and maintenance of airway	Position patient Give suction if required Use adjuncts if required If patient tolerates oral airway, may require intubation
B	Rate Air entry Effort of breathing Colour Percussion Listening	Give oxygen 15 L via trauma mask **Reassess**

C	Rate
	BP and pulse pressure
	Peripheral and central pulses:
	  Are the pulses present?
	  Check amplitude
	Skin perfusion:
	  Capillary refill time (>2 seconds)
	  Temperature
	  Colour
	  Mottling
		Obtain access
		Monitor
		Support
		Consider fluid challenge

D	Glasgow Coma Scale (GCS) score: worrying if it
	  drops by 2 points or more
	  Eyes (E) = 4
	  Verbal (V) = 5
	  Motor (M) = 6
	AVPU:
	  Alert
	  Responds to voice
	  Responds to pain
	  Unresponsive
	If AVPU is recorded as P or below (equal to a
	  GCS of approximately 8 or less), airway
	  protection may be required
		Seek **help**!!!
		Airway may be at risk

E	Exposure	Examine patient Carry out top-to-toe assessment

BP, blood pressure.
*This assessment has to be swift and efficient if it is to be effective. Problems **must** be dealt with as they arise. **Always** reassess after every action and if the patient's condition changes, start ABCDE again.

without a glossopharyngeal reflex). Airway adjuncts should be used only by personnel experienced in their use; if senior, expert help is required, it should be called for immediately.
- If the airway is completely obstructed, the patient may develop a 'see-saw' pattern of respiration, with a silent chest. A see-saw respiratory pattern is confirmed by the abdomen moving in as the chest moves out and vice versa. **This is an extreme clinical emergency and will require immediate, advanced airway management; an anaesthetist should be contacted immediately, according to local protocol.**

Breathing

- When breathing is being assessed, the respiratory rate should be observed and particular attention should be paid to the effort of breathing displayed by the acutely ill patient. Tachypnoea and the use of accessory muscles of respiration should be noted and reported immediately, as these are worrying signs.
- Other observations of breathing should include listening into the chest with a stethoscope and percussion of the chest by trained personnel.
- Any patient with an acute breathing problem should be given high-flow oxygen initially (O'Driscoll et al. 2017).

Circulation

- The nurse should observe the patient for signs of circulatory failure; an initial observation will determine if the patient is sweaty, clammy, pale and so on.
- The patient's pulse should be recorded, noting the rate, regularity and volume, *to indicate cardiovascular function* (*see* Ch. 5).
- A blood pressure recording (*see* Ch. 5) will *determine the effectiveness of the cardiovascular system.* In patients with cardiovascular compromise, a manual blood pressure should be recorded, as electronic devices may be inaccurate.
- Changes in pulse and blood pressure should be reported to medical staff, according to local policy.
- If the patient is clearly deteriorating and an adequately experienced clinician is available, the circulation should be accessed with intravenous cannulae *to aid quick and easy administration of medication.*
- If the equipment is available, the patient should be monitored with a cardiac monitor and pulse oximetry *to provide objective physiological measurements.*

Disability

- Disability relates to the neurological status of the patient.
- *A quick and easy way to determine how well the brain is being perfused is to assess the patient using the AVPU score.* This translates to the following:
  - the patient is **A**lert
  - the patient responds to **V**oice
  - the patient responds to **P**ain
  - the patient is **U**nresponsive
- If a patient's condition deteriorates from one level to a lower one, this is indicative of a significant change in neurological status and should not be overlooked. An AVPU recording of 'P' or less approximately correlates to a Glasgow Coma Scale score of less than 8 and means that the patient is unable to protect their own airway fully. *Expert help is required immediately.*

Exposure

- A top-to-toe examination of the patient *provides an opportunity to identify any obvious cause of their deteriorating condition.*
- Unnecessary exposure of the patient should be avoided *to preserve the dignity of the patient.*

3. CARDIAC ARREST AND RATIONALE FOR IN-HOSPITAL CPR

Cardiac arrest is the abrupt cessation of cardiac output and is the ultimate medical emergency (Riley 2013). CPR is an emergency exercise that aims to restore effective circulation and ventilation following cardiac arrest.

Causes of cardiac arrest include:
- heart attack
- drowning
- choking
- bleeding
- drug overdose
- hypoxia.

CONFIRMING CARDIAC ARREST

When sudden cardiac arrest occurs, cerebral blood flow is reduced to almost zero, which can cause seizure-like activity in the victim (Perkins et al. 2015). As this could be mistaken for epilepsy, it is important for nurses to adopt a high index of suspicion of cardiac arrest in the presence of seizures (Perkins et al. 2015). The sequence of steps used to confirm a diagnosis of cardiac arrest can be remembered using the mnemonic 'Dr's ABC'.

- **Danger:** remove any obvious danger to the rescuer.
- **Response:** check the response of the patient by shaking them and asking, 'Are you alright?' (Fig. 8.1). If the casualty does not respond, proceed as follows.
- **Shout:** and summon **help.**
- **Airway:** open the airway using the head tilt–chin lift manoeuvre (Fig. 8.2); if an obvious obstruction is visible, remove this with suction or forceps. Dentures should remain in situ if they are well-fitting, as this creates a good seal during assisted ventilation.
- **Breathing:** while maintaining an open airway, position your ear over the mouth and nose, and direct your eyes towards the chest to look for chest movement. Listen for breath sounds and feel for expired air (Fig. 8.3). *Take no more than 10 seconds to do this.* If the breathing is abnormal (occasional, noisy, laboured gasps), act as if it is absent. This type of breathing pattern is also referred to as 'agonal gasps' and will be evident in 40% of patients. **Do not** confuse this with normal respiration.

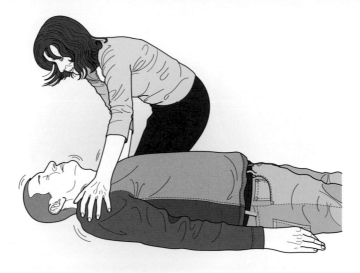

Fig. 8.1 Shake and shout to check for response.

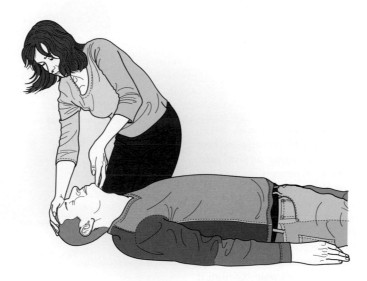

Fig. 8.2 Open the airway.

- Circulation: check by looking for obvious signs of life (movement, swallowing and so on). If you are experienced in clinical assessment, you may wish to combine the breathing check with a carotid pulse check. *This combined assessment should take no longer than 10 seconds* (Perkins et al. 2015).
The diagnosis of cardiac arrest is confirmed by:
- a sudden loss of consciousness or seizure-like activity

- absent or abnormal breathing (e.g. slow, laboured, gasping).

As soon as the diagnosis is confirmed, ensure that appropriately experienced clinicians are alerted and the emergency equipment is gathered. In hospital, this will be the cardiac arrest team or equivalent. With as little delay possible, begin chest compressions. This may involve sending a second person for help, *to make best use of the elapsing*

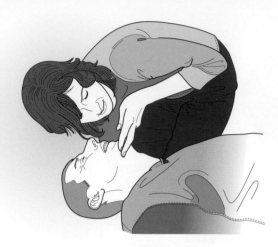

Fig. 8.3 Look, listen and feel for signs of life.

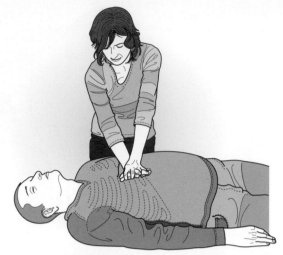

Fig. 8.4 Place hands on centre of chest, one on top of the other.

time and gain support from skilled personnel (Perkins et al. 2015).

GUIDELINES AND RATIONALE FOR THIS NURSING PRACTICE

Chest Compression

High-quality chest compressions significantly improve the chances of a successful outcome (Gwinnutt et al. 2015). These should be started immediately and interruptions kept to a minimum throughout, *to achieve higher survival rates* (Christenson et al. 2009). Ideally, if enough rescuers are available, the person delivering chest compressions should be alternated every 2 minutes (McDonald et al. 2013), *to prevent rescuer fatigue reducing the quality of chest compressions* (Foo et al. 2010). This should be planned and clearly communicated between rescuers *to keep chest compression interruptions to an absolute minimum and improve the chances of a successful outcome* (Gwinnutt et al. 2015).

- Place the patient in a supine position on a firm, flat surface *to permit easy access to the patient's chest and airway.*
- Expose the chest and place the one hand on top of the other, on the centre of the chest, at the lower half of the sternum (breastbone) (Fig. 8.4). The rescuer should maintain straight arms with their elbows locked, lean over the casualty with the shoulder positioned in line with the heel of the hand, and keep the fingers off the ribs *to ease the delivery of chest compressions while preventing damage to the ribs* (Fig. 8.5).

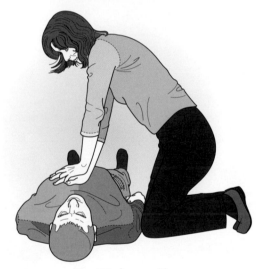

Fig. 8.5 Arm position.

- Press down on the chest by 5–6 cm, aiming for a rate of 100–120/minute, and ensure that the chest recoils completely between each compression *to optimize coronary artery perfusion, cardiac output and myocardial flow* (Niles et al. 2011). Give 30 compressions (Gwinnutt et al. 2015).

Ventilation

The ratio of chest compressions to ventilation for adults is 30:2. After delivering 30 compressions, two ventilations should be delivered with supplementary oxygen, using the most appropriate equipment available. In some cases, this

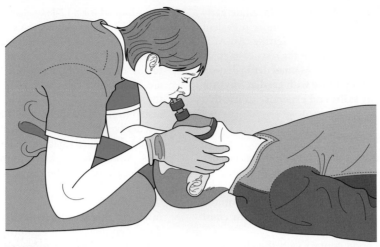

Fig. 8.6 Pocket mask in use.

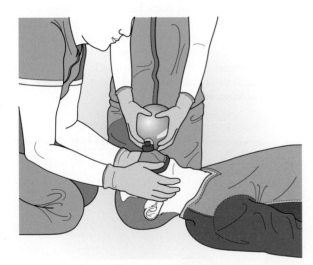

Fig. 8.7 Bag–valve–mask technique.

may be a pocket mask (Fig. 8.6); however, a bag–valve–mask device with reservoir bag will provide higher concentrations of oxygen (Fig. 8.7). The oxygen should be connected and switched to 15 L/minute while chest compressions are ongoing, *to minimize interruptions to chest compression and make the most effective use of time* (Parry and Higginson 2016).

- While maintaining an open airway, one person must use two hands to hold a correctly fitting mask in position using a head tilt–chin lift or jaw thrust manoeuvre, *to maintain an open airway.* The mask should cover the patient's mouth and nose, without overhanging the chin

or covering the eyes, *to optimize oxygen delivery and prevent damage to the eyes* (Parry and Higginson 2016).

- A second person should then squeeze the bag for 1 second to deliver a tidal volume of 500–600 mL of air, which should be enough to create chest movement similar to a normal breath (Perkins et al. 2015). *Tidal volumes greater than this can result in inflation of the stomach, which presents a risk of regurgitation in an unprotected airway.*
- The chest should fall fully prior to the second breath being delivered, *to avoid hyperventilation.*
- Immediately after the second breath, recommence chest compressions without waiting for the chest to fall, *to maintain coronary artery perfusion pressure.*
- The combination of compressions to ventilation should be in a ratio of 30:2. This is achievable with a minimum of two members of staff: one to hold the mask in position while opening the airway, and one to combine delivery of chest compressions with ventilation. Ideally, however, three people should be available: one to hold the mask in position while opening the airway, one to deliver chest compressions and a third to squeeze the bag for ventilation of the patient.
- Once an airway is secured with an endotracheal tube, chest compressions should continue uninterrupted at a rate of 100/minute and the patient should be ventilated at a rate of 10 breaths/minute *to improve coronary perfusion pressure* (Soar et al. 2015) (*see* Fig. 8.9 later).

Defibrillation

Early CPR and defibrillation can more than double the chances of survival from a cardiac arrest caused by a shockable rhythm (Perkins et al. 2015). To facilitate early defibrillation, access to AEDs is becoming more prevalent both in hospital and in the community setting. An AED provides voice and/or visual prompts for the rescuer to guide them through its use (Simpson 2017). **Manual defibrillation should be carried out only by those with cardiac rhythm recognition skills, and the skills and expertise to use this equipment.**

Automated External Defibrillation

- While chest compressions continue, another rescuer should switch on the AED and follow the prompts.
- Prepare to attach the adhesive electrode pads to the patient's bare chest while chest compressions continue (Simpson 2017), *to minimize interruptions to chest compressions.*
- The pads must be in good contact with the chest wall. Carefully and smoothly place them on the chest, ensuring there are no air bubbles, *to optimize delivery of electrical current to the myocardium.* It may be necessary quickly to remove any chest hair that is present (Deakin et al. 2005); however, absence of a razor should not delay defibrillation (Simpson 2017).
- One pad is positioned under the right clavicle (collar bone) and the other on the left side of the chest in the mid-axillary line (approximately where the V6 electrode

is positioned for a 12-lead electrocardiogram) (Soar et al. 2015). This is known as the sternal-apical position and is the standard site for pad placement (Fig. 8.8).
- Some AED pads are integral and already connected to the machine; if this is not the case, once the pads are in place on the chest, plug the pad connector into the AED.
- Listen to the voice prompts; if a shock is indicated, the rescuer will be instructed to deliver this.
- Unless the casualty has immediately regained consciousness, which is unlikely, immediately resume chest compressions after the shock is delivered (Fig. 8.9).

Safety Issues

- In an institutional setting, there may be difficulty accessing the patient because of equipment and furniture. If this is the case, the immediate area should be cleared as quickly as possible *to enhance access to the patient and promote staff and patient safety*.
- If the patient is on the floor, kneel by their side; if they are in bed, alter the bed height to suit the rescuer. If the patient is on a chair, they should be lowered to the floor, adhering to the local moving and handling policy.
- When delivering a defibrillatory shock, ensure that no other rescuers are touching the patient, *to prevent the risk of electrocution.*

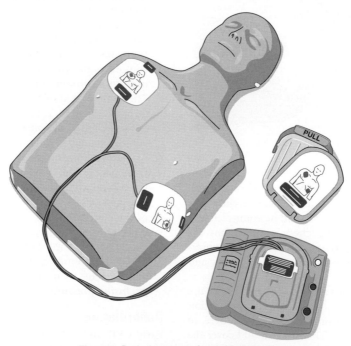

Fig. 8.8 Pad placement for defibrillation.

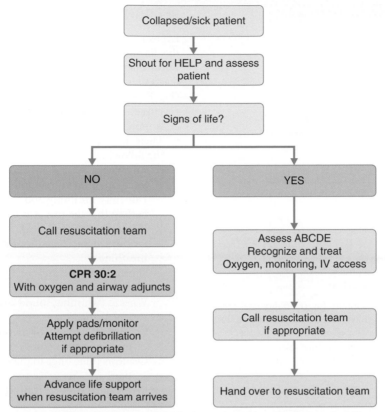

Fig. 8.9 In-hospital resuscitation algorithm. *ABCDE,* airway, breathing, circulation, disability, exposure; *CPR,* cardiopulmonary resuscitation; *IV,* intravenous. Reproduced with permission from Resuscitation Council (UK): In-Hospital Resuscitation, London, 2015a, RCUK.

- The oxygen-rich environment during resuscitation attempts can present a small fire risk during defibrillation. Free-flowing oxygen devices should therefore be moved at least 1 metre away from the patient's chest (Soar et al. 2015).

4. HEALTHCARE PROVIDER CPR IN THE PRIMARY CARE ENVIRONMENT

The guidelines described above for in-hospital CPR should be followed with some alterations (Fig. 8.9):
- Telephoning for help will require contacting the emergency medical services (dial 999 or 112) *to provide skilled personnel assistance.*
- Begin CPR and send for an AED as soon as possible.
- If you are trained and able to, you should combine chest compression with rescue breaths; it may be advisable to carry a pocket mask for this purpose.

- If you are unable to deliver or are not trained in rescue breathing, deliver compression-only CPR at a rate of 100–120/minute.
- Resuscitation should continue until expert help arrives, the casualty displays signs of life or the rescuer becomes exhausted.

5. RESPIRATORY ARREST

A respiratory arrest exists when the patient is not breathing but has a pulse. Respiratory arrest can be a primary event or can occur after the return of spontaneous circulation (ROSC) following cardiac arrest. In this situation, there is no requirement for chest compressions, as the heart is functioning as a pump and can circulate oxygenated blood. However, the lack of oxygen during respiratory arrest can lead to cardiopulmonary arrest and it is therefore vital to oxygenate the patient as promptly as possible. The

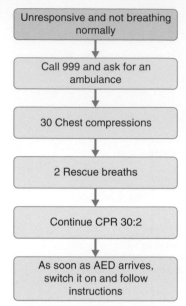

```
┌─────────────────────────────┐
│ Unresponsive and not        │
│ breathing normally          │
└─────────────────────────────┘
              ↓
┌─────────────────────────────┐
│ Call 999 and ask for an     │
│ ambulance                   │
└─────────────────────────────┘
              ↓
┌─────────────────────────────┐
│ 30 Chest compressions       │
└─────────────────────────────┘
              ↓
┌─────────────────────────────┐
│ 2 Rescue breaths            │
└─────────────────────────────┘
              ↓
┌─────────────────────────────┐
│ Continue CPR 30:2           │
└─────────────────────────────┘
              ↓
┌─────────────────────────────┐
│ As soon as AED arrives,     │
│ switch it on and follow     │
│ instructions                │
└─────────────────────────────┘
```

Fig. 8.10 Adult basic life support for out-of-hospital cardiopulmonary resuscitation (*CPR*). *AED,* automated external defibrillator. Reproduced with permission from Resuscitation Council (UK): Adult Basic Life Support and Automated External Defibrillation, London, 2015b, RCUK.

patient's airway should be maintained in an open position and they should be ventilated at a rate of 10 breaths/minute using a bag–valve–mask device with supplementary oxygen. The pulse should be checked after every minute (10 breaths); should the pulse disappear, CPR should be commenced immediately at a ratio of 30 compressions to two ventilations (Fig. 8.10).

6. ANAPHYLAXIS

Anaphylaxis is a clinical emergency and potentially a life-threatening condition (Muraro et al. 2014); it is caused by a generalized or systemic hypersensitive reaction to an allergen or trigger (Alvarez-Perea et al. 2017), such as insect stings, nuts, foods or medication (Resuscitation Council (UK) 2012).

Anaphylaxis can be difficult to diagnose but usually has an acute and sudden onset that can vary in severity and, on occasion, may spontaneously resolve (Simons et al. 2009). It is characterized by a rapidly developing problem with the patient's airway and/or breathing and/or circulation, and usually coexists with skin and/or mucosal changes (Resuscitation Council (UK) 2012).

RECOGNITION

Exposure to a known allergen or trigger can help confirm the diagnosis; however, diagnosis is not always straightforward. The following criteria suggest that an anaphylactic reaction is highly likely (Resuscitation Council (UK) 2012) (Fig. 8.11):

- Onset of symptoms is sudden and deterioration is rapid.
- There are life-threatening problems with some or all of the following:
  - Airway:
    Swelling of the throat and tongue
    Difficulty breathing and swallowing
    Feeling that the throat is closing over
    Hoarseness
    Stridor (high-pitched sound on inspiration)
  - Breathing:
    Shortness of breath
    Tachypnoea
    Wheeze (whistling sound on expiration)
    Patient tiring
    Confusion (caused by hypoxia: a low amount of oxygen in the tissues)
    Cyanosis (blue tinge to the skin): a late and worrying sign
    Respiratory arrest (breathing stops)
  - Circulation:
    Signs of shock: pale, clammy
    Tachycardia
    Hypotension
    Reduced conscious level
    Signs of myocardial ischaemia/angina
    Cardiac arrest
  - Disability
    Feeling of 'impending doom'
    Anxiety, panic
    Decreased conscious level caused by airway, breathing or circulation problem
    Changes in the skin and/or mucosa, which can take the form of flushing, urticaria or angioedema (see 'Exposure')
  - Exposure:
    Skin changes: often the first presenting sign and evident in 80% of anaphylactic reactions
    Skin, mucosal or both skin and mucosal changes in the form of a rash or erythema (a generalized red rash)
    Urticaria (also called hives, nettle rash, weals or welts)
    Angioedema (similar to urticaria but involving swelling of deeper tissues, e.g. eyelids and lips, sometimes in the mouth and throat)

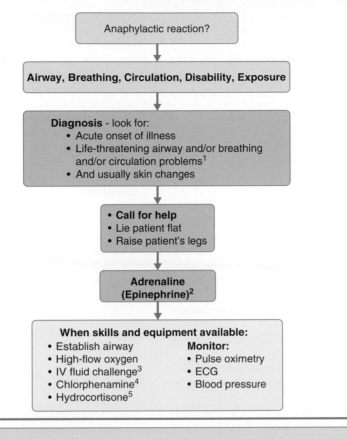

Anaphylactic reaction?

Airway, Breathing, Circulation, Disability, Exposure

Diagnosis - look for:
- Acute onset of illness
- Life-threatening airway and/or breathing and/or circulation problems[1]
- And usually skin changes

- **Call for help**
- Lie patient flat
- Raise patient's legs

Adrenaline (Epinephrine)[2]

When skills and equipment available:

- Establish airway
- High-flow oxygen
- IV fluid challenge[3]
- Chlorphenamine[4]
- Hydrocortisone[5]

Monitor:
- Pulse oximetry
- ECG
- Blood pressure

[1]**Life-threatening problems:**

Airway:	swelling, hoarseness, stridor
Breathing:	rapid breathing, wheeze, fatigue, cyanosis, SpO_2 <92%, confusion
Circulation:	pale, clammy, low blood pressure, faintness, drowsiness/coma

[2]**Adrenaline** *(give IM unless experienced with IV adrenaline)*
IM doses of 1:1000 adrenaline (repeat after 5 min if no better)
- Adult   500 micrograms IM (0.5 mL)
- Child more than 12 years: 500 micrograms IM (0.5 mL)
- Child 6–12 years: 300 micrograms IM (0.3 mL)
- Child less than 6 years: 150 micrograms IM (0.15 mL)

Adrenaline IV to be given **only by experienced specialists**
Titrate: Adults 50 micrograms; Children 1 microgram/kg

[3]**IV fluid challenge:**
Adult - 500–1000 mL
Child - crystalloid 20 mL/kg

Stop IV colloid
if this might be the cause
of anaphylaxis

	[4]**Chlorphenamine** (IM or slow IV)	[5]**Hydrocortisone** (IM or slow IV)
Adult or child more than 12 years	10 mg	200 mg
Child 6–12 years	5 mg	100 mg
Child 6 months to 6 years	2.5 mg	50 mg
Child less than 6 months	250 micrograms/kg	25 mg

Fig. 8.11 Anaphylaxis algorithm. *ECG,* electrocardiogram; *IM,* intramuscular; *IV,* intravenous, Reproduced with permission from Resuscitation Council (UK): Emergency Treatment of Anaphylactic Reactions: Guidelines for Healthcare Providers, London, 2012, RCUK.

Other presenting symptoms, which can include gastrointestinal symptoms (e.g. abdominal pain, vomiting, diarrhoea).

If in any doubt about the diagnosis, get help immediately.

TREATMENT

As with any patient who is experiencing acute deteriorating physiology, the ABCDE approach outlined earlier in the chapter should be employed and expert help called immediately. Life-threatening problems must be treated without delay and the patient's response to this treatment closely monitored. While the skills and expertise required to treat anaphylaxis may be beyond your current level or the scope of your clinical practice, you should know the steps in the process and be able to assist if required. While the information here presents a step-by-step process, in reality some steps may happen concurrently when there are enough personnel (see Fig. 8.10).

- Call for help, *as the patient's condition can deteriorate rapidly*.
- Remove the trigger, if it is still there and it is possible to do so.
- Monitor the patient's vital signs and attach pulse oximetry, electrocardiography (ECG) and blood pressure monitors as soon as possible.
- Lay the patient flat and elevate their legs if their blood pressure is low, *to reduce the work of the heart and optimize the circulation.*
- Locate and retrieve the emergency equipment *to allow prompt treatment*.
- Prepare 500 mcg intramuscular (IM) adrenaline (epinephrine) for administration (the concentration is 1:1000, which can be repeated after 5 minutes if the patient has not improved).
- **Never administer IV adrenaline (epinephrine) in cases of anaphylaxis**.
- As soon as skills are available, treat using ABCDE:
  - **A:** Establish a patent airway.
  - **B:** As this is an emergency, deliver high-flow oxygen (O'Driscoll et al. 2017). If asthma symptoms are evident, these should be treated with bronchodilators.
  - **C:** Prepare and deliver a fluid challenge (500–1000 mL of saline or Hartmann's solution in an adult).
  - **D:** Observe conscious level (AVPU).
  - **E:** Record vital signs and attach monitoring for pulse oximetry and ECG. Prepare for administration of antihistamine (chlorphenamine) and steroids (hydrocortisone).

PATIENT/CARER EDUCATION: KEY POINTS

During a resuscitation attempt, it may be that relatives will request to stay and observe the resuscitation, depending on the circumstances (Boyd 2000). In this case, it is considered best practice to allocate an experienced member of the interprofessional team to answer questions and act as a communicator between the clinical team and family (National Clinical Guideline Centre 2015).

Following a successful resuscitation, the patient and relatives must be given information about the event and be permitted to discuss their feelings and anxieties about the emergency. Other patients within the clinical area will also need to be given an explanation of the events to assist in relieving some of their own anxieties.

A training programme on basic resuscitation techniques may be required for relatives and carers of patients who are considered high-risk.

REFERENCES

Alvarez-Perea, A., Tanno, L.K., Baeza, M.L., 2017. How to manage anaphylaxis in primary care. Clinical and translational allergy 7 (1), 45.

Boyd, R., 2000. Witnessed resuscitation by relatives. Resuscitation 43 (3), 171–176.

Christenson, J., Andrusiek, D., Everson-Stewart, S., et al., 2009. Chest compression fraction determines survival in patients with out-of-hospital ventricular fibrillation. Circulation 120 (13), 1241–1247.

Cullinane, M., Findlay, G., 2005. National Confidential Enquiry into Patient Outcome and Death. An Acute Problem. Available from: https://www.ncepod.org.uk/2005aap.html.

Deakin, C.D., Nolan, J.P., European Resuscitation Council, 2005. European Resuscitation Council guidelines for resuscitation 2005. Section 3. Electrical therapies: automated external defibrillators, defibrillation, cardioversion and pacing. Resuscitation 67 (Suppl. 1), S25–S37.

Deakin, C.D., Nolan, J.P., Soar, J., et al., 2010. European Resuscitation Council Guidelines for Resuscitation 2010 Section 4. Adult advanced life support. Resuscitation 81 (10), 1305–1352.

Foo, N.P., Chang, J.H., Lin, H.J., Guo, H.R., 2010. Rescuer fatigue and cardiopulmonary resuscitation positions: a randomized controlled crossover trial. Resuscitation 81 (5), 579–584.

Gwinnutt, C., Davies, R., Soar, J., 2015. In-Hospital Resuscitation. Available at: http://www.resus.org.uk/resuscitation-guidelines/in-hospital-resuscitation.

Hodgetts, T.J., Kenward, G., Vlackonikolis, I., et al., 2002. Incidence, location and reasons for avoidable in-hospital cardiac arrest in a district general hospital. Resuscitation 54 (2), 115–123.

Jevon, P., 2010. ABCDE: the assessment of the critically ill patient. British Journal of Cardiac Nursing 5 (6), 268–272.

McDonald, C.H., Heggie, J., Jones, C.M., et al., 2013. Rescuer fatigue under the 2010 ERC guidelines, and its effect on cardiopulmonary resuscitation (CPR) performance. Emergency Medicine Journal 30 (8), 623–627.

Marshall, S., Harrison, J., Flanagan, B., 2009. The teaching of a structured tool improves the clarity and content of interprofessional clinical communication. BMJ Quality & Safety 18 (2), 137–140.

Muraro, A., Roberts, G., Worm, M., et al., 2014. Anaphylaxis: guidelines from the European Academy of Allergy and Clinical Immunology. Allergy 69 (8), 1026–1045.

National Clinical Guideline Centre (2015). Care of dying adults in the last days of life. Clinical Guideline NG31. Commissioned by the National Institute for Health and Care Excellence.

Niles, D.E., Sutton, R.M., Nadkarni, V.M., et al., 2011. Prevalence and hemodynamic effects of leaning during CPR. Resuscitation 82 (Suppl. 2), S23–S26.

Nursing and Midwifery Council, 2018. The Code: Professional Standards of Practice and Behaviour for Nurses, Midwives and Nursing Associates. NMC, London. Available at: https://www.nmc.org.uk/globalassets/sitedocuments/nmc-publications/nmc-code.pdf.

O'Driscoll, B.R., Howard, L.S., Earis, J., Mak, V., 2017. BTS guideline for oxygen use in adults in healthcare and emergency settings. Thorax 72 (Suppl. 1), ii1–ii90.

Parry, A., Higginson, R., 2016. How to use a self-inflating bag and face mask. Nursing Standard 30 (19), 36–38.

Perkins, G.D., Handley, A.J., Koster, R.W., et al., 2015. European Resuscitation Council Guidelines for Resuscitation 2015: section 2. Adult basic life support and automated external defibrillation. Resuscitation 95, 81–99.

Resuscitation Council (UK), 2012. Emergency Treatment of Anaphylactic Reactions: Guidelines for Healthcare Providers. Resuscitation Council (UK). Available from: https://www.resus.org.uk/anaphylaxis/emergency-treatment-of-anaphylactic-reactions/.

Resuscitation Council (UK), 2015a. In-Hospital Resuscitation. Resuscitation Council (UK). Available from: https://www.resus.org.uk/resuscitation-guidelines/in-hospital-resuscitation/.

Resuscitation Council (UK), 2015b. Adult Basic Life Support and Automated External Defibrillation. Resuscitation Council (UK). Available from: https://www.resus.org.uk/resuscitation-guidelines/adult-basic-life-support-and-automated-external-defibrillation/.

Riley, J., 2013. Breathing and circulation. In: Brooker, C., Waugh, A. (Eds.), Foundations of Nursing Practice: Fundamentals of Holistic Care, second ed. Mosby Elsevier, London, pp. 397–430.

Simons, F.E.R., Clark, S., Camargo, C.A., Jr., 2009. Anaphylaxis in the community: learning from the survivors. The Journal of Allergy and Clinical Immunology 124 (2), 301–306.

Simpson, E., 2016. In-hospital resuscitation: recognising and responding to adults in cardiac arrest. Nursing Standard 30 (51), 50.

Simpson, E., 2017. How to use an automated external defibrillator following out-of-hospital cardiac arrest. Nursing Standard 31 (32).

Smith, G., Pitcher, D., 2015. Prevention of Cardiac Arrest and Decisions About CPR. Resuscitation Council (UK). Available from: https://www.resus.org.uk/resuscitation-guidelines/prevention-of-cardiac-arrest-and-decisions-about-cpr/#in.

Soar, J., Nolan, J.P., Böttiger, B.W., et al., 2015. European resuscitation council guidelines for resuscitation 2015: section 3. Adult advanced life support. Resuscitation 95, 100–147.

Waugh, A., Grant, A., 2014. Ross & Wilson Anatomy and Physiology in Health and Illness E-Book. Elsevier Health Sciences.

❓ SELF-ASSESSMENT

1. In relation to an ABCDE approach, what does each of the letters mean?
2. What are the common causes of cardiac arrest?
3. When sudden cardiac arrest occurs, what might cause seizure-like activity in the patient?
4. How do you confirm cardiac arrest?
5. When delivering chest compressions, what rate and depth should you use?
6. What do the letters AED stand for?
7. What is the difference between respiratory arrest, cardiac arrest and cardiorespiratory arrest?
8. List the common causes of anaphylaxis.

Cardiovascular Risk Assessment

INDICATIONS AND RATIONALE FOR PERFORMING A CARDIOVASCULAR RISK ASSESSMENT

Cardiovascular disease (CVD) is the leading cause of death globally (World Health Organization 2017). Within the UK, CVD is recognized as being a significant cause of mortality and morbidity, accounting for nearly a third of all deaths and making CVD a major public health concern (National Institute for Health and Care Excellence 2014). Furthermore, the British Heart Foundation (2017) recognizes that CVD remains the largest cause of mortality and morbidity in the UK, with the highest associated costs, to both the NHS and the economy, of all of the long-term conditions. It is therefore argued that preventative strategies are essential.

Cardiovascular disease is a collective term for a range of disorders that affect the heart and blood vessels, and are related to atherosclerosis (thickening of the lining of the blood vessels with plaques of atheroma, or fatty deposits; National Institute for Health and Care Excellence 2014; UK National Screening Committee 2012). Some of the most common CVDs are coronary heart disease (CHD), cerebrovascular disease (stroke and transient ischaemic attack, TIA) and peripheral arterial disease (PAD).

Although progress has been made in recent years to reduce death from CVD, many cardiovascular deaths remain preventable. Assessment of cardiovascular risk is an essential step in addressing this important public health issue, allowing health resources to be allocated to individuals who are at the highest risk and who are most likely to benefit from a risk reduction. Furthermore, assessment of CVD risk can help practitioners to determine who should be prescribed medication such as statins (cholesterol-lowering medications) in order to reduce the risk of cardiovascular events.

The nurse has an important role in assessing an individual's CVD risk and thereafter providing tailored health education, treatment or onward referral as necessary. Furthermore, the Nursing and Midwifery Council's publication, *The Code* (2018), recognizes that it is a duty of the nurse to promote well-being, prevent ill health and meet the changing health and care needs of people during all life stages.

HEALTH PROMOTION AND APPROACHES TO CARDIOVASCULAR DISEASE PREVENTION

Health promotion is an umbrella term that encompasses health education, illness prevention and health protection. It is increasingly important for nurses to be active in promoting health, with Wills & Jackson (2014) recognizing that this should embrace a person-centred approach that involves listening to patients and seeks to involve them in their own health decisions.

There are three main levels of health promotion: primary prevention, secondary health promotion and tertiary health promotion (Wills & Jackson 2014). Primary prevention aims to prevent the onset of specific diseases through risk reduction (e.g. reducing cardiovascular risk through smoking cessation in an individual who does not already have CVD). Secondary health promotion aims to help individuals who already have a particular disease to modify risk factors in order to improve health (e.g. reducing cardiovascular risk through a dietary advice and weight loss programme for overweight individuals who have already had a heart attack). Tertiary health promotion aims to reduce the disability arising from a particular condition and to improve an individual's function, life expectancy and quality of life (Wills & Jackson 2014) (e.g. a health education and well-being programme for individuals living with heart failure – commonly a consequence of coronary disease).

In cardiovascular risk assessment, primary prevention involves estimating the CVD risk for patients who do not already have existing CVD, in order to identify modifiable risk factors and to offer interventions aimed at reducing the likelihood of the individual having a future cardiovascular event. CVD risk assessment tools, such as QRISK2, ASSIGN and JBS3 (*see* later), are indicated only for individuals who do not already have a diagnosis of heart disease or stroke.

The topic of cardiovascular risk assessment is large and this chapter is designed to provide an overview of some of the key issues related to the nursing practice. The nurse should engage in further reading in relation to health promotion approaches and follow local and national guidelines.

CARDIOVASCULAR RISK FACTORS AND RISK ESTIMATION

The underlying cause of CVD is atherosclerosis. Cardiovascular risk factors are therefore related to the risk of individuals developing atheroma and the extent and rate of this development. Risk factors may be largely categorized as non-modifiable, including age, gender, family history of CVD, and ethnicity; or modifiable, such as smoking, raised blood pressure and cholesterol (National Institute for Health and Care Excellence 2014). Further to this, a number of other special factors can strongly influence CVD risk, including social deprivation and comorbidity (National Institute for Health and Care Excellence 2014).

The calculation of absolute cardiovascular risk forms the foundation of most CVD prevention strategies. In this sense, 'absolute' risk (also known as global risk or total risk) is defined as the percentage chance of an individual having a cardiovascular event over a specified period of time, usually 10 years (Scottish Intercollegiate Guideline Network (SIGN) 2017). For example, a 10-year risk of 20% means that the individual has a 1 in 5 chance of having a CVD event within the next 10 years.

A number of different cardiovascular risk assessment tools exist. These can be extremely valuable in assessing risk;

however, it is important to note that no risk assessment tool can perfectly predict absolute cardiovascular risk (SIGN 2017; National Institute for Health and Care Excellence 2014).

The National Institute for Health and Care Excellence (NICE) (2014) recommends that, for primary prevention of CVD in primary care, a systematic strategy should be used to identify individuals who are likely to be at high risk. The guidelines advocate the use of the QRISK2 assessment tool to estimate CVD risk for the primary prevention of CVD in individuals under the age of 85 years, with a number of important caveats (NICE 2014). More recently, the Joint British Societies' consensus paper (2015) recommends the use of the JBS3 assessment tool, which is adapted from the QRISK2 tool to include measures of social class and family history of premature CVD. In Scotland, however, the ASSIGN score is preferred, as this has been adapted specifically to Scotland's population (SIGN 2017). Nurses should be aware of the expectations of CVD risk assessment within their own locality, as set out by national and local policy, and ensure that their nursing practice aligns with this.

In England, eligible adults aged between 40 and 74 should be invited every 5 years to attend for a full formal CVD risk assessment as part of the NHS health check (Public Health England 2016). In Scotland, SIGN (2017) recommends that all adults aged 40 years or above, and individuals of any age with a first-degree relative who had premature atherosclerotic CVD or familial dyslipidaemia, should be invited for a CVD risk assessment at least every 5 years. These health checks are normally administrated and conducted through primary care services. Elsewhere, in 2009 a Cardiovascular Service Framework was established in Northern Ireland, and in Wales the National Service Framework for Cardiac Disease was published (Department of Health, Social Services and Public Safety 2009; Welsh Government 2009). Both of these take a similar approach to cardiovascular risk assessment.

OUTLINE OF THE PROCEDURE

Cardiovascular risk assessment involves obtaining measurements and information from an individual in relation to their status and exposure to cardiovascular risk factors (Loades 2017). In many health and social care settings, the nurse may be responsible for conducting CVD risk assessments, e.g. in primary care it is often the practice nurse who undertakes this role.

GUIDELINES AND RATIONALE FOR THIS NURSING PRACTICE

Obtaining a clinical history together with measurement of relevant risk factors is key to the process of CVD risk assessment. Effective communication is an essential part of this nursing practice and nurses should use everyday language, avoiding jargon and medical terminology (NICE 2014). Sufficient time should be allocated to the consultation to allow full discussion of the results with the individual, offering tailored health education messages and providing an opportunity to ask questions. Furthermore, the nurse should be aware of potential psychosocial issues during the CVD risk assessment, as they can influence management decisions and future lifestyle choices (SIGN 2017).

- Ensure privacy for the consultation, as some of the information discussed may be sensitive to the individual, *to ensure privacy, confidentiality and dignity.*
- Explain the nursing practice to the individual, ensuring that they understand the purpose of the consultation and that they are happy to discuss various CVD risk factors and lifestyle choices. They should also understand that some clinical measurements will be taken as part of the assessment. Do this *to obtain informed consent and cooperation* (Nursing and Midwifery Council 2018).

Taking a Clinical History and Recording Clinical Measurements

- This process will involve obtaining information about the individual's age, gender, lifetime smoking habit (including number of cigarettes smoked daily), family history of CVD, ethnicity and socioeconomic status (SIGN 2017; Public Health England 2016). Although physical activity levels are not risk factors included in the QRISK2,

ASSIGN and JBS3 tools, SIGN (2017) recommends that the health professional should discuss physical activity as part of the consultation, as this can help to prioritize interventions in those who are not meeting current recommended levels. Do this *to identify and address any potential areas for health improvement.*

- If appropriate (i.e. the individual does not have a pre-existing diagnosis of heart disease, stroke or type 1 diabetes), a valid and reliable risk assessment tool should be used to guide the consultation (e.g. QRISK2, ASSIGN or JBS3). This is in order *to obtain an assessment of the individual's CVD risk that is as accurate as possible.*
- Measurements of the parameters outlined in Table 9.1 should be obtained as part of the CVD risk assessment.
- The clinical data obtained from the assessment should be entered into the assigned CVD risk estimation tool (QRISK2, ASSIGN or JBS3), usually using a computer or tablet, as per local policy. As many fields should be completed as possible (NICE 2014) *to obtain an assessment of the individual's absolute CVD risk that is as accurate as possible.*
- Combining the information obtained from taking a clinical history (i.e. age, gender, smoking history, family history of CVD, ethnicity and socioeconomic status) together with the clinical measurements/assessments (i.e. blood pressure, weight and body mass index, cholesterol level, diabetes, rheumatoid arthritis, renal function) should allow the nurse to build a cardiovascular risk

TABLE 9.1 Parameters to Be Measured as Part of the CVD Risk Assessment

Risk Factor	Measurement/Assessment	Rationale for Measurement
Blood pressure (BP; *see* Ch. 5)	Accurately measured according to NICE guidelines. The mean of two measurements of systolic BP should be used (Scottish Intercollegiate Guideline Network (SIGN) 2017)	High BP increases the risk of stroke, heart and kidney disease (Edmunds 2014) Reducing systolic BP by just 12 mmHg and diastolic by 6 mmHg can reduce the risk of heart disease by 20% and stroke by 40% (UK National Screening Committee 2012)
Weight and body mass index (BMI)	Accurately obtained using calibrated equipment	Individuals with a BMI of greater than 30 kg/m^2 have a 40-fold increase in risk of developing diabetes (strongly linked to increased cardiovascular risk) They also have a two- to threefold increase in risk of developing coronary heart disease and stroke, compared to those with a normal BMI (SIGN 2017)

Continued

TABLE 9.1	**Parameters to Be Measured as Part of the CVD Risk Assessment—cont'd**	
Risk Factor	**Measurement/Assessment**	**Rationale for Measurement**
Cholesterol	Total cholesterol, high-density lipoprotein (HDL – 'good cholesterol') and triglyceride levels obtained from a random non-fasted sample	Epidemiological evidence shows that populations with higher levels of cholesterol have more atherosclerosis; the higher the cholesterol level, the larger the risk of a coronary event (SIGN 2017) There is strong evidence to support the fact that lowering low-density lipoprotein (LDL – 'bad cholesterol') reduces cardiovascular risk (SIGN 2017)
Diabetes	Where there is a known diagnosis of diabetes, this should be recorded SIGN (2017) recommends against formal risk estimation using a tool for individuals who have a diagnosis of diabetes, as they should already be considered to be at high cardiovascular risk and therefore automatically eligible for preventative measures NICE (2014), however, suggests that the QRISK2 assessment tool can be used for individuals with type 2 diabetes but not those with type 1 Where individuals do not have a diagnosis of diabetes but do have risk factors for this (e.g. obesity), validated tools should be used to screen for the condition: fasting blood glucose, glycated haemoglobin (HbA$_{1c}$) (SIGN 2017)	Diabetes approximately doubles the risk of cardiovascular events for those that have the condition (SIGN 2017) Earlier diagnosis and management of diabetes improves patient outcomes Statin therapy for individuals with diabetes is associated with a significant reduction in all-cause mortality and heart attacks (SIGN 2017)
Rheumatoid arthritis	Information obtained through history-taking and review of clinical notes	Individuals with rheumatoid arthritis are at a significantly increased risk of cardiovascular events (SIGN 2017)
Kidney function	A blood test to assess estimated glomerular filtration rate (eGFR) should be checked to assess for kidney disease Individuals with an eGFR of less than 60 mL/min per 1.73 m^2 (and/or those with albuminuria) – indicative of kidney disease – should be automatically considered to be at high CVD risk and therefore do not require formal risk assessment (SIGN 2017; NICE 2014). They should be offered aggressive interventions to reduce their risk of cardiovascular events (SIGN 2017)	Individuals with chronic kidney disease (CKD) are at significantly increased risk of cardiovascular events (SIGN 2017)

profile for a particular individual. An integral part of this is the absolute CVD risk, as estimated by the QRISK2, ASSIGN or JBS3 tool. Do this *to identify and address potential areas for health improvement and to guide recommendations for specific interventions.*

- The information obtained should be recorded carefully in the medical/nursing notes *to ensure accurate record-keeping in line with your professional requirements* (Nursing and Midwifery Council 2018).

- The cardiovascular risk profile should be communicated to the patient in simple, jargon-free language so that they are able to understand their absolute risk of CVD (NICE 2014). Do this *to allow patients to make informed lifestyle choices to reduce cardiovascular risk, and to be fully involved in the process.*

- Where necessary, the information should be shared with the multidisciplinary team so that clinical decisions can be made based on the assessment. For example, a doctor may prescribe a statin to reduce cardiovascular risk for certain patients, or treatment may be given where a new diagnosis of diabetes is established. Do this *to offer patients optimal evidence-based treatments tailored to their clinical need.*

PATIENT/CARER EDUCATION: KEY POINTS

Patient and carer education is central to cardiovascular risk assessment, and the health education information available to patients to reduce their cardiovascular risk is vast. This may include guidance on modifiable risk factors, such as diet, physical activity levels, smoking and alcohol intake, e.g. advising patients to increase physical activity levels, lose weight, reduce alcohol intake or stop smoking. The nurse should be familiar with this information and ensure that it is delivered to patients in a way that they can easily understand. The nurse should also be familiar with local and national policy and guidelines in relation to health promotion and the facilities available for patients locally.

REFERENCES

British Heart Foundation, 2017. Heart and Circulatory Diseases Statistics 2017. Available at: https://www.bhf.org.uk/what-we-do/our-research/heart-statistics/heart-statistics-publications/cardiovascular-disease-statistics-2017.

Department of Health, Social Services and Public Safety, 2009. Cardiovascular Health and Wellbeing Service Framework. DHSSPS, Belfast.

Edmunds, L., 2014. Back to basics: assessing cardiovascular risk. (Report). Practice Nurse 44 (4), 12.

JOINT BRITISH SOCIETIES, 2014. Joint British Societies' consensus recommendations for the prevention of cardiovascular disease (JBS3). Heart (British Cardiac Society) 100 (Suppl. 2), ii67.

Loades, J., 2017. Cardiovascular disease prevention: where are we now? Practice Nurse 47 (9).

National Institute for Health and Care Excellence, 2014. Cardiovascular disease: risk assessment and reduction, including lipid modification. Available at: https://www.nice.org.uk/.

Nursing and Midwifery Council, 2018. The Code: Professional Standards of Practice and Behaviour for Nurses, Midwives and Nursing Associates. NMC, London. Available at: https://www.nmc.org.uk/globalassets/sitedocuments/nmc-publications/nmc-code.pdf.

Public Health England, 2016. NHS Health Check. Best practice guidance. Available at: https://www.healthcheck.nhs.uk/commissioners_and_providers/guidance/national_guidance1/.

Scottish Intercollegiate Guideline Network, 2017. Risk estimation and the prevention of cardiovascular disease, SIGN 149. Available from: https://www.sign.ac.uk.

UK National Screening Committee, 2012. The Handbook for Vascular Risk Assessment, Risk Reduction and Risk Management. University of Leicester, Leicester.

Welsh Government, 2009. National Service Framework for Cardiac Disease. Welsh Government, Cardiff.

Wills, J., Jackson, L., 2014. Health promotion and public health. In: Wills, J. (Ed.), Fundamentals of Health Promotion for Nurses, second ed. Wiley Blackwell, Chichester.

World Health Organization, 2017. Cardiovascular Diseases Fact Sheet. Available at: http://www.who.int/news-room/fact-sheets/detail/cardiovascular-diseases-(cvds).

SELF-ASSESSMENT

1. Why is cardiovascular risk assessment important?
2. List five modifiable risk factors that can affect an individual's cardiovascular risk profile.
3. What group of medications may be prescribed to help reduce an individual's cholesterol level, and why is this important?
4. How might you discuss weight loss with an individual with a high BMI in terms of their absolute cardiovascular risk?

10

Care After Death

LEARNING OUTCOMES

By the end of this chapter, you should be able to:
- care for a deceased person.

BACKGROUND KNOWLEDGE REQUIRED

- Revision of local policy on the care of a deceased person
- Review of the religious and spiritual rites of care for a deceased person
- Revision of 'Fundamental Care' (see Ch. 19) and 'Oral Hygiene' (see Ch. 27)

◎ EQUIPMENT

- Disposable gloves and apron
- Equipment as for 'Fundamental Care' (see Ch. 19)
- Equipment as for 'Oral Hygiene' (see Ch. 27)
- Clean sheets
- Continence pad and disposable pants
- Dressing pack, tape and occlusive dressings if wounds present
- Shroud or disposable gown
- Disposable body bag if advised (refer to local trust policy)
- Two patient identification bands appropriately completed with the patient's full name and other details
- Two notification of death cards
- Mortuary sheet, or an additional sheet if this is not available
- Gauze bandage
- Trolley for equipment
- Receptacle for patient's clothing
- Receptacle for patient's valuables
- Patient clothing list book
- Patient valuables list book
- Receptacle for soiled linen
- Receptacle for soiled disposable items

INDICATIONS AND RATIONALE FOR CARE OF A DECEASED PERSON

Before transfer to the mortuary or undertaker's premises, a deceased patient requires care that may be delivered by a professional carer, an undertaker or the appropriate person identified by the spiritual beliefs of the deceased (Martin & Bristowe 2015). This care demonstrates continued respect for the patient as an individual (Nursing and Midwifery Council 2018). This care was formerly referred to as 'last offices'; however, 'care after death' is the preferred term in a multicultural society, reflecting all aspects of care at the time of death and including support for family members and others identified as important to the deceased (Wilson 2015).

GUIDELINES AND RATIONALE FOR THIS NURSING PRACTICE

Details of the practice can vary, according to the patient's cultural background and religious practice; an awareness of specific requirements prior to, during or after death is therefore essential (Swift 2015; Public Health England 2016).

A patient who dies suddenly and unexpectedly will require a post-mortem examination (NHS Scotland 2005). Hand-washing should take place before commencement and on completion of the practice.

- Inform the medical practitioner when a patient is thought to have died *to confirm the diagnosis of death and comply with the legal requirements before the issue of a death certificate.* An experienced registered nurse assessed as competent may also be permitted to verify the death of a patient or resident within the agreed local policy (Wilson et al. 2017).
- Ensure privacy for the patient and relatives *to prevent further distress to those persons present.*

- Ensure that the patient's relatives, if they are not present, are notified of the death. *This will allow the expressed wishes of the deceased to be implemented and funeral arrangements to be initiated.*
- Ensure that relatives are adequately and kindly informed about immediate practicalities (Wilson 2015).
- Assist and support bereaved relatives, *as the professional carer is in a key position at this time* (Hills & Albarran 2010).
- Check nursing documentation for patient and family preferences for care after death, including an advanced care plan if present (Mullick et al. 2013), *to ensure patient- and family-centred care provision* (McCormack & McCance 2016).
- Inform the charge nurse or deputy and portering staff, or, if in the patient's home, assist the carer to contact the undertaker *to make the initial arrangements for the transfer of the body to the mortuary or undertaker's premises.*
- Collect and prepare the equipment *to ensure that all the equipment is available.*
- Wash your hands and apply an apron and gloves *to reduce the potential of cross-infection* (Pattison 2008).
- Remove all the upper bed linen, leaving a sheet to cover the patient, *to give easy access to the body.*
- Lay the patient flat, face up, with limbs in a natural position and arms by their side. **Rigor mortis occurs 2–4 hours following death; positioning the body after this time is difficult.**
- Remove any *nursing or medical equipment in order to reduce the 'clinical' appearance of the room.*
- Gently close the eyelids *to protect the tissues, should the deceased or relatives have given permission for corneal donation, and also to improve the facial appearance.*
- Clean the patient's mouth and replace any dentures *to enhance the aesthetic appearance of the deceased and maintain hygiene.*
- Support the mandible in a closed position using a light pillow.
- Remove all tubes and drains, unless otherwise instructed, *to reduce the hazard to health:*
  - redress all wounds with a waterproof dressing, *thereby reducing the potential problem of leakage of body fluids*; any drains or tubes left in position should also be covered with a padded waterproof dressing
  - drains, tubes and dressings may be left in position during this practice if a patient dies unexpectedly, within 24 hours of surgery or receiving an anaesthetic, or within 24 hours of involvement in some form of trauma (Scottish Government 2017).
- Wash the patient as for 'Fundamental Care' (*see* Ch. 19), *for general hygiene purposes.*

- A male patient may be shaved *for aesthetic reasons; check the local policy.*
- All jewellery, once removed, should be listed in the patient valuables book in the presence of two nurses, *to maintain security for the deceased's belongings.* In the community, personal belongings should not be removed by the nurse unless a witness is present. Any action should be documented and signed.
- Apply identification bands and cards to the appropriate limbs and parts of the body as per local policy, *to ensure continued identification of the deceased.*
- Apply an incontinence pad or disposable napkin *to reduce the health hazard from further body fluid leakage for staff who are in contact with the body.*
- Place the shroud, or fresh bedclothes at home, in position *to enhance the appearance, should relatives wish to view the deceased.*

Institution

- Wrap the body in the sheet, ensuring complete coverage, and secure the sheet with adhesive tape or a gauze bandage *to prevent exposure of the deceased during transfer to the mortuary.*
- Fix an identification card or notification of death card to the sheet using adhesive tape, *to aid future identification.*
- If there is a risk of infection, the body may be placed in a body bag. The bag is labelled 'danger of infection', along with the name of the infection.
- List the patient's clothing *to create a receipt for future use.*
- Place this clothing and the patient's valuables in a secure place *to ensure safekeeping until removal by the relatives.*
- Dispose of equipment safely *to reduce any health hazard.*
- Inform portering staff that the body is ready for collection *to permit the body to be cooled as soon as possible after death, thus slowing the decomposition process.*
- On arrival of the portering staff with the mortuary trolley, ensure the privacy of the other patients *to attempt to prevent further distress.*
- Other patients should be informed kindly and honestly that the patient has died and given support when needed (Wilson 2015).
- Document the nursing practice appropriately *to provide a written record of the care given.*

Community

- Cover the patient with a sheet *for aesthetic purposes.* Unless requested otherwise by the carer, leave the face uncovered.

- Following the removal of the body, arrange for the collection of any residual equipment, ***thereby returning the home environment to 'normal'***.
- Document the nursing practice appropriately ***to provide a written record of the care given.***
- In undertaking this practice, nurses are accountable for their actions, the quality of care delivered and record-keeping according to *The Code* (Nursing and Midwifery Council 2018).

 PATIENT/CARER EDUCATION: KEY POINTS

It is important for families and carers to be aware of what to do after a death and what support groups are available to them (Scottish Government 2017). The bereaved relatives will require sensitive and compassionate care (Hills & Albarran 2010). Any request to see the deceased should be met as soon as possible, as this may assist the relatives during the grieving process; care should be taken to ensure that the patient looks as peaceful as possible, that the environment is cleared of equipment and that a chair is available.

Nurses and other professionals should receive education and training on all aspects of care after death (Wilson 2015). The nurse may also need to assist and support their colleagues prior to, during and after the nursing practice (de Swardt & Fouche 2017). An opportunity for debriefing should be provided (Hockley 2014).

REFERENCES

De Swardt, C., Fouche, N., 2017. "What happens behind the curtains?" An exploration of ICU nurses' experiences of post mortem care on patients who have died in intensive care. Intensive and Critical Care Nursing 43, 108–115.

Hills, M., Albarran, J.W., 2010. After death 1: caring for bereaved relatives and being aware of cultural differences. Nursing Times 106 (27), 19–20.

Hockley, J., 2014. Learning, support and communication for staff in care homes: outcomes of reflective debriefing groups in two care homes to enhance end of life care. International Journal of Older People Nursing 9 (2), 118–130.

Martin, S., Bristowe, K., 2015. Last Offices: nurses' experiences of the process and their views about involving significant others. International Journal of Palliative Nursing 21 (4), 173–178.

McCormack, B., McCance, T., 2016. Person-Centred Practice in Nursing and Health Care Theory and Practice, second ed. Wiley–Blackwell, Chichester.

Mullick, A., Martin, J., Sallnow, L., 2013. An introduction to advance care planning in practice. British Medical Journal 347, 60–64.

NHS Scotland, 2005. Post-Mortem Examination of an Adult. Scottish Government, Edinburgh.

Nursing and Midwifery Council, 2018. The Code: Professional Standards of Practice and Behaviour for Nurses, Midwives and Nursing Associates. NMC, London. Available at: https://www.nmc.org.uk/globalassets/sitedocuments/nmc-publications/nmc-code.pdf.

Pattison, N., 2008. Care of patients who have died. Nursing Standard 22 (28), 42–48.

Public Health England, 2016. Faith at End of Life: A Resource for Professionals, Providers and Commissioners Working in Communities. Public Health England, London.

Scottish Government, 2017. What to do After a Death in Scotland: Practical Advice for Times of Bereavement, eleventh ed. Scottish Government, Edinburgh.

Swift, C., 2015. NHS Chaplaincy Guidelines: Promoting Excellence in Pastoral, Spiritual & Religious Care. NHS England, London.

Wilson, J., 2015. Care After Death: Guidance for Staff Responsible for Care After Death. Hospice UK, London.

Wilson, J., Laverty, D., Cooper, M., 2017. Care After Death: Registered Nurse Verification of Expected Adult Death (RNVoEAD) Guidance. Hospice UK, London.

WEBSITES

https://www.mariecurie.org.uk/professionals/palliative-care-knowledge-zone/individual-needs/faith-end-life *Marie Curie*

rcnendoflife.org.uk/the-patient-journey/culture-and-spirituality-2/ *Royal College of Nursing*

 SELF-ASSESSMENT

1. What equipment is required for care after death?
2. How would you describe the procedure of care after death to a colleague?
3. What is essential to prevent cross-infection during this procedure?
4. How should the nurse deal with the deceased patient's personal belongings?

11

Catheterization: Urinary

There are four parts to this chapter:
1. Catheterization
2. Catheter care
3. Bladder irrigation
4. Administration of catheter maintenance solutions

The concluding boxes, 'Patient/carer education: key points' and 'Self-assessment', refer to the four practices collectively.

LEARNING OUTCOMES

By the end of this chapter, you should be able to:
- prepare the patient for these four nursing practices
- collect and prepare the equipment
- carry out catheterization, catheter care and bladder irrigation
- administer catheter maintenance solutions.

BACKGROUND KNOWLEDGE REQUIRED

- Revision of the anatomy and physiology of the urinary system and external genitalia
- Revision of 'Wound Care' (see Ch. 40)
- Revision of local policy regarding catheterization, catheter bags and administration of catheter maintenance solutions

1. CATHETERIZATION

INDICATIONS AND RATIONALE FOR URETHRAL CATHETERIZATION

It is estimated that healthcare-associated infections (HAIs) cost the NHS over £1 billion each year (Mantle 2015). More importantly, patient safety is compromised when these infections occur, which in turn increases the use of NHS resources (Taylor 2018). Mantle (2015) further asserts that urinary tract infection (UTI) is among the top six common HAIs (alongside meticillin-resistant *Staphylococcus aureus* (MRSA), *Clostridium difficile*, respiratory tract infections, wound infections and poor hand hygiene), and these account for 80% of all HAIs across healthcare settings. The most common site for HAI is the urinary tract, and between 43% and 56% are associated with an indwelling urinary catheter (Mantle 2015; Loveday et al. 2014).

The risk of catheter-associated urinary tract infection (CAUTI) in both short- and long-term catheter use is well documented (National Institute for Health and Care Excellence 2014); the risk increases with the length of time the catheter remains in place (Loveday et al. 2014). Due to the invasive nature of urinary catheterization, the National Institute for Health and Care Excellence (NICE) (2013) states that practitioners must be competent before undertaking the nursing procedure. This competency should minimize the risks to the patient of discomfort, pain and CAUTI.

Catheter insertion is an aseptic technique that requires a full clinical assessment; it should be performed only when there is an identified clinical need or when the insertion of a catheter is likely to improve the patient's quality of life. Shackley et al. (2017) suggest that 30%–50% of urinary catheterizations take place without a robust clinical indication and a comprehensive assessment is therefore essential. This is important because patients having a catheter inserted as part of their clinical care are in significant danger of acquiring a UTI. The risk of UTI is associated with the method and duration of catheterization, the quality of catheter care and host susceptibility (Pratt et al. 2007). The use of indwelling catheterization should be a last resort, and Mantle (2015), the European Association of Urology Nurses (2012) and NICE (2012) agree that intermittent catheterization (IC) or intermittent self-catheterization (ISC) is considered to be the gold standard for reducing infection. This is also a recognized alternative to indwelling urinary catheterization.

Urinary catheters can be inserted to:
- re-establish a flow of urine in urinary retention
- provide a channel for drainage when micturition is impaired
- empty the bladder preoperatively

- allow the monitoring of fluid balance in a seriously ill patient
- facilitate bladder irrigation procedures
- administer intravesical medication
- dilate a stricture by insertion of a catheter
- relieve urinary incontinence when all other forms of nursing intervention have failed (although it should be considered as a last resort).

◎ EQUIPMENT

Catheterization pack content varies but should include:
- Sterile drape
- Bowl with swabs
- Pair of sterile gloves

Additional Items
- Sterile catheter: you may need a selection of appropriate catheters and it is advisable to ensure this is available
- Sterile anaesthetic lubricating gel or water-based lubricant as per local policy (6 mL for females and 11 mL for males)
- Syringe
- Disposable towel
- Disposable pad for bed protection
- Universal specimen container
- Bactericidal alcohol hand disinfection
- Catheter drainage bag or sterile receptacle for urine
- Personal protective equipment
- Suitable trolley or adequate surface for equipment
- If requested, a sterile specimen collector appropriately labelled with a completed laboratory form and plastic specimen bag for transportation
- Disposal bag for waste

CATHETER SELECTION

Catheter Type

This is dependent on the reason for catheterization and the length of time the catheter needs to remain in the bladder (Fig. 11.1). Selection of the correct catheter also depends on catheter material, size, length, balloon volume and drainage system (Association for Continence Advice 2007). Careful assessment of the most appropriate material, size and balloon capacity will ensure that the catheter selected is as effective as possible, complications are minimized, and patient comfort and quality of life are promoted. Catheters should be used in accordance with the manufacturer's recommendations in order to avoid product liability (Dougherty et al. 2015).

Catheter Material and Duration of Use

The key criterion for selecting the appropriate material and type of catheter is the length of time the catheter is expected to remain in place (Pellowe 2009; NICE 2012).

A variety of materials are available. When choosing a catheter, the following should be considered:
- ease of use
- allergy to latex
- patient comfort.

Intermittent Catheters

- Polyvinyl chloride (PVC) non-coated catheters: these are quite rigid and require lubrication prior to insertion.
- Hydrophilic-coated catheters: these are impregnated with a coating that lubricates the catheter throughout the catheterization process. Hydrophilic catheters may require activation with water.

Short-Term Catheters (1–28 days)

- Polytetrafluoroethylene (PTFE)-coated latex catheters: the coating is applied to the latex catheter to render the latex inert and reduce irritation. These catheters are normally used for short to mid-term durations, although it is important to check the manufacturer's recommendations. They may be suitable for long-term catheterized patients requiring a catheter change more frequently than every 4 weeks.

Long-Term Catheters (up to 12 weeks)

- Silicone elastomer-coated latex catheters: latex core catheters coated with silicone do not provide smooth internal and external surfaces, which are resistant to encrustation.
- Hydrogel-coated latex catheters: latex core catheters coated with a hydrophilic polymer coating provide very smooth internal and external surfaces, which are resistant to encrustation. They are also inert and well tolerated by the urethral mucosa.
- Silicone catheters: these are made by an extrusion process that produces a thin-walled catheter with a large D-shaped lumen. Due to the inert nature of the silicone, they can reduce irritation and are suitable for those with a latex allergy. However, they are relatively stiff and some patients find them uncomfortable. Silicone permits gas diffusion, and balloons may deflate and allow the catheter to fall out prematurely. For patients with a latex allergy, only 100% silicone catheters are latex-free; there is, however, a risk of diffusion of water from the balloon and so the water in the balloon must be checked regularly (Association for Continence Advice 2007).

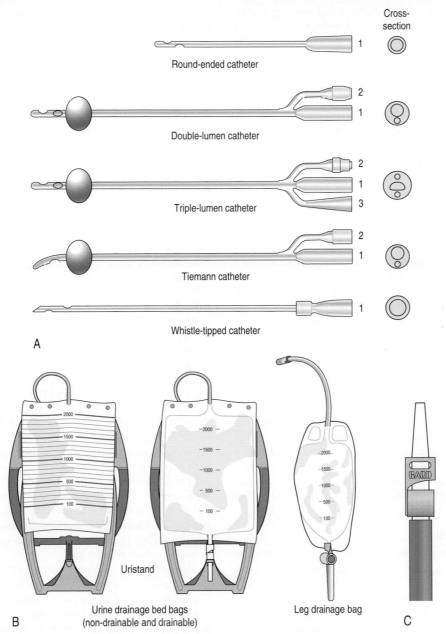

Cross-section

Round-ended catheter

Double-lumen catheter

Triple-lumen catheter

Tiemann catheter

Whistle-tipped catheter

A

Uristand

Urine drainage bed bags
(non-drainable and drainable)

Leg drainage bag

B   C

Fig. 11.1 Catheterization. (A) Examples of catheters. *1*, Channel for urine flow; *2*, channel for balloon inflation; *3*, channel for irrigating fluid flow. (B) Types of drainage bag. (C) Catheter valve.

Catheter Size

The external diameter of the catheter is measured in Charrière units (Ch). One Ch equals one-third of a millimetre (mm); therefore 12 Ch = 4 mm. (French gauge, or Fg, units are the same as Charrière units.) For routine drainage in an adult, select the smallest Charrière size that will ensure adequate drainage, as larger sizes will cause urethral trauma and irritation of the bladder mucosa (Pellowe 2009) (*see* Fig. 11.1). The larger sizes are usually used for clot drainage and stricture dilation. In any other situation, their use should be questioned. A suitable catheter size for female and male patients is 12–14 Ch (or Fg), although catheters for females range from 10–14 Ch, and those for males from 12–16 Ch (or Fg). Intermittent non-retaining self-catheters are usually size 10–12 Ch (or Fg).

Catheter Balloon Size

A 10 mL balloon size should be used, except in specialist uro-surgery situations. A larger balloon size may not fully inflate, causing bypassing and local bladder trauma. A larger balloon size also raises the point of drainage and a residual pool may form, resulting in bypassing and bacteria (Bardsley 2005). The balloon should be inflated only with sterile water. Do not use tap water to inflate the balloon, as it may introduce bacteria into the bladder. Saline may cause crystal formation in the inflation channels. It is important for manufacturer's guidelines to be followed at all times.

Balloons are available in three sizes:
- 5 mL paediatric balloons
- 10 mL balloons for routine drainage
- 30 mL balloons, which should **not** be routinely used; these are for post-prostatectomy use and must be employed only on the specific instruction of, and as directed by, a urologist.

The weight of water in larger balloons may lead to dragging/pulling of the catheter. The larger balloon may also cause bladder spasm and discomfort because it will rest against the sensitive part of the lower bladder, known as the trigone, causing spasm, bypassing, pain, haematuria and possible erosion of the bladder wall. **Never** insert more or less water into the balloon than is specified by the manufacturer, as over-inflation will **not** prevent a catheter being expelled. Under-inflation results in balloon distortion, with the risk that the catheter may become dislodged from the bladder; therefore it is not best practice to deflate and reinflate the balloon for troubleshooting (Dougherty et al. 2015).

Catheter Length

Catheters are manufactured in female and male lengths, the female being 26 cm and the male being 41–45 cm (European Association of Urology Nurses 2012). However, a male catheter length can be used for females if the female patient is bed-bound. Also, if the female patient is obese, using the standard male length can help with drainage (European Association of Urology Nurses 2012).

The female-length catheter (short length) should **never** be used for males, as inflation of the balloon within the urethra can be traumatic and may cause severe trauma to the prostatic urethra (National Patent Safety Agency 2009).

Catheter Bags and Choice of Drainage System

The following should be taken into consideration when selecting products:

Ambulant patients will probably prefer leg bags. These are available in 350, 500 and 750 mL volumes, with short, medium or long tubing. It is important to ensure that the volume and tubing length are specified on prescription, remembering that leg bags are usually worn by women on the thigh and by men on the calf. There are many different types of tap to facilitate drainage and this is one of the most important factors to take into account when selecting a drainage bag, as patients whose manual dexterity is compromised may not be able to operate certain types.

Choose a length that will prevent kinking or dragging of the catheter and tubing. The bags should have a drainage tap (lever type) to facilitate emptying. Patients with an indwelling catheter will need to use a leg bag by day and a night bag at night. The night bags should be attached to the leg bag using a clean procedure and the bags should be non-drainable (one use only); the only exception is for bed-bound patients. Here, a reusable night bag can be chosen rather than a leg bag. The bags must be used in accordance with the manufacturer's instructions. The leg bag is not disconnected from the catheter unless it is due to be changed: this is normally every 5–7 days, in accordance with the manufacturer's instructions. Night bags should be placed on a stand and **never** on the floor or lying in a receptacle, e.g. a bucket. The stand should be positioned to prevent any kinking of the catheter and tubing.

It is important for the night bag to be attached using the 'closed system' technique, i.e. the night bag is attached to the leg bag, and the valve on the leg bag is opened to allow free drainage. A belly bag is also available for patients with suprapubic catheters. It is called a belly bag as it is designed to be worn around the waist by males or females who have an indwelling urinary catheter or suprapubic catheter. It is manufactured for users with bilateral amputations (NHS Quality Improvement Scotland 2004) or with a spinal injury. Specialist bags such as belly bags can also be used in place of a leg bag.

Bag selection also depends on the rationale for catheter use, patient preference and the patient's manual dexterity. The leg bag should be supported either by leg straps or by a variety of other accessories such as net sleeves. The importance of catheter stability is stressed by Dougherty et al. (2015) as promoting patient comfort and limiting the potential complications of catheter migration and a subsequent need for recatheterization. The choice of drainage system must be dictated by the intended duration, patient mobility and dexterity, patient choice and clinical decision. More frequent disconnections will break the closed system and increase the risk of infection. A study carried out by Madeo et al. (2009) demonstrated that use of a sealed system reduced CAUTI by 41%. The urine bag should be emptied frequently enough to maintain urine flow and prevent reflux (National Institute for Health and Care Excellence 2012).

Catheter Valves

There is evidence to show that catheter valves are preferred by patients and should always be considered where appropriate (Yates 2008). There is no significant difference in rates of urinary infection; however, there is evidence to show that patients using catheter valves may suffer less from catheter encrustation and catheter blockage, and that the valves also help to prevent bladder neck trauma. This is thought to be due to emptying the bladder periodically via a catheter valve, which produces a 'flushing' effect that may help reduce the build-up of bacterial biofilm and encrustation (Raheem et al. 2011). Woodward (2013) suggests that the use of a catheter valve may allow for the normal action of the bladder (filling and emptying periodically) and that this action can help maintain the sensation of bladder fullness and bladder tone. However, she also suggests that there is a shortage of empirical evidence from physiological studies to support these assertions.

There are a number of valves available, and these should be selected for ease of use, prevention of leaks and compatibility with the patient's system. They should be used in accordance with the manufacturer's guidance and local NHS continence formulary, and should be changed using a clean technique. Some individuals may not be suitable for a catheter valve. All patients require an individual assessment prior to the use of a catheter valve and they also need the mental capacity to remember to release the valve at regular intervals. People with an overactive bladder, renal impairment and ureteric reflux may not be suitable for a catheter valve (Dougherty et al. 2015). Patients with reduced bladder capacity are also not recommended for catheter valve use (NHS Business Services Authority 2013).

GUIDELINES AND RATIONALE FOR THIS NURSING PRACTICE

Female Patients

The nurse should obtain a history from the patient and fully assess the patient's needs before the procedure. Prior to the catheterization, provide the patient with a verbal explanation of what will happen, as well as giving written information. Catheters and drainage bags should be shown to the patient beforehand to facilitate understanding and choice of drainage bag and bag valve (Loveday et al. 2014). Patients, relatives and carers should also be given information regarding the reason for the catheter, as well as the plan for review and renewal. If discharged with a catheter, the patient should be given written information on its management.

- Explain the procedure to the patient, including risks and benefits, *to obtain consent and cooperation.*
- *Ascertain if any problems have been experienced with previous catheterizations.*
- *Check for allergies to latex or lidocaine (anaesthetic gel).* Lidocaine hydrochloride 2%, chlorhexidine gluconate solution 0.25% is a sterile local anaesthetic and lubricant for the urethral mucosa. It can prevent injury to the urethra and as a consequence reduces the subsequent risk of urethral damage; it **must be used for catheterizing both male and female patients.** Lidocaine hydrochloride 2%, chlorhexidine gluconate solution 0.25% facilitates a reduction in pain on insertion and helps reduce the risk of associated infection.
- Collect and prepare the equipment *to ensure that all equipment is available and ready for use.*
- Ensure the patient's privacy *to reduce anxiety.*
- Always observe the patient throughout the procedure *to note any signs of distress.*
- Prepare and help the patient to assume the supine position with the knees bent, the hips flexed, and the feet resting on the bed approximately 70 cm apart. *This position provides good access to, and visualization of, the genitalia.*
- Place a procedure pad underneath the patient's sacral area *to prevent any spillage of fluids on to the patient's bed linen/clothing.*
- Arrange the lighting *to assist with good visualization of the genitalia.*
- Decontaminate your hands and clean a trolley, arranging the equipment on the trolley.
- Put on an apron and decontaminate your hands again; then prepare the sterile field. *These measures act as a barrier between the nurse's skin and the patient's tissues, thus reducing the incidence of contamination* (National Institute for Health and Care Excellence 2012; NHS Quality Improvement Scotland 2004).
- Open and arrange the equipment, maintaining sterility at all times, *to reduce contamination.*
- Add the other sterile equipment, ensuring that you do not contaminate the sterile field, including sterile gloves, sterile gauze and clinical waste bag.
- Decontaminate your hands using soap and water or alcohol hand rub.
- Put on non-sterile gloves.
- Remove the cover that is maintaining the patient's privacy and position a disposable pad under the patient's buttocks. In some catheter packs there is a sterile drape and this should be used to cover the patient's thighs; a small hole can be made in the drape in order to access the genitalia.
- If a catheter is already in situ, attach a syringe to the catheter port and allow the balloon contents to

drain slowly prior to removing and disposing of the catheter.

- Using a non-dominant hand, cleanse the labia minora by separating them and using a swab, as this will allow visualization of the urethral orifice. The cleansing agent is determined by local health policy but is usually sterile normal saline (0.9%). Cleanse using single downward strokes from front to back *to prevent the contamination of the urethral meatus with bowel flora.*
- One hand should be used to maintain labial separation until catheterization is completed.
- Insert the nozzle of the anaesthetic lubricating jelly into the urethra. Squeeze the gel into the urethra and then remove the nozzle and discard. Allow 5 minutes for the anaesthetic to take effect *to ease the passage of the catheter.* Slow insertion of the lubricant gel reduces urethral trauma and patient discomfort.
- For a female patient, 6 mL of anaesthetic gel or water-based lubricant should be used, following the recommended manufacturer's guidance. This should be inserted and left in situ for the recommended time before commencing the catheter insertion procedure. The European Association of Urology Nurses (2012) and Mangnall (2013) state that best practice evidence suggests that the risk of urethral trauma can be reduced in both male and female patients by using a sterile single-use lubricant during catheter insertion. European Association of Urology Nurses (EAUN) (2012) also suggests that the risk of infection associated with urethral trauma may be reduced by using a lubricant containing local anaesthetic. According to the *British National Formulary* (Joint Formulary Committee 2015), anaesthetic gel is contraindicated in cardiac patients with liver problems or epilepsy. The effect of using the anaesthetic gel also reveals the location of the urethral meatus for catheterization. Nurses must allow the time specified by manufacturers for the anaesthetic gel to work.
- Remove gloves and decontaminate your hands using soap and water or alcohol rub.
- Put on sterile gloves.
- Place the catheter in the receiver between the patient's legs; alternatively, attach it to the urine drainage bag.
- **Use aseptic technique at all times.**
- Place a small amount of lubricating jelly or anaesthetic gel on the tip of the catheter; *providing additional gel prevents trauma to the urethra.*
- Using the dominant hand, introduce the catheter tip into the urethral orifice in an upward and backward direction that *follows the anatomical route of the female urethra* (Fig. 11.2).
- Advance the catheter until 5–6 cm has been inserted and urine flows.

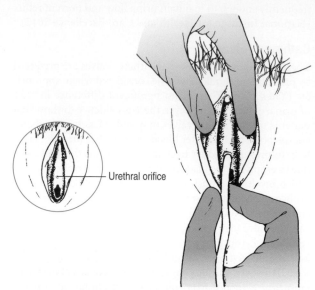

Fig. 11.2 Catheterization: inserting a catheter into the female urethra. Reproduced with permission from Roper N, Logan W, Tierney A: The Elements of Nursing, 2nd edn. Edinburgh, 1985, Churchill Livingstone.

- If no urine is present, remove the catheter and start the procedure again.
- If urine is present, advance the catheter 6–8 cm *to ensure the catheter is correctly positioned in the bladder and prevent the balloon from being inflated in the urethra.*
- If the catheter is not intended to be left in, remove it once the flow of urine has ceased; do so by gently pulling back on the catheter.
- If the catheter is to be retained, having advanced the catheter 6–8 cm and ensured that the catheter is draining well, inflate the balloon according to the manufacturer's instructions with 10 mL of sterile water; *the inflated balloon will keep the catheter in situ.*
- If the patient complains of pain, there is a risk that the inflating balloon may still be in the urethra. Stop the inflation and withdraw the fluid already inserted into the balloon. Advance the catheter 6–8 cm and repeat the inflation. *The length of the urethra can vary from patient to patient; therefore it is important to adjust practice to meet the needs of the individual and prevent complications.*
- Ask the patient to report any discomfort and observe them closely for signs of distress.
- Withdraw the catheter slightly (resistance can be felt when the balloon locates the bladder neck opening) and connect the drainage bag system/catheter valve (Fig. 11.3).

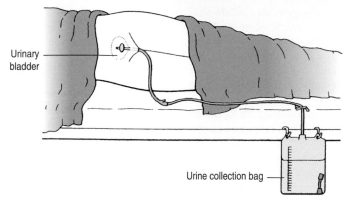

Fig. 11.3 Closed bladder drainage system showing the drainage bag below the level of the bladder.

- Failure to stabilize a catheter can lead to dislodgement and, in some cases, actual expulsion of the catheter. (A 'G' strap or a Conveen Aquasleeve can be found in the local continence/catheter formulary; *see* later.) Ensure careful management of all points of entry to prevent the development of ascending infection.
- Ensure that the patient is left comfortable and the genital area is dry and clean.
- Observe for urine draining into the bag and measure the amount drained.
- Dispose of the equipment safely and according to local policy.
- Remove personal protective equipment.
- Record and document nursing actions, size of catheter inserted, water infill and the expiry date and batch number of the catheter *to assist in implementing any action, should an adverse reaction to the practice be noted.*

If using a standard-length catheter, support it by using a specially designed support strap or adhesive fixation device on the thigh. Ensure that the catheter does not become taut when the patient is mobilizing. Ensure that the catheter lumen is not occluded. Anchor the catheter to avoid pulling or traction of the catheter, which can damage the urethra, and use recommended accessories such as a G strap. Best practice indicates that a strap/adhesive fixation should be used to anchor the catheter to prevent urethral and bladder neck trauma, as poorly stabilized catheters can also lead to catheter movement, inflammation and pain.

Pink (2013) highlights the fact that catheters that are not stabilized can lead to irritation of the detrusor, resulting in bladder spasm in patients with an overactive bladder. The detrusor muscle is commonly known as the bladder. When the bladder is filling with urine, the detrusor muscle remains relaxed and stretches to hold the urine. When it is time to urinate, the detrusor muscle contracts to allow the urine to come out. If the detrusor muscle is not working normally, micturition will be affected. If the detrusor muscle is overactive, it tries to squeeze the urine out, even when the patient is not ready to urinate. This can feel like pain in the bladder area. If the squeeze of the detrusor muscle is strong enough, it can push urine out, even if the patient is not ready to urinate. This is sometimes referred to as an overactive bladder or detrusor overactivity. If the detrusor muscle does not squeeze or is overstretched, it can be difficult to expel urine, even when the patient is trying to urinate. This is sometimes referred to as retention of urine. Individuals who suffer from an overactive bladder may also have difficulty with catheter patency, as the overactivity of the bladder reacts to the catheter. This can also lead to the individual experiencing bypassing of the catheter or increased spasms.

The Code (Nursing and Midwifery Council 2018) states, under the heading 'Preserve Safety', that nurses must make sure that patient and public safety is protected. Nurses must work within the limits of their competence, exercising a professional 'duty of candour' and raising concerns immediately whenever situations are encountered that could potentially put patients or public safety at risk. It is essential to recognize and understand this, and to work within the limits of your own competence. Information and advice provided to patients and families/carers should be evidence-based and nurses' knowledge and skills must be updated to ensure safe and effective practice at all times.

Male Patients

This procedure is carried out by medical staff or nurses who have undertaken and achieved the required level of competency. Female nurses catheterizing male patients may require a chaperone; seek advice and refer to local health policy.

- Explain the nursing procedure to the patient, including risks and benefits, *to obtain consent and cooperation.*

- Ensure that the patient has no allergy to latex or lidocaine gel. Lidocaine hydrochloride 2%, chlorhexidine gluconate solution 0.25% is a sterile local anaesthetic and lubricant for the urethral mucosa. It can prevent injury to the urethra and as a consequence reduces the subsequent risk of urethral damage; it **must be used for catheterizing both male and female patients.** Lidocaine hydrochloride 2%, chlorhexidine gluconate solution 0.25% facilitates a reduction in pain on insertion and helps reduce the risk of associated infection.
- Collect and prepare the equipment *to ensure that all equipment is available and ready for use.*
- Ensure the patient's privacy *to reduce anxiety.*
- Always observe the patient throughout the procedure *to note any signs of distress.*
- Prepare and help the patient to assume the supine position *to provide access to, and visualization of, the genitalia.*
- Place a procedure pad underneath the patient's buttock *to prevent any spillage of fluids on to the patient's bed linen/clothing.*
- Arrange the lighting *to assist with good visualization of the genitalia.*
- Wash hands and apply gloves, which *acts as a barrier between the nurse's skin and the patient's tissues, thus reducing the incidence of contamination.*
- Withdraw the patient's foreskin with the non-dominant hand. Maintain this position until the catheter insertion is completed *to prevent recontamination of the urethral meatus by the foreskin after cleansing.* **Do not fully retract a phimotic foreskin** (a phimotic foreskin is a condition where the foreskin is too tight to be pulled back over the head of the penis, or glans).
- Using the dominant hand, cleanse the glans penis and urethral meatus with saline and gauze *to prevent the introduction of microorganisms into the urethra and/ or bladder.* Cleanse the urethral meatus and glans in a circular motion, moving out from the centre.
- Holding the penis upright, apply a small amount of lubricating gel to the tip of the meatus and then insert the nozzle of the anaesthetic gel into the urethra. Squeeze the gel in and slowly remove the nozzle and discard. Instil 11 mL of anaesthetic gel. Wait 5 minutes before catheter insertion and follow the manufacturer's guide *to allow the anaesthetic time to act.*
- Remove gloves and decontaminate the hands, using soap and water or alcohol rub.
- Put on sterile gloves.
- Take hold of the penis behind the glans, raising it until almost totally extended. Maintain a grasp of the penis until the procedure is finished.
- Position the sterile receiver and, with the non-dominant hand, gently grasp the shaft of the penis, raising it straight

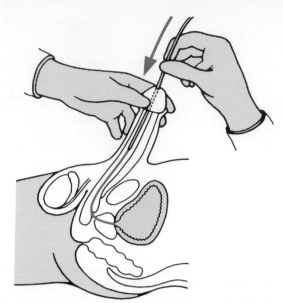

Fig. 11.4 Catheterization: inserting a catheter into the male urethra.

up *to aid the passage of the catheter along the length of the urethra.*
- **As the male urethra is longer than the female urethra,** insert the lubricated catheter into the urethral meatus for approximately 15–25 cm until a flow of urine is established (Fig. 11.4). If resistance is felt at the external sphincter, increase the traction on the penis slightly and apply a steady gentle pressure on the catheter. Ask the patient to strain gently as if passing urine or coughing (Dougherty et al. 2015).
- Continue as for the female patient until the anchoring of the catheter.
- When urine begins to flow, advance the catheter almost to its bifurcation *to ensure the catheter is correctly positioned in the bladder and prevent the balloon from being inflated in the urethra.*
- Gently inflate the catheter with 10 mL of sterile water as per the manufacturer's guidance.
- Ask the patient to report any pain or distress.
- Withdraw the catheter slightly (resistance can be felt when the balloon locates with the bladder neck opening).
- Clean and replace the foreskin over the glans penis *to prevent the development of paraphimosis.*
- Connect the catheter to the drainage system/catheter valve for anchoring of the catheter (see 'Female patients' earlier).
- Ensure that the patient is left comfortable as possible, *to maintain the quality of this nursing practice.*

- Dispose of the equipment safely and according to local policy *to reduce any health hazard.*
- Record and document nursing actions, size of catheter inserted, water infill and the expiry date and batch number of the catheter *to assist in implementing any action, should an adverse reaction to the practice be noted.*

As for female catheterization, adhere to the principles of *The Code* (Nursing and Midwifery Council 2018).

CATHETER-ASSOCIATED URINARY TRACT INFECTION

Catheterization carries a risk of infection and CAUTI accounts for 40% of hospital infections (Andreessen et al. 2012). Maintenance of the urine drainage system is important to reduce the risk of catheter-associated infection. The microorganisms can reach the bladder in two ways: from urine in the urine bag and from the space between the catheter and urethral mucosa (Ostaszkiewicz & Paterson 2011). To reduce infection, there should be minimal interruption between the catheter and the connection to the drainage bag. Nursing staff should minimize the number of times the urine bag is disconnected from the catheter, avoid taking too many urine samples, avoid frequent changes of the drainage bag and should follow the manufacturer's guidance on product use (Fig. 11.5).

Depending on the local continence/catheter formulary and/or choice, closed drainage systems can be selected that hold a closed integral catheter and drainage bag; however, the choice of product should be user-driven and based on advice from the nurse. It is important to remember this when the nurse educates and prepares the patient about who requires catheterization. The nurse should be aware of the products available in the catheter formulary. A continence/catheter formulary is a list of products used in urinary catheterization that are available on NHS prescription. Each region will have a continence/catheter formulary and this will vary from region to region (refer to your local formulary).

Key Factors to Consider Relating to CAUTI

- The nurse should consider the clinical reason for catheterization and if the catheter will be in situ over the short or the long term, mainly as a greater length of time may increase the opportunity to acquire an infection.
- Selection of the correct catheter type, material and drainage system should be considered
- The procedure for catheterization should be performed using an aseptic technique.
- Education should be provided for care staff and for the family, to prevent CAUTI occurring and to ensure that the individual can manage the catheter successfully.

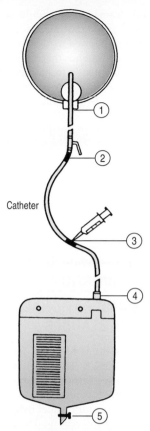

Catheter

Fig. 11.5 Points at which pathogens can enter a closed urinary drainage system. *1*, The urethral orifice; *2*, the connection between the catheter and the drainage tube; *3*, the point at which a urine sample is taken; *4*, the connection between the drainage tube and collecting bag; *5*, the drainage bag outlet. Reproduced with permission from Roper N, Logan W, Tierney A: The Elements of Nursing, 2nd edn. Edinburgh, 1985, Churchill Livingstone.

2. CATHETER CARE

INDICATIONS AND RATIONALE FOR CATHETER CARE AND CLEANSING OF THE EXPOSED PART OF THE CATHETER

Washing the urethral meatus with unperfumed soap and water during the daily bathing or showering routine is now recommended as best practice. Vigorous meatal cleansing may increase the risk of infection. Patients with a catheter in situ should be instructed on personal hygiene and measures to prevent ascending infection.

Catheters and drainage bag should be positioned to prevent backflow of urine into the bladder (*see* Fig. 11.3). The bag should not be allowed to fill beyond three-quarters full. NICE (2012) recommends that the urine drainage bag should be emptied frequently to maintain urine flow and prevent reflux using a clean procedure. The drainage bag should also be changed when clinically indicated.

◎ **EQUIPMENT**

If undertaken by the nurse:
- Gloves/apron
- Disposable wipes
- Unperfumed soap and water
- Flat surface for equipment
- Receptacle for soiled disposable items

---

3. BLADDER IRRIGATION

INDICATIONS AND RATIONALE FOR IRRIGATING THE BLADDER

Bladder irrigation is the continuous washing out of the bladder with sterile fluid, usually 0.9% normal saline. It is performed only in a specialized clinical environment, e.g. a urology department. Moslemi & Rajaei (2010) recommend using three-way catheters for bladder irrigation. One lumen is used to drain urine, another is used to inflate the catheter balloon and the final lumen carries the irrigation solution (*see* Fig. 11.1). This solution is used to prevent and wash out blood clots post prostatectomy. The rate of infusion is dependent on the patient's urine colour. If the urine is heavily blood-stained, then the rate of fluid needs to be fast; if there is little bleeding, then the rate of infusion can be slowed down or stopped.

Other indications for use of bladder irrigation include:
- drug installation
- prevention of haematuria following chemotherapy
- pre- or postsurgical procedures
- removal of sediment in the bladder.

◎ **EQUIPMENT**

- Sterile gloves and apron
- Sterile catheter pack
- Sterile irrigation fluid: 0.9% normal saline at 38.7°C
- Sterile disposable irrigation set
- Infusion stand
- Sterile drainage bag with tap or sterile jug
- Trolley for equipment
- Receptacle for disposal of equipment

GUIDELINES AND RATIONALE FOR THIS NURSING PRACTICE

- Explain the practice to the patient *to gain consent and cooperation.*
- Collect and prepare all equipment *to ensure the equipment is ready for use.*
- Ensure the patient's privacy *to reduce anxiety.*
- Observe the patient throughout the procedure *to note signs of distress.*
- Wash hands and apply sterile gloves and apron, *to reduce cross-infection* (National Institute for Health and Care Excellence 2012).
- Help the patient into a comfortable position that will also *allow the nurse easy access during the practice.*
- Cleanse the irrigation inlet arm of the catheter with cleansing solution *to reduce cross-infection.*
- Insert the irrigation set connecter into the cleansed inlet arm of the catheter *to permit the introduction of the irrigation fluid.*
- Attach the urine drainage bag if a drain bag is already in situ. *This will act as a collecting container for the returned irrigation fluid.*
- Empty the drainage bag *to allow accurate monitoring of the volume of returned irrigation fluid and urine output.*
- Open the valve of the irrigation set and regulate the flow to the prescribed rate, *complying with medical practitioner's prescription.*
- Renew the irrigation fluid as stated on the patient's prescription and empty the drainage bag *as required to maintain the bladder irrigation.*
- Ensure the patient is left feeling comfortable as possible, *to maintain the quality of the nursing practice.*
- Remove the gloves and apron.
- Dispose of the equipment safely and as per local health policy.
- Document the nursing practice, monitor the after-effects and report any abnormal findings immediately, providing a written record to assist in the implementation of any action, should an abnormality or adverse reaction to the practice be noted.

---

4. ADMINISTRATION OF CATHETER MAINTENANCE SOLUTIONS

Encrustation is common problem for those with long-term catheters (Yates 2018). It is important that nurses are proactive in the management of individuals with a long-term catheter in situ and that assessment is a continual process. Recurrent catheter blockage will have an impact on patients' quality of life; it also has consequences for time and resources for nursing practice. According to Yates (2018), half of all individuals with a catheter will experience catheter blockage due to encrustation. Encrustation is caused by microorganisms in the urine that produce an enzyme. The enzyme breaks down urea to form ammonia, which results in the urine becoming alkaline. When this happens, mineral salts, calcium phosphate and magnesium ammonium phosphate (struvite) are deposited on to the catheter surface, causing encrustation (Yates 2018). Studies suggest that there is an association between high urinary pH (alkaline) and encrustation and blocking, but there is no evidence that monitoring urinary pH can be used to predict catheter blockage (Rigby 2004).

Catheters can also bypass due to reduced oral intake, constipation, bladder spasm and CAUTIs. Bladder spasm occurs when the bladder mucosa becomes clamped around the catheter, occluding the eyes of the catheter (Yates 2018). Urine cannot drain effectively and therefore follows the path of least resistance, leaking down the sides of the catheter and causing the patient to experience an episode of incontinence. There will usually be urine in the drainage bag, and catheter drainage should return to normal flow once the spasm has decreased. A blockage of the catheter will not resolve spontaneously; evidence suggests that, if blocked, a catheter should be removed and a new one inserted. On removal of the blocked catheter, the nurse should inspect it for evidence of encrustation and deposits.

If the patient is having recurring blockages, the nurse should be proactive in managing the problem. Individuals with a catheter that blocks frequently are sometimes referred to as 'pH blockers'; the number of catheter blockages can be recorded using a catheter diary. Documenting the insertion of the new catheter and when the blocking occurs informs the nurse of the average time the catheter remains problem-free. Encrustation occurs due to higher urine pH. If the catheter blocks every 2 weeks and the pH is alkaline, then the insertion of an acidic catheter maintenance solution (CMS) is recommended. Care should be taken to ensure that the chosen solution has components aimed at reducing irritation of the bladder wall. Loveday et al. (2014) suggest that CMSs should not be used to prevent CAUTIs and that CMSs must not be used to unblock a catheter. A blocked catheter should be replaced.

CMSs include:
- Normal saline 0.9%: neutral solution pH 7, recommended for flushing of debris and small blood clots. It will not remove encrustation.
- Solution G: citric acid 3.2% pH 4, intended to dissolve crystals that form within the lumen of the catheter. It contains magnesium oxide to prevent bladder irritation.

- Solution R: stronger citric acid 6% pH 2, intended to dissolve more persistent crystals due to its acidic nature. It should be used only after solution G has been tried and has been found to be ineffective.

CMSs were originally introduced to prevent or reduce the occurrence of CAUTIs. In recent years the usage has been aimed primarily at minimizing the effects of recurrent encrustation and blockage (Hagen et al. 2010). Although they are still described in the literature as CMSs, the newer term 'catheter patency solutions' has been suggested.

The installation of any solution into a urinary catheter is not without risk. In order to administer the solution, the drainage bag needs to be disconnected from the catheter, and this could increase the risk of UTI (National Institute for Health and Care Excellence 2012). In administering CMSs, the nurse must follow the manufacturer's guidance.

The bladder mucosa plays an important role in the defence against UTI. During the instillation process, the nurse should use minimal force, as this will reduce damage to the bladder mucosa. Both neutral and acidic solutions can cause irritation to the bladder wall.

CMSs come in volumes of 50 mL or 100 mL. Studies have shown that two sequential 50 mL rinses are more effective than either one 50 mL or one 100 mL rinse (Yates 2012).

There is no clear evidence of how often a CMS should be administered for it to be effective for catheter patency. The administration and frequency of delivery of CMSs depend on the clinical judgement of the registered nurse, considering the risks and benefits to the patient.

A Cochrane review (Hagen et al. 2010) and NICE guidelines (2012) both concluded that there was insufficient evidence to guide clinical practice regarding all aspects of using CMSs for long-term indwelling urinary catheters. Therefore the risks or benefits to patients are as yet unclear.

INDICATIONS AND RATIONALE FOR ADMINISTERING CATHETER MAINTENANCE SOLUTIONS

CMSs are prescription-only medications and should be treated in the same way as any prescription-only medication. The solution should be prescribed for each individual patient as per prescribing guidelines. CMSs have been developed to reduce the build-up of encrustation. They can reduce the risk of catheter blockage associated with encrustation, and allow the catheter to remain patent and last till the expiry date. This can then reduce the episodes of catheter changes. Other indications include their use if there has been no drainage of urine for a few hours, if drainage is very slow and sluggish, or if the patient has lower abdominal pain.

When Not to Use

The nurse must adhere to local policies on the use of CMSs and must also be mindful of when **not** to use them. They should not be used if the patient presents with:

- spinal cord injury when there is a risk of developing an episode of autonomic dysreflexia
- known or suspected cancer of the lower urinary tract
- a recent UTI
- recent radiotherapy to the lower urinary tract
- recent urological surgery or vesicovaginal fistula
- any allergy to the products used in the CMS.

The procedure of administering a CMS requires an aseptic technique because of the use of sterile solutions. Non-sterile gloves can be used when undertaking the procedure; however, it is important not to touch the key parts with anything that is not sterile. Key parts are the sites where harmful microorganisms can be introduced into the body and include the disconnected end of the catheter tubing and the tip of the CMS bag to be attached to catheter tubing. These areas need to remain sterile.

◎ EQUIPMENT

- Two pairs of non-sterile gloves
- Disposable plastic apron
- Sterile single-use CMS at room temperature
- New leg bag/overnight bag/catheter valve
- Procedure pad
- Trolley/adequate surface for equipment
- Receptacle for disposal of waste/equipment

GUIDELINES AND RATIONALE FOR THIS NURSING PRACTICE

- Explain the procedure to the patient *to obtain consent and cooperation*; document these in the nursing notes/care plan.
- Wash your hands as per local policy and infection control policy *to minimize infection* (National Institute for Health and Care Excellence 2012).
- Put on an apron and disposable non-sterile gloves.
- Collect and prepare the equipment required *to ensure that all equipment is available and ready for use.*
- Check that the medication administration chart is completed *to ensure that the correct CMS has been prescribed.*
- Check that the solution has not expired. *The choice of CMS depends on local health policy and assessment.*
- When using a twin container solution, warm the CMS to body temperature before use, while it is still in its packaging, *to minimize discomfort to the patient.*

- Prepare the working area *to provide a clean working surface.*
- Assist the patient into a suitable position.
- If the patient already has a urethral catheter in situ, place the disposable nursing procedure pad under the patient's buttocks and thighs, and cover the genital area *to provide patients with dignity and comfort, and to ensure that urine does not leak on to clothing/bed linen.*
- Empty the leg/night bag *to minimize the risk of cross-infection* (National Institute for Health and Care Excellence 2012).
- Remove gloves, wash hands and put on the second pair of disposable non-sterile gloves.
- Peel apart the outer package from the CMS and the new leg bag/night bag/catheter valve.
- Disconnect the leg bag night bag/catheter valve from the catheter. Place the leg bag/night bag/catheter valve in a receiver for disposal while continuing to hold the catheter *to prevent leakage of urine.*
- Remove the protective cap from the CMS, being careful not to touch the connecting end. Immediately insert the CMS into the end of the catheter *to minimize the risk of cross-infection*
- Instil the CMS as per the manufacturer's guidance *to reduce the risk of damage to the bladder mucosa.*
- Disconnect the catheter maintenance solution from the catheter and dispose of the CMS while continuing to hold the catheter *to minimize the risk of cross-infection.*
- Remove the protective cap from the new sterile leg/night bag/catheter valve without touching the connection. Insert the leg/night bag/catheter valve into the end of the catheter *to facilitate drainage of urine.*
- Secure the drainage system, i.e. leg bag holder or straps, *to prevent tension being exerted on the catheter by weight or urine.*
- Remove the gloves and wash your hands as per local infection control policies/hand hygiene *to minimize the risk of cross-infection* (National Institute for Health and Care Excellence 2012).
- Document the procedure, including type of solution, rationale for use of the CMS, amount of fluid instilled, batch number, colour, odour and appearance of the urine, frequency, and length of time it took to instil the CMS *to record and evaluate the procedure.*
- Observe the patient throughout the procedure, noting any signs of distress, pain or discomfort, particularly if the patient has a small-capacity bladder. If using a concertina container, be wary of exerting too much pressure on the container and observe for symptoms or signs of distress or shock.
- In patients with spinal cord injury, signs of autonomic dysreflexia can include skin mottling, pupil dilation,

changes in blood pressure – usually high blood pressure, perspiration and headache.

- Document the nursing practices and monitor the after-effects. Report any abnormal findings immediately, providing a written record and assisting in the implementation of any action, should an abnormality or adverse reaction to the practice be noted.
- As discussed previously for catheterization, adhere to the principles of *The Code* (Nursing and Midwifery Council 2018).

ADDITIONAL INFORMATION

Those patients who require catheterization will have their fluid intake and output monitored. In addition to observing the amount of urine passed, the nurse should report any abnormalities in urine, such as colour; pale pink or red, through to brown, is suggestive of blood in the urine (haematuria). Blood or sediment in the urine can indicate a problem in the renal or urinary system. Certain foods and medications can also affect the colour of the urine. Purple bag syndrome can occur in those who are long-term catheter users. It is thought to be associated with high-level trypto-phan (amino acid), present in the gut for longer due to constipation or slow gut transit. Tryptophan is broken down by the enzyme tryptophanase in the gastrointestinal tract. This produces indole, which is absorbed into the blood by the intestines and passes to the liver. The liver converts it to indoxyl sulphate, which is excreted in the urine. Individuals with purple bag syndrome are known to have levels of bacteria in their urine; however, the condition may not be a symptom of infection.

PATIENT/CARER EDUCATION: KEY POINTS

Patients and carers must be educated in the correct infection control procedures. Having a urinary catheter in situ can affect a patient's self-esteem and alter body image. Nurses and carers should demonstrate sensitivity to the needs of patients by supporting them through the transition. Sensitive topics, such as sexual activity, also need to be addressed and nurses should offer practical advice verbally and also in leaflet form.

It is important for nurses to use the teach-back method to ensure that all aspects of catheterization and after-care are understood by the patient and family member/carer. Using the teach-back method confirms that all information provided by the healthcare professional is being understood by getting people to 'teach back' what has been discussed and what instruction has been given. This consists of more than saying 'do you understand?' and is more of a check on how you have explained things than on the patient/client's understanding.

Whether the patient is at home or is being discharged from the hospital, they require catheter supplies, sufficient day and night bags, leg straps, and information on how to obtain regular supplies by prescription. A number of pharmacy outlets will also provide prescription services and door-to-door delivery of products.

Prior to discharge, patients and carers must be taught the care of the catheter, such as prevention of catheter kinking, positional issues and securing of the drainage bag. Prevention of constipation, good hand-washing technique and dietary and fluid intake should also be reinforced.

REFERENCES

Andreessen, L., Wilde, M.H., Herendeen, P., 2012. Preventing Catheter Associated urinary tract infections in acute care: the bundle approach. Journal of Nurse Care Quality 27 (3), 209–217.

Association for Continence Advice, 2007. Notes on good practice. Association for Continence Advice. London.

Bardsley, A., 2005. Use of lubricant gels in urinary catheterisation. Nursing Standard 20 (8).

Dougherty, L., Lister, S., West-Oram, A. (Eds.), 2015. The Royal Marsden Manual of Clinical Nursing Procedures: Student Edition, ninth ed. Marsden NHS Foundation Trust. Wiley and Sons, (Chapter 5).

European Association of Urology Nurses, 2012. Evidence based guidelines for best practice in Urological Health Care.

Catheterisation. Indwelling Catheters in Adults Urethral & Suprapubic. www.uroweb.org/guidelines/online-guidlines.

Hagen, S., Sinclair, L., Cross, S., 2010. Washout polices in long term indwelling urinary catheterisation in adults. The Cochrane Database of Systematic Reviews (3), CD004012.

Joint Formulary Committee, 2015. British National Formulary. 68. BMJ Group and Pharmaceutical Press, London.

Loveday, H.P., Wilson, J.A., Pratt, R.J., et al., 2014. EPIC 3: national evidence based guidelines for preventing healthcare associated infections in NHS hospitals in England. Journal of Hospital Infection 86 (Suppl. 1), S1–S70.

Madeo, M., Barr, B., Owen, E., 2009. A study to determine whether the use of pre-connect urinary catheters reduces the incidence of nosocomial urinary tract infections. Journal of Infection Prevention 10 (2), 79–80.

Mangnall, J., 2013. Changing a urethral or suprapubic catheter: the patient's perspective. British Journal of Community Nursing 18 (12), 591–596.

Mantle, S., 2015. Reducing HCAI – what the commissioner needs to know. NHS England, London.

Moslemi, M.K., Rajaei, M., 2010. An improved delivery system for bladder irrigation. Therapeutics and Clinical Risk Management 6, 459–462. 10.2147/TCRM.S13525.

National Institute for Health and Care Excellence, 2012. Clinical Guidelines 139. Healthcare associated infections: prevention and control in primary care. NICE, London.

National Institute for Health and Care Excellence, 2013. Urinary Incontinence: The Management of Urinary Incontinence in Women. Clinical Guideline 171. NICE, London.

National Institute for Health and Care Excellence, 2014. Infection Prevention and Control Quality Standard QS61. NICE, London.

National Patient Safety Agency, 2009. Female Urinary Catheters Causing Trauma to Adult Males – Rapid Response Report. Archived from: http://webarchive.nationalarchives.gov.uk/20170906180051/http://www.nrls.npsa.nhs.uk/alerts/?entryid45=59897&cord=ASC&p=3.

NHS Business Services Authority, 2013. NHS Electronic Drug Tariff: Catheter Valves. Available at: http://tinyurl.com/oswbeb8.

NHS Quality Improvement Scotland, 2004. Best Practice statement – Urinary catheterisation and Catheter Care. Edinburgh: NHS Quality Improvement Scotland.

Nursing and Midwifery Council, 2018. The Code: Professional Standards of Practice and Behaviour for Nurses, Midwives and Nursing Associates. NMC, London. Available at: https://www.nmc.org.uk/globalassets/sitedocuments/nmc-publications/nmc-code.pdf.

Ostaszkiewicz, J., Paterson, J., 2011. Nurses' advice regarding sterile or clean urinary drainage bags for individuals with a long term indwelling urinary catheter. Journal of Wound Ostomy and Continence Nurses Society/WOCN 39 (1), 77–83.

Pellowe, C., 2009. Using evidence-based guidelines to reduce catheter related urinary tract infections in England. Journal of Infection Prevention. 10 (2), 44–48.

Pink, J., 2013. Urinary Incontinence and the importance of catheter fixation. Journal of Community Nursing 27, 524–529.

Pratt, R.J., Pellowes, C., Wilson, J., et al., 2007. EPIC 2 National evidence based guidelines for preventing hospital associated infection in NHS Hospitals in England. British Journal of Hospital Infection 65 (Suppl. 1), 1–59.

Raheem, O.A., Casey, R.G., D'Arcy, F.T., Lynch, T.H., 2011. The safety and efficacy of the indwelling valve catheters in the long-term catheterised patients: a systematic comparative study. Current Urology 5 (4), 173–178.

Rigby, D., 2004. pH testing in catheter maintenance the clinical debate. British Journal of Community Nursing 9 (5), 189–194.

Shackley, D.C., Whytock, C., Parry, G., et al., 2017. Variation in the prevalence of urinary catheters: a profile of national health service patients in England. British Medical Journal Open 7 (6), e013842.

Taylor, Julie, 2018. Reducing the incidence of inappropriate indwelling urinary catherisation. Journal of Community Nursing 32 (3), 50–56.

Woodward, S., 2013. Catheter Valves: a welcome alternative to leg bags. British Journal of Nursing 22 (11), 650–654.

Yates, A., 2008. Urinary catheters part 6-catheter valves. Nursing Times 104 (44), 24–25.

Yates, A., 2012. Management of long-term urinary catheters. Nursing and Residential Care 14 (4), 172–178.

Yates, A., 2018. Using patency solutions to manage urinary catheter blockage. Nursing Times 114 (5), 18–21.

WEBSITES

https://www.bladderandbowel.org/ Bladder and Bowel Community

http://www.healthcareimprovementscotland.org Healthcare Improvement Scotland

http://www.healthliteracyplace.org.uk NHS The Health Literacy Place – tools and techniques on the teach-back method

https://www.ics.org International Continence Society

https://www.sign.ac.uk/assets/sign88.pdf SIGN Guideline 88: Management of Suspected Bacterial Urinary Tract Infection in Adults: A National Clinical Guideline

SELF-ASSESSMENT

1. Identify five reasons for the insertion of an indwelling catheter.
2. Name four risk factors increasing the risk of catheter-associated urinary tract infection in patients.
3. Describe the various types of catheter available.
4. What is the best size of catheter to use and why? Consider the different patient groups when answering this question.
5. What are the indications for using a catheter maintenance solution?

Chest Auscultation

INDICATIONS AND RATIONALE FOR CHEST AUSCULTATION

Auscultation of the chest is one of the oldest diagnostic procedures, used traditionally by physicians to diagnose a variety of pulmonary and cardiac diseases. It is an inexpensive, non-invasive and safe procedure, which is easy to carry out and which constitutes a vital part of respiratory examination (Sarkar et al. 2015). Along with detailed history-taking, inspection, palpation and percussion, auscultation is a crucial part of clinical examination.

As air moves through the bronchial tree it produces sounds that travel to the chest wall; this allows for the assessment of the lungs and pleural space. The auscultation process involves listening to airflow, produced by breathing, through the tracheobronchial tree and to differentiate normal breath sounds from abnormal sounds. In listening to breath sounds it is important to distinguish normal respiratory sounds from abnormal ones, e.g. crackles, wheezes and pleural rubs. Breath sounds change as the air moves from the large airways to the small airways, and also as air moves through fluid, mucus or narrowed airways.

THE STETHOSCOPE

Some stethoscopes used for clinical examination have both a bell and a diaphragm, and it is essential to understand the correct use of these (Fig. 12.1). The diaphragm is superior at picking up high-pitched sounds, whereas the bell is more sensitive at picking up low-pitched sounds. Most of the sounds that reach the chest wall are of low frequency and are usually best heard by using the bell of the stethoscope, with the diaphragm being reserved for listening to higher-pitched sounds such as pleural friction rubs (Innes et al. 2018). Some authors however, advocate the use of the diaphragm in chest auscultation (Hogan-Quigley et al. 2012; Willis 2017).

GUIDELINES AND RATIONALE FOR THIS NURSING PRACTICE

Auscultation Sequence

The sequence used to perform chest auscultation is shown in Figs 12.2 and 12.3; this is the suggested pattern to use for moving the stethoscope from one side to the other *to compare right and left lungs.*

Breath Sounds

Breath sounds are classified according to:
- intensity
- pitch
- location
- duration
- characteristics.

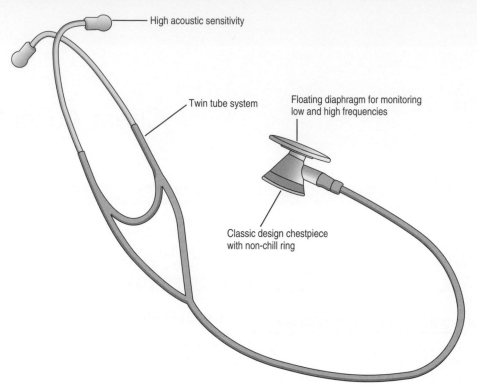

High acoustic sensitivity

Twin tube system

Floating diaphragm for monitoring
low and high frequencies

Classic design chestpiece
with non-chill ring

Fig. 12.1 Anatomy of a stethoscope.

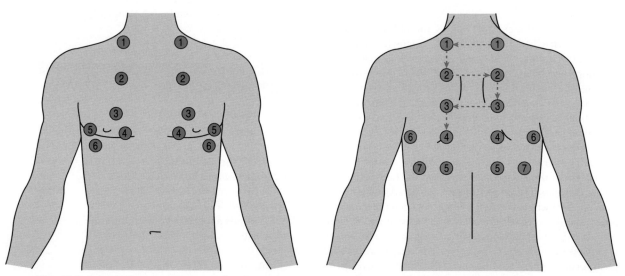

Fig. 12.2 Auscultation sequence: anterior view.

Fig. 12.3 Auscultation sequence: posterior view.

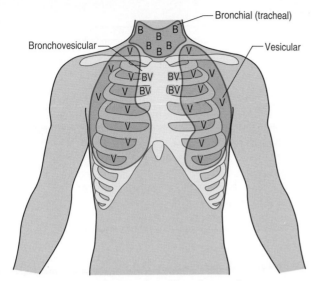

Bronchial (tracheal)

Bronchovesicular

Vesicular

Fig. 12.4 Location of breath sounds.

The purpose of auscultation is to assess the flow of air through the tracheobronchial tree *and assess the condition of the lungs and pleural space.* The process of auscultation involves:

- listening to breath-generated sounds
- listening for extra sounds (referred to as adventitious sounds)
- listening to a spoken or whispered voice sound if any abnormalities are detected.

Normal breath sounds are described as:

- vesicular – soft, low-pitched sounds heard on inspiration and one-third of the way through expiration before fading
- bronchovesicular – inspiratory and expiratory sounds of equal length, separated by a pause; at times these breath sounds are medium in volume and pitch
- bronchial breath sounds – loud, high-pitched sounds with the expiratory component lasting longer than the inspiratory component (Fig. 12.4) (Hogan-Quigley et al. 2012; Willis 2017; Innes et al. 2018).

Performing Auscultation

- Auscultation should be carried out in a quiet environment and preferably in a sitting position *to facilitate an accurate assessment.* Auscultation should never be done through the clothing, *as this will muffle the sound.*
- Ask the patient to take deep breaths through an open mouth, *as breathing through the nose changes the pitch*

of the sounds. If the patient has profuse chest hair, either wet the hair or press more firmly the stethoscope *to prevent the hair from causing crackles.*

- Using the diaphragm of the stethoscope, start auscultation using the sequences shown in Figs 12.2 and 12.3 *to ensure a consistent and comprehensive approach.*
  - Start anteriorly at the apices, moving side to side to compare the symmetrical areas of each lung.
  - Listen to each area for at least one full breath (inspiration and expiration).
- Exercise caution and be aware of possible discomfort for the patient from breathing too quickly and deeply, *as they may feel lightheaded.* Allow the patient to rest as required.
- Listen to the quality of the breath sounds and the pitch, intensity and the length of the inspiratory and expiratory sounds *to gain a full assessment.*
- Listen for any extra (adventitious) sounds too *that may indicate other health problems.*

EXTRA (ADVENTITIOUS) BREATH SOUNDS

Detecting extra breath sounds is important, as it can assist in the diagnosis of either cardiac or respiratory conditions. The most common types of extra breath sound are crackles (sometimes termed rales), wheezes and rhonchi.

Crackles

Crackles are interrupted, non-musical sounds; they can be described as fine crackles, which are soft and high-pitched in nature, or coarse crackles, which are louder and have a low pitch. If the crackles do not clear after asking the patient to cough, listen carefully for:

- intensity, pitch and duration
- number of crackles
- timing in relation to the respiratory cycle (inspiratory crackles/expiratory crackles)
- location of the crackles.

Wheezes and Rhonchi

These are continuous and musical in nature, with wheezes being high-pitched and rhonchi being low-pitched. If wheezes and rhonchi are heard, listen carefully and note:

- location of the sounds
- timing of the sounds in relation to the respiratory cycle (heard on inspiration/expiration or both)
- whether the sounds change with deep breathing or coughing.

When you have finished your auscultation, make patient comfortable and clean the bell and diaphragm of your stethoscope.

PATIENT/CARER EDUCATION: KEY POINTS

It is important to inform the patient about the reasons for chest auscultation so as to gain their cooperation during the assessment.

Once the practice is complete, ensure the nurse-call buzzer is close to hand, should any assistance be required.

REFERENCES

Hogan-Quigley, B., Palm, M., Bickley, L., 2012. Bates' Nursing Guide to Physical Examination and History Taking: Guide to Physical Exam & History Taking. Wolters Kluwer Health. Lippincott Williams and Wilkins, London.

Innes, J.A., Dover, A.R., Fairhurst, K., 2018. MacLeod's Clinical Examination, fourteenth ed. Elsevier, London.

Sarkar, M., Madabhavi, I., Niranjan, N., Dogra, M., 2015. Auscultation of the respiratory system. Annals of Thoracic Medicine 10 (3), 158–168.

Willis, L.N., 2017. Health Assessment Made Incredibly Visual, third ed. Wolters Kluwer, Philadelphia.

WEBSITES

https://www.easyauscultation.com/lung-sounds *Easy Auscultation*

SELF-ASSESSMENT

1. What are the indications for auscultating a patient's chest?
2. How would you prepare the patient for this practice?
3. Can you describe the auscultation process?
4. What types of normal and abnormal breath sound might you hear on auscultation?

Chest Drainage: Underwater Seal or Chest Drainage System

There are three parts to this chapter:
1. Insertion of an underwater seal chest drain or chest drain system
2. Changing a chest drainage collection system
3. Removal of an underwater seal chest drain

LEARNING OUTCOMES

By the end of this chapter, you should be able to:
- support and prepare the patient for each of the three procedures outlined above
- collect and prepare the equipment required for insertion of a chest drain, changing a chest drain collection system and removal of an underwater seal chest drain
- change a chest drainage collection system safely
- assist the medical practitioner with insertion of an underwater seal chest drain
- remove an underwater seal chest drain safely
- provide safe care to the patient who has an underwater seal chest drain.

BACKGROUND KNOWLEDGE REQUIRED

- Revision of the anatomy, physiology and pathology of the respiratory system, including the structures of the chest wall
- Revision of aseptic technique (see Ch. 40)
- Revision of local health authority or National Health Service (NHS) hospital policy on management of a chest drain

1. INSERTION OF AN UNDERWATER SEAL CHEST DRAIN

INDICATIONS AND RATIONALE FOR INSERTION OF AN UNDERWATER SEAL CHEST DRAIN

Abnormal collections of air or fluid in the pleural cavity can cause compression of the lung tissue, which reduces the surface area for gas exchange and increases the patient's work of breathing (Dougherty & Lister 2015). Air or fluid can accumulate within the pleural cavity due to traumatic injuries, malignancy or post-thoracic surgery, or after spontaneous collapse of the lung causing impaired ventilation (Coombs et al. 2013).

Chest drainage refers to a closed system that allows air or fluid to pass in one direction, from the pleural cavity into an underwater drainage collection system (Fig. 13.1) or flutter valve system (Welch & Black 2017) (Fig. 13.2). Chest drainage is indicated to drain air (pneumothorax), blood (haemothorax), both blood and air (haemopneumothorax), pus (pyothorax) or lymph (chylothorax) from the pleural cavity, to enable the lung to expand and improve the patient's capacity for ventilation (Welch & Black 2017).

The choice of drainage system will depend on the clinical status and underlying condition of the patient, the viscosity and volume of the drainage expected and whether the drain is being inserted within the perioperative, ward or outpatient area. Underwater drainage collection systems are widely used and require patients to be monitored on an inpatient basis, however drainage collection systems can limit patient mobilization and are at risk of being knocked over, causing the lung to collapse (Harris et al. 2010). The flutter valve system is useful for draining air, although it has a tendency to occlude when draining fluid; thus it should not be used for this purpose (Havelock et al. 2010). Flutter valves have the advantage of allowing the patient to mobilize.

Contemporary underwater seal drains are single-use, sterile, plastic drainage collection systems containing either a single chamber with an underwater seal, or three chambers: one for fluid collection, one for suction and an underwater seal chamber (Durai et al. 2010) (Fig. 13.3).

The drain insertion site is determined by the clinical status of the patient. In most cases the site will be the fourth or fifth intercostal space in the mid-axillary line (Coombs et al. 2013). Decisions regarding the insertion site should always be guided by clinical examination of the patient and observation of the chest X-ray (Havelock et al. 2010). The

only exception to this is if the patient develops a tension pneumothorax, a medical emergency where quick insertion of the drain takes priority (Welch & Black 2017). Thoracic ultrasound guidance is recommended to guide the insertion of drains into clearly defined collections of fluid (i.e. pleural effusions), if the patient's clinical condition is not immediately life-threatening (Havelock et al. 2010).

Position of the Patient

The patient's clinical status will determine the optimal position for chest drain insertion. Fig. 13.4 illustrates three positions: Fig. 13.4B shows the favoured position, with the patient sitting upright over a bedside table with a pillow to rest on (Havelock et al. 2010).

OUTLINE OF THE PROCEDURE

Using an aseptic technique, the medical practitioner cleanses the patient's skin with an appropriate solution, eg chlorhexidine gluconate 2% in 70% alcohol, or as per local skin preparation policy. The selected site of entry for the chest drain is injected with a local anaesthetic, allowing 2–3 minutes for this to take effect. The method of drain insertion will vary, depending on the size of drain required. Excessive force should be avoided to prevent damage to intrathoracic structures.

There are two recommended methods for chest tube insertion. The first is the Seldinger technique, where an introducer is used to advance a small-bore tube into the pleural cavity (Coombs et al. 2013). The second involves blunt dissection of the subcutaneous tissue and intercostal muscles using artery forceps, followed by insertion of a large-bore tube (Durai et al. 2010). Insertion of large-bore tubes is more uncomfortable for the patient but allows for drainage of viscous fluids like blood or pus with less risk of the drain occluding (Coombs et al. 2013).

Once the chest tube is in place, the medical practitioner connects the drain to the drainage collection system that

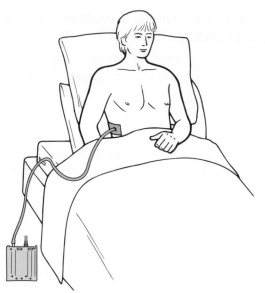

Fig. 13.1 Patient with a chest drain in the pleural cavity, attached to a drainage system.

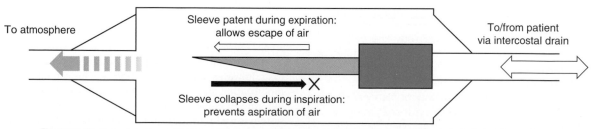

To atmosphere

Sleeve patent during expiration: allows escape of air

Sleeve collapses during inspiration: prevents aspiration of air

To/from patient via intercostal drain

Fig. 13.2 Flutter valve. From Mallett J, Albarran J, Richardson A (eds): Critical Care Manual of Clinical Procedures and Competencies. Chichester, 2013, John Wiley & Sons, Fig. 5.14.

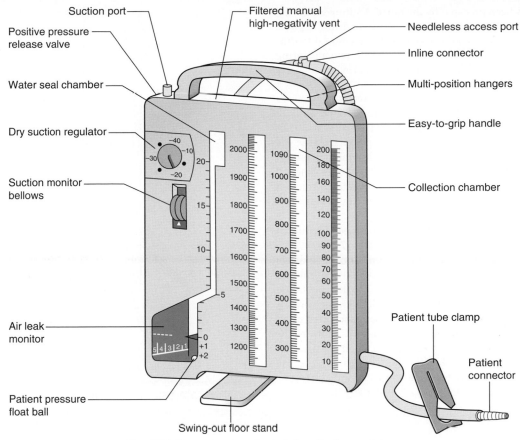

Suction port

Positive pressure release valve

Water seal chamber

Dry suction regulator

Suction monitor bellows

Air leak monitor

Patient pressure float ball

Filtered manual high-negativity vent

Needleless access port

Inline connector

Multi-position hangers

Easy-to-grip handle

Collection chamber

Patient tube clamp

Patient connector

Swing-out floor stand

Fig. 13.3 Three-chamber chest drain collection container.

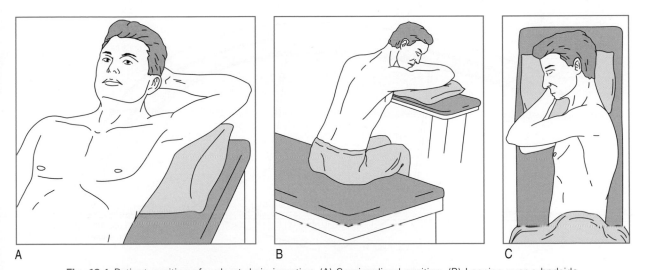

A   B   C

Fig. 13.4 Patient positions for chest drain insertion. (A) Semi-reclined position. (B) Leaning over a bedside table, arms supported with a pillow. (C) Lateral decubitus position. From Havelock T, Teoh R, Laws D, et al.: Pleural procedures and thoracic ultrasound: British Thoracic Society pleural disease guideline, Thorax 65:i61–i76, Fig. 3, 2010.

has already been prepared by the nurse. A suture is inserted to seal off the entry site and secure the drain firmly in place. For large-bore drains, a horizontal 'mattress suture' is recommended (Havelock et al. 2010), along with two anchoring sutures either side of the tube (Rashid et al. 1998; Dougherty & Lister 2015) (Fig. 13.5).

Purse-string sutures are no longer recommended, as they leave a circular rather than a linear wound and are painful for the patient on removal (Havelock et al. 2010). A simple sterile transparent dressing is placed over the site to prevent infection of the incision site; thick dressings should be avoided (Havelock et al. 2010). An omental dressing is recommended at the insertion site, to traction the drainage tube to the patient's chest wall (Fig. 13.6) (Coombs et al. 2013).

Following insertion, a chest X-ray is obtained to confirm the position of the tube (Welch & Black 2017).

Suction can be added to a single-chamber chest drainage system to augment the negative pressure created by the underwater seal, aiding lung expansion. The decision to use suction is determined by medical practitioner; pressures of 10–20 cm H_2O can be prescribed. Suction is achieved using a high-volume/low-pressure vacuum wall unit. High-pressure/high-volume suction units *used* for airway management must not be used with chest drains because the pressures generated are too high and could inflict harm or pain on the patient (Dougherty & Lister 2015).

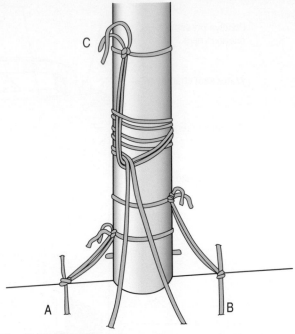

Fig. 13.5 Horizontal mattress suture and anchoring suture. A and B are tied to close the wound; C is tied around the tube to secure it. From Rashid MA, Wikstrom T, Ortenwall P: A simple technique for anchoring chest tubes, European Respiratory Journal 12: 958–959, Fig. 2, 1998.

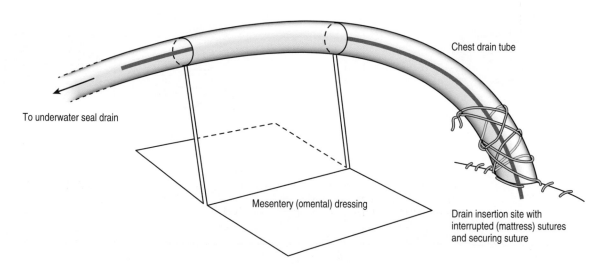

Fig. 13.6 Omental dressing providing traction of a large-bore chest drain to the chest wall to prevent kinking and to reduce pain. From Mallett J, Albarran J, Richardson A (eds): Critical Care Manual of Clinical Procedures and Competencies. Chichester, 2013, John Wiley & Sons, Fig. 5.13.

⊚ EQUIPMENT

- Trolley
- Sterile chest drain pack including sterile drapes, sterile scalpel and Spencer Wells forceps (contents dependent on local policy)
- Sterile disposable scalpel blade
- Sterile gloves (appropriately sized) and surgical gown (worn by the medical practitioner)
- Personal protective equipment, including non-sterile gloves, apron and safety goggles (as required) for the assisting nurse
- Skin cleansing solution, e.g. chlorhexidine gluconate 2% in 70% alcohol (Chloraprep™) or as per local skin preparation policy
- Local anaesthetic, e.g. lidocaine 1% or 2%
- Pre-medication and/or analgesia, as prescribed
- Syringes: 2 × 10 mL and appropriately sized needles (21 gauge and 23 gauge)
- Sterile needle and black silk suture
- Sterile chest drain (appropriately sized, with introducer if small-bore)
- Sterile underwater chest drainage collection system (container and tubing)
- Bottle of sterile water
- Sterile dressing and tape to create an omental dressing
- Sterile scissors
- Two pairs of tubing clamps
- Receptacle for soiled disposable items
- Sharps disposal container
- Monitoring equipment and oxygen (as prescribed)
- High-volume/low-pressure suction and tubing (if required)
- National Early Warning System (NEWS) chart

GUIDELINES AND RATIONALE FOR THIS NURSING PRACTICE

- Explain the procedure to the patient *to obtain informed consent* (Nursing and Midwifery Council 2018). Care should be person-centred and patients should be encouraged to be active partners in their care (McCormack & McCance 2016). *Written consent should be obtained by the medical practitioner if the patient's clinical condition allows* (Havelock et al. 2010).
- Wash your hands *to prevent cross-infection* (World Health Organization 2018; Health Protection Scotland 2016).
- The assisting nurse should wear personal protective equipment (disposable apron, non-sterile gloves, safety goggles), as deemed appropriate, *to prevent cross-infection*

and to break the chain of infection (NHS Education for Scotland 2017).
- Protect the patient's privacy *to help maintain dignity.*
- Administer a pre-medication, if prescribed, *to help to reduce the patient's anxiety;* administer analgesia as prescribed *to minimize pain during and after the procedure.* A patient with an indwelling chest drain must have adequate analgesia to enable them to perform deep breathing exercises and to cough, *thus preventing development of a chest infection* (Dougherty & Lister 2015).
- Collect all of the equipment required *to maintain efficiency of practice and patient safety.*
- Help the patient into an optimal position *to allow best access to the site for insertion of the drain* (*see* Fig. 13.4).
- On a sterile trolley, lay out the sterile chest drain insertion equipment, including the sterile chest drain pack: sterile drapes, sterile disposable scalpel and Spencer Wells forceps (contents dependent on local policy). *Chest drain insertion should be carried out under strict asepsis* (Havelock et al. 2010).
- Observe the patient throughout this activity *to detect signs of discomfort, distress or adverse haemodynamic or respiratory effects.* Attach cardiac monitoring equipment and an oxygen saturation probe *to detect deterioration in the patient's condition rapidly.* Provide oxygen as prescribed.
- Ensure that the chest drainage collection equipment is assembled correctly. The chest drain container will be primed with the required volume of water to create an underwater seal. The drain should be ready to be connected to the drainage container when required, *to maintain efficient practice.*
- Assist the medical practitioner to scrub for this aseptic procedure *to prevent cross-contamination of the chest insertion site.* The medical practitioner should be assisted into a disposable sterile gown, and appropriately sized sterile gloves should be provided.
- At the drain insertion site, the medical practitioner will cleanse the patient's skin, using an appropriate solution, e.g. chlorhexidine gluconate 2% in 70% alcohol (Chloraprep™), or as per local skin preparation policy. Sterile drapes will be applied to the area of insertion.
- Local anaesthetic, e.g. lidocaine 1%–2%, will be drawn up and infiltrated into the skin surrounding the insertion site, using appropriately sized syringes and needles *to prevent pain and discomfort.*
- The medical practitioner will make an incision into the chest wall at the insertion site and use the chest drain insertion kit to insert an appropriately sized chest drain into the patient. A sterile needle and black silk suture will be used to ensure that the drain is appropriately

secured with tube anchoring and horizontal mattress sutures (*see* Fig. 13.5).

- Attach the drain to the chest drain tubing and container and seal all connections *to ensure that they are airtight, as this is necessary for maximum functioning of the drain.*
- Ensure that the chest drainage collection container is always placed below the level of the patient's chest *to prevent reflux into the pleural cavity* (Havelock et al. 2010) (*see* Fig. 13.1). Ensure that the chest drainage collection container is supported in the stand provided by the manufacturer, *to prevent the chest drainage container falling over.*
- *To allow the apparatus to start functioning*, release the clamps when the drain is connected and you are satisfied that there are no air leaks at the connections.
- Check that the apparatus is functioning; the fluid should be oscillating in the long underwater tube in synchrony with the patient's respiratory pattern, indicating patency of the tube.
- If a large-bore tube is used, apply a sterile transparent dressing to the wound site *to help to prevent infection and to facilitate observation of the site.* Use the scissors to fashion an omental dressing. Apply the omental dressing, *to secure the tube to prevent kinking of the drain and to minimize pain at the insertion site* (*see* Fig. 13.6).
- If suction is required, connect the chest drainage system to a high-volume/low-pressure suction unit and set to the pressure prescribed by the medical practitioner. Observe the patient, the chest drain and low-pressure suction unit (Havelock et al. 2010).
- Ensure that the patient is left feeling as comfortable as possible, *to maintain the quality of this practice.*
- Decontaminate equipment and dispose of waste safely, in accordance with local policy *to reduce risks to health and safety.*
- Remove all personal protective equipment and dispose of it safely, in accordance with local policy, *to prevent cross-infection* (NHS Education for Scotland 2017).
- Document the procedure appropriately, monitor the after-effects and report any abnormal findings immediately *to ensure safe practice and enable prompt, appropriate medical and nursing intervention to be initiated* (Nursing and Midwifery Council 2018).
- Ensure that a further chest X-ray is ordered by the medical practitioner and assist the patient with this, *to ensure that the chest drain is in the correct position.* Further chest X-rays may be carried out over the ensuing hours/days *to monitor reinflation of the lung.*
- Ensure that the patient is nursed in an area where they can be observed. Nursing staff must be competent in the management of a patient with a chest drain. Adhere to local policy; **nursing staff must be reminded to keep the drain below the insertion site at ALL times** (Havelock et al. 2010).
- Give immediate care: assess the patient using the 'ABCDE' approach (*see* Ch. 18). Observe and monitor the patient's vital signs (respiratory rate/depth/pattern, oxygen saturations, heart rate, blood pressure, temperature, pain assessment and level of consciousness) (Jevon & Ewens 2012). Document observations on the patient's NEWS chart *to assess the patient's response to the intervention.* Use SBAR (situation, background, assessment, recommendation) to communicate any signs of deterioration to the medical practitioner.
- Observe and record the volume, type and consistency of drainage *to monitor the patient's progress and maintain accurate fluid balance.* For pleural effusions, a maximum of 1.5 L should be drained in the first hour (Havelock et al. 2010). Frequency of drain observations will be dictated by the patient's clinical condition; adhere to local policy.
- Observe and record whether the fluid is bubbling, if this is evident. Oscillation will cease when the lung reinflates. Bubbling in the drain is abnormal and indicative of a leak, possibly due to a bronchopleural fistula; in this instance, **contact the medical practitioner immediately and do not clamp the drain, as this may cause a tension pneumothorax** (Havelock et al. 2010).
- Ensure that a pair of safety clamps is available at the patient's bedside for use in case of accidental disconnection only. **Chest drains should never be routinely clamped for transfer or positional changes.** Clamping can generate high levels of positive pressure, resulting in a tension pneumothorax (Havelock et al. 2010).
- In partnership with the patient, assess, plan, implement and evaluate their care with reference to evidence-based practice, *to ensure that high-quality, safe care is provided.* Care should be patient-centred (McCormack & McCance 2016). An underwater chest drain will restrict the patient's ability to achieve their activities of daily living independently, and care planning should promote the patient's independence (Holland 2008).
- Observing the 'five moments of hand hygiene', decontaminate your hands at appropriate intervals, *to break the chain of infection* (World Health Organization 2018).
- In undertaking this practice, nurses are accountable for their actions, the quality of care delivered and record-keeping in accordance with the standards outlined within *The Code* (Nursing and Midwifery Council 2018).

2. CHANGING A CHEST DRAINAGE COLLECTION SYSTEM

INDICATIONS AND RATIONALE FOR CHANGING A CHEST DRAINAGE COLLECTION SYSTEM

The chest drainage collection system must be changed when the level in the drainage container approaches three-quarters full *to enable the equipment to continue functioning efficiently*, as increased volume in the drainage container may cause resistance to drainage.

> ### ⊚ EQUIPMENT
>
> - Appropriate personal protective equipment: non-sterile gloves, apron, safety goggles (as required)
> - Sterile chest drainage collection system (bottle and tubing)
> - Chest drain clamps × 2
> - 500 mL of sterile water or normal saline
> - Cap for closing used chest drain collection system
> - Receptacle for soiled disposable items (as per local policy)
> - NEWS chart

GUIDELINES AND RATIONALE FOR THIS NURSING PRACTICE

- Explain the procedure to the patient *to obtain informed consent* (Nursing and Midwifery Council 2018). Care should be person-centred and patients should be encouraged to be active partners in their care (McCormack & McCance 2016).
- Wash your hands *to prevent-cross infection* (World Health Organization 2018; Health Protection Scotland 2016).
- Wear personal protective equipment, as appropriate, *to prevent cross-infection and to break the chain of infection* (NHS Education for Scotland 2017).
- Collect and prepare the equipment *to maintain efficiency of practice.*
- Observe the patient throughout this activity *to detect signs of discomfort, distress or adverse effects.*
- Clamp off the chest drain for the shortest time possible. Place one clamp close to the chest wall *to prevent air from entering the chest drain from the atmosphere and causing a pneumothorax*; place the other clamp below the connection to the drainage tubing *to prevent any backflow of air or fluid.*

- Disconnect the tubing.
- Connect the fresh chest drainage collection system (bottle and tubing).
- Ensure that all the connections are airtight and that the drainage bottle is below chest level *to ensure that it will function correctly.*
- Release the clamps and check the oscillation of the fluid in the underwater tube *to confirm that the apparatus is functioning correctly.*
- Ensure that the patient is left feeling as comfortable as possible, *to maintain the quality of this practice.*
- Apply the cap to seal the used chest drainage bottle and to prevent spillage of body fluid. Dispose of the used bottle in an appropriate receptacle, adhering to local infection control guidelines and procedures (NHS Education for Scotland 2017).
- Decontaminate equipment and dispose of waste safely, in accordance with local policy, *to reduce risks to health and safety.*
- Remove all personal protective equipment and dispose of it safely, in accordance with local policy, *to prevent cross-infection* (NHS Education for Scotland 2017).
- Document the procedure appropriately, monitor the after-effects and report any abnormal findings immediately *to ensure safe practice and enable prompt, appropriate medical and nursing intervention to be initiated* (Nursing and Midwifery Council 2018).
- Record observations and recordings of vital signs on the patient's NEWS chart, following the procedure *to observe for any changes in the patient's condition.*
- Continue observation and monitoring of drainage *to monitor the patient's progress and maintain fluid balance.*
- In undertaking this practice, nurses are accountable for their actions, the quality of care delivered and record-keeping in accordance with the standards outlined within *The Code* (Nursing and Midwifery Council 2018).

3. REMOVAL OF AN UNDERWATER SEAL CHEST DRAIN

INDICATIONS AND RATIONALE FOR REMOVAL OF AN UNDERWATER SEAL CHEST DRAIN

Underwater seal drainage is a temporary measure and the drain is removed when:
- radiological examination demonstrates that the patient's lung has fully reinflated
- air or fluid no longer drains
- the patient's respiratory function has improved.

GUIDELINES AND RATIONALE FOR THIS NURSING PRACTICE

Two nurses, one of whom must be qualified, or a nurse and a medical practitioner are required to carry out this practice.

- Explain the aim of the nursing practice to the patient *to gain consent* (Nursing and Midwifery Council 2018).
- Fully explain the procedure to the patient, providing time for rehearsal/practice of the required techniques *to enable the patient to engage with the procedure;* patients should be encouraged to be active partners in their care.
- Ensure the patient's privacy *to maintain dignity and a sense of self.*
- Administer analgesia, as prescribed by the medical practitioner, in advance of the procedure *to manage pain effectively.*
- Collect the equipment *to maintain efficiency of practice.*
- Prepare and assist the patient into an upright position in bed, supported with pillows, *to allow clear access to the drain site* (Allibone 2015).
- Observe the patient throughout this activity *to detect any signs of discomfort and distress.*
- Prepare and set up the trolley for the procedure.
- Both nurses should wash their hands *to prevent cross-infection* (World Health Organization 2018; Health Protection Scotland 2016).
- Both nurses should wear personal protective equipment, as appropriate, *to prevent cross-infection and to break the chain of infection* (NHS Education for Scotland 2017).
- Remove the dressing and visualize the sutures at the drain site; identify the mattress sutures (which are closing the wound) and the anchor sutures (which are securing the tube) (*see* Fig. 13.5). The anchor sutures will be cut and removed, and the mattress sutures will be tightened to close the wound as the tube is removed (Dougherty & Lister 2015).

- Nurse 1 should loosen the ends of the mattress suture, while nurse 2 cuts the anchor suture with the disposable suture cutter and loosens the chest drain tube gently, *to prepare for removal of the chest drain* (Dougherty & Lister 2015).
- Nurse 2 assertively coaches the patient to take a deep inhalation followed by exhalation. The patient is asked to do this three times; then, on the fourth breath, the patient is instructed to hold their breath (at the end of inspiration) whilst performing the Valsalva manoeuvre, as nurse 1 smoothly and firmly removes the chest drain (Dougherty & Lister 2015). The aim is *to increase the patient's intrapulmonary pressure to prevent atmospheric air from entering the pleural cavity once the drain is removed* (Welch & Black 2017).
- As soon as the drain is removed from the incision site, nurse 1 quickly pulls the ends of the mattress sutures and ties them securely *to close the wound and form an airtight seal* (Allibone 2015).
- As soon as this is achieved, nurse 2 coaches the patient to breathe normally again.
- Clean the area around the wound with 0.9% sodium chloride, using the dressing pack, and apply an occlusive dressing (as per local policy).
- Assist the patient into a comfortable position.
- Dispose of all waste in accordance with local policy, *to protect the health and safety of all patients, visitors and staff.*
- Order a chest X-ray *to ensure that both lungs are fully expanded.*
- Ensure that the patient is left feeling as comfortable as possible, *to maintain the quality of this practice.*
- Observe the patient for any deterioration in respiratory function caused by reaccumulation of air or fluid in the pleural cavity. Observe the drain insertion site for surgical emphysema.
- Assess the patient using the 'ABCDE' approach (*see* Ch. 18). Observe and monitor the patient's vital signs (respiratory rate/depth/pattern, oxygen saturations, heart rate, blood pressure, temperature, pain assessment and level of consciousness) (Jevon & Ewens 2012). Document on the patient's NEWS chart *to assess the patient's response to the intervention.* Use SBAR (situation, background, assessment, recommendation) to communicate any signs of deterioration to the medical practitioner immediately.
- Document the nursing practice. Continue to monitor the after-effects and report any abnormal findings immediately *to provide a written record and assist in the implementation of any action, should an abnormality or adverse reaction to the practice be noted.*
- During and at the end of the procedure, ensure that all practitioners observe the 'five moments of hand hygiene'

by decontaminating their hands at appropriate intervals, ***to break the chain of infection*** (World Health Organization 2018).

- In undertaking this practice, nurses are accountable for their actions, the quality of care delivered and record-keeping in accordance with the standards outlined within *The Code* (Nursing and Midwifery Council 2018).

 PATIENT/CARER EDUCATION: KEY POINTS

The patient should be given clear information about the procedure to ensure that they are able to give informed consent and to encourage their participation in care. Written educational leaflets should be available (Havelock et al. 2010).

The patient and carers should be informed of the need to keep the drainage system below the level of the chest. Specific information about mobilizing safely should also be given.

The patient should be encouraged to report any problems, such as pulling of the tube or increased dyspnoea.

Adequate pain relief should be available to the patient. Patients should be informed of the nursing observations that will be made when the chest drain is in place to alleviate anxiety.

REFERENCES

Allibone, L., 2015. How to remove a chest drain. Nursing Standard 30 (6), 34–36.

Coombs, M., Dyos, J., Waters, D., Nesbett, I., 2013. Assessment, monitoring and interventions for the respiratory system. In: Mallett, J., Albarran, J., Richardson, A. (Eds.), Critical Care Manual of Clinical Procedures & Competencies. John-Wiley & Sons, Chichester.

Dougherty, L., Lister, S., 2015. The Royal Marsden Manual of Clinical Nursing Procedures. Wiley-Blackwell., Oxford.

Durai, R., Hoque, H., Davies, T., 2010. Managing a chest tube and drainage system. AORN Journal 91 (2), 275–283.

Harris, A., O'Driscoll, R., Turkington, P., 2010. Survey of major complications of intercostal chest drain insertion in the UK. Postgraduate Medical Journal 86 (68), 68–72.

Havelock, T., Teoh, R., Laws, D., Gleeson, F., on behalf of the BTS Pleural Disease Guideline Group, 2010. Pleural procedures and thoracic ultrasound: British Thoracic Society pleural disease guideline. Thorax 65, i61–i76.

Health Protection Scotland, 2016. Standard infection control precautions literature review: hand hygiene: hand washing, version 2. National Health Services Scotland. Available from: http://www.nipcm.hps.scot.nhs.uk/documents/sicp-hand-hygiene-hand-washing-in-the-hospital-setting/.

Holland, K., 2008. Applying the Roper-Logan-Tierney Model in Practice, 2nd ed. Churchill Livingstone, Oxford.

Jevon, P., Ewens, B., 2012. Monitoring the Critically Ill Patient. Blackwell, Oxford.

McCormack, B., McCance, T., 2016. Person-Centred Practice in Nursing and Health Care - Theory and Practice, second ed. John Wiley & Sons, Chichester.

NHS Education for Scotland, 2017. Personal protective equipment. Available from: https://www.nes.scot.nhs.uk/education-and-training/by-theme-initiative/healthcare-associated-infections/training-resources/personal-protective-equipment-(ppe).aspx.

Nursing and Midwifery Council, 2018. The Code: Professional Standards of Practice and Behaviour for Nurses, Midwives and Nursing Associates. NMC, London. Available from: https://www.nmc.org.uk/globalassets/sitedocuments/nmc-publications/nmc-code.pdf.

Rashid, M., Wikstom, T., Ortenwall, P., 1998. A simple technique for anchoring chest tubes. European Respiratory Journal 12, 958–959.

Welch, J., Black, C., 2017. Respiratory problems. In: Adam, S., Osborne, S., Welch, J. (Eds.), Critical Care Nursing Science and Practice, third ed. Oxford University Press, Oxford.

World Health Organization, 2018. Five moments for hand hygiene. Available from: https://www.who.int/gpsc/tools/Five_moments/en/.

? SELF-ASSESSMENT

1. Outline the indications for chest drain insertion.
2. Consider what you would say to a patient to prepare them for chest drain insertion.
3. What aspects of the procedure might pose an infection control risk?
4. What observations should be carried out on the patient who has a chest drain in place?
5. What are the indications for chest drainage removal?

Diagnostic Investigations

INDICATIONS AND RATIONALE FOR COLLECTING SPECIMENS

A specimen may be required:
- *to aid the diagnosis of disease*
- *to monitor the effect of treatment*
- to permit laboratory culture *to identify pathogenic microorganisms and determine drug sensitivity*
- *to carry out screening in health to facilitate cancer diagnosis, staging and typing.*

GUIDELINES AND RATIONALE FOR THIS NURSING PRACTICE

- Explain the nursing practice to the patient *to gain consent and cooperation*. Patients should be encouraged to be active partners in care.
- Ensure the patient's privacy *to help to maintain dignity and a sense of self.*
- The nurse and the patient (if the patient is involved in the collection of the specimen) should wash their hands before and after specimen collection *to reduce the risk of cross-infection* (Health Protection Scotland 2012).
- Ensure that standard infection control precautions, including the use of personal protective equipment, are observed *to reduce the risk of transmission of infectious agents from both recognized and unrecognized sources of infection* (National Institute for Health and Care Excellence 2012).
- Collect the specimen at the most appropriate time *to facilitate obtaining accurate results*. This time will vary depending on the specimen; the optimum time for the collection of a specimen of urine for culture, for example, is from the first voiding of the bladder in the morning.
- *To avoid interference with accurate results*, ensure that no substance that might cause an inaccurate result has been used prior to collection. A specimen of sputum, for example, could be adversely affected by the patient using an antiseptic mouthwash before giving the specimen.
- Ensure that sufficient quantities of the specimen have been collected *to assist the laboratory staff in preparing the specimen for analysis, which will lead to accurate results.*
- Avoid contamination of the specimen by the hands of the nurse or patient, *as this could invalidate the results of the culture and be a hazard to the individual's health.*
- Follow standard blood and body substance isolation precautions when placing a specimen into the container and take precautions to avoid contamination of the

outside of the container with the specimen substance (Association for Perioperative Practice 2016).

- Ensure that the patient is left feeling as comfortable as possible after the specimen is collected.
- Dispatch the labelled specimen container to the laboratory immediately with the completed form; **any delay may alter the reliability of any results obtained**. If a delay is unavoidable, the specimen can usually be stored in a specimen refrigerator until it can be sent for analysis.
- Document this nursing practice appropriately, monitor the after-effects and report any abnormal findings immediately *to facilitate the instigation of appropriate measures to relieve the problem.*
- In undertaking this practice, nurses are accountable for their actions and the quality of care delivered; they must keep clear and accurate records in accordance with *The Code* (Nursing and Midwifery Council 2018).

SWAB COLLECTION

◎ SPECIFIC EQUIPMENT

- Microbiology swab
- Disposable gloves and apron
- Sterile water for a nose swab
- Sterile vaginal speculum for a vaginal swab
- Sterile lubricating jelly for a vaginal swab
- Spatula for a throat swab

Specific Guidelines and Rationale for this Nursing Practice

Wound Swabs

- Obtain a specimen before the wound is washed *to ensure that the specimen material is not contaminated by the washing agent.*
- Rotate the swab in the wound *to obtain a sufficient quantity for examination.*

Throat Swabs

- Help the patient to sit in an appropriate position *to facilitate a good view of the tonsils and pillars of the fauces.*
- Depress the patient's tongue with a spatula *to facilitate access to the site.*
- Gently rub the swab over the tonsillar area and pillars of the fauces for 3–5 seconds (Health Protection Scotland 2016).
- Avoid touching any other area of the mouth as the swab is being removed *to ensure that the specimen will not be contaminated.*

Ear Swabs

- Help the patient to sit in a comfortable position with the head slightly tilted to the unaffected side.
- Gently pull the patient's pinna upwards and backwards to straighten the external canal. Do this *to facilitate the insertion of the swab and to obtain a specimen of the discharge.*
- Insert the swab into the external canal and rotate it gently *to ensure that the swab is well coated with the discharge.*

Nasal Swabs

- Help the patient to sit in a comfortable position *to allow access to the nasal cavity.*
- Moisten the swab in sterile water before insertion into the nose *to make the procedure more comfortable for the patient,* as the nasal cavity can be dry.
- Insert the swab into one nostril, rotating it gently and moving it upwards towards the tip of the nose. Repeat the procedure on the other nostril, using the same swab.

Vaginal Swabs

- Help the patient into an appropriate position *to allow access to the vagina.*
- Gently insert a lubricated speculum into the vagina to separate the vaginal walls and *to allow the area to be swabbed to be visualized.*
- Introduce the swab into the high vaginal area and rotate it gently. A charcoal-based transport medium is frequently used for vaginal swabs.

Penile Swabs

- Help the patient into a comfortable position *to allow access to the penis.*
- Retract the foreskin *to allow the area that is to be swabbed to be visualized.*
- Rotate the swab gently in the urethral meatus *to collect a sample of the secretions.*
- Reposition the foreskin completely.

FAECES

◎ SPECIFIC EQUIPMENT

- Disposable gloves and apron
- Bedpan
- Sterile spatula
- Sterile container
- Receptacle for soiled disposable items

Specific Guidelines and Rationale for this Nursing Practice

- Ask the patient to empty their bladder first and then to defaecate into a clean bedpan; do this *to ensure that the faecal matter does not become contaminated with urine, as this could affect the analysis results.*
- Use a spatula or implement provided to fill about one-third of the specimen container with faecal material.
- If the faeces are being tested for occult blood, follow the instructions on the packaging in which the occult blood testing equipment is supplied.

URINE

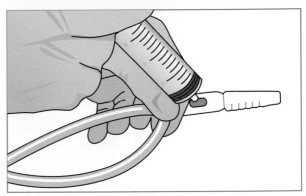

Fig. 14.1 Collecting a specimen of urine when a catheter is in position.

SPECIFIC EQUIPMENT

- Sterile container
- Disposable gloves and apron
- Bedpan or urinal: may be necessary
- Sterile receiver: may be necessary to receive the specimen
- Washing equipment: to wash the surrounding tissue
- Midstream specimens of urine: a sterile tin-foil bowl
- Catheter specimens of urine: a sterile syringe and alcohol-impregnated swab
- 24-hour urine collection: a large plastic/glass sterile container with a lid

Specific Guidelines and Rationale for this Nursing Practice

- *To facilitate the collection of a midstream specimen of urine,* ask the patient to wash and dry their hands and undertake cleaning of their genitalia with soap and water, 0.9% sodium chloride or a disinfectant-free solution (Dougherty & Lister 2015).
- Instruct the patient to begin passing urine (15–30 mL) directly into the toilet (or bedpan/urinal) and then, without any interruption in flow, the patient should collect the middle section of the stream directly into a broad-necked sterile container. Transfer the specimen into the sterile specimen container.
- *To facilitate the collection of a catheter specimen of urine,* clean the sampling port on the tubing of the catheter drainage bag with a swab containing 2% chlorhexidine in 70% isopropyl alcohol and allow it to dry (Shepherd 2017). Using an aseptic, non-touch technique, insert the tip of a 10 mL syringe into the sampling port and withdraw the required amount of urine into the syringe (Fig. 14.1). Transfer it to the sterile container.

- To commence a 24-hour collection, ask the patient to void their bladder and discard the urine *to ensure that the patient and staff know the exact time the collection commences.* Collect all the urine passed in the next 24 hours.

CERVICAL SMEAR

This procedure should be undertaken only by healthcare professionals that are competent to do so and have undergone the appropriate training (National Institute for Health and Care Excellence 2017).

SPECIFIC EQUIPMENT

- Disposable gloves
- Lubricating gel
- Vaginal speculum
- Cervex-Brush
- Specimen pot for liquid-based cytology (fixation vial)
- Disposable modesty sheet
- Medical wipes/tissues

Specific Guidelines and Rationale for this Nursing Practice

- Lay the modesty sheet over the patient's pubic area. Help the patient into the most appropriate position *to facilitate collection of the specimen.*
- Put on the disposable gloves.
- Lubricate the speculum, avoiding the tip, *so as not to contaminate the cervix.*
- Gently and slowly, insert the speculum side on into the vagina.

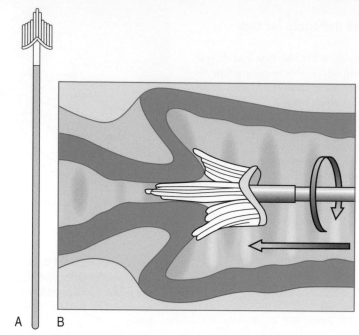

A   B

Fig. 14.2 Cervical smear. (A) Cervex-Brush. (B) Correct use of cervix brush.

- Open and close the speculum slightly or change the angle of insertion *to bring the cervix into view* (Public Health England 2016).
- Using the Cervex-Brush, insert the central bristles into the endocervical canal so that the shorter bristles are in full contact with the ectocervix. Rotate the brush five times in a clockwork direction (Fig. 14.2).
- Immediately and vigorously, rinse the brush in the fixative vial, *to ensure that all the material reaches the liquid.* Seal and label the vial.

- Withdraw the speculum gently, allowing the blades to close once they are clear of the cervix.
- Offer tissues to the patient for her to clean the outside of her vagina and then provide privacy for dressing.
- Allow the patient time to recover from this procedure before sitting her upright because handling the cervix can cause a feeling of faintness as the result of a vasovagal response.

PATIENT/CARER EDUCATION: KEY POINTS

In partnership with the patient and/or carer, ensure that they are competent to carry out any practices required. Information should be given on an appropriate point of contact for any concerns that may arise.

The actions associated with this practice may challenge the cultural norms of the patients and their carers. The nurse should be sensitive to these issues when discussing this practice with the patient and carers. For intimate procedures the nurse should offer the patient the option of having an impartial observer (a chaperone) present wherever possible.

An explanation of the method of, and reasons for, collecting the specimen will help the patient to understand how and why the practice is necessary. This is particularly important if the patient is in the community and the specimen is being collected in their home. If the specimen is collected at home, the patient will need clear instructions on the storing of the specimen and where and when to deliver it, so that it arrives at the laboratory in optimum condition.

REFERENCES

Association for Perioperative Practice, 2016. Standards and Recommendations for Safe Perioperative Practice, fourth ed. AfPP, Harrogate.

Dougherty, L., Lister, S., 2015. The Royal Marsden Manual of Clinical Nursing Procedures. Wiley-Blackwell, Oxford.

Health Protection Scotland, 2012. National Infection Prevention and Control Manual. Available at: http://www.nipcm.hps.scot.nhs.uk/.

Health Protection Scotland, 2016. Protocol for CRA MRSA Screening National Rollout in Scotland. HPS, Edinburgh. Available at: https://www.hps.scot.nhs.uk/resourcedocument.aspx?resourceid=1639.

Human Tissue Act, 2004. Available from: https://www.legislation.gov.uk/ukpga/2004/30/contents.

National Institute for Health and Care Excellence, 2012. Healthcare-associated infections: prevention and control in primary and community care. NICE, London. Available at: https://www.nice.org.uk/guidance/cg139/chapter/1-Guidance#standard-principles.

National Institute for Health and Care Excellence, 2017. Clinical Knowledge Summaries - Cervical screening. NICE, London. Available at: https://cks.nice.org.uk/cervical-screening#!scenario.

Nursing and Midwifery Council, 2018. The Code: Professional Standards of Practice and Behaviour for Nurses, Midwives and Nursing Associates. NMC, London. Available at: https://www.nmc.org.uk/globalassets/sitedocuments/nmc-publications/nmc-code.pdf.

Public Health England, 2016. NHS Cervical Screening Programme Guidance for the training of cervical sample takers. NHS, London. Available at: https://assets.publishing.service.gov.uk/government/uploads/system/uploads/attachment_data/file/577158/NHS_Cervical_Screening_Progamme_-_guidance_for_cervical_sample_takers.pdf.

Shepherd, E., 2017. Specimen collection 2: obtaining a catheter specimen of urine. Nursing Times 113 (8), 29–31.

WEBSITES

https://www.dh.gov.uk *Department of Health – advice and national publications*

https://www.ips.uk.net *Infection Prevention Society*

https://www.nes.scot.nhs.uk *NHS Education for Scotland – publications and web-based materials*

https://www.nmc.org.uk *Nursing and Midwifery Council – publications*

https://www.rcn.org.uk *Royal College of Nursing – publications*

 SELF-ASSESSMENT

1. List and discuss three reasons for specimen collection.
2. What measures can the nurse employ to ensure that accurate results from the collected specimen are obtained?
3. How you would explain to a patient how to collect a midstream urine specimen at home?

Electrocardiogram Set-up and Recording

INDICATIONS AND RATIONALE FOR ECG MONITORING

An electrocardiograph is a heart monitor that measures and records the time sequence of the electrical activity generated by the heart muscle (Oster 2014). An ECG is a time/voltage graph that provides a recording of the heart's electrical activity (Woodrow & Davies 2009). Patients who are having their heart monitored in this way merit being in a high-observation area (Higgins 2011).

There are two main approaches:
- continuous cardiac monitoring, which provides a constant, real-time, one-dimensional view of the heart's electrical rhythm
- a 12-lead ECG, which provides a three-dimensional view of the electrical activity of the heart.

The terminology used in relation to ECG monitoring can occasionally be confusing. While the word 'lead' would normally be associated with a wire, in terms of ECG monitoring it refers to the view of the electrical activity of the heart (Woodrow & Davies 2009). Adhesive electrodes are placed on the surface of the skin at specific points, to which wires are connected (Resuscitation Council (UK)

2016). These wires then transmit electrical information (Woodrow & Davies 2009) to the ECG machine (for a 12-lead ECG) or ECG monitor (for continuous cardiac monitoring).

While the electrical activity of the heart can be associated with overall heart health, it is important to note that other factors must be considered and that more detailed, specialized investigations are required to assess the health of the heart fully.

The indications for continuous monitoring of the ECG include:
- any acute critical illness, *to detect a deterioration or complications promptly*
- peri- and post-cardiac arrest *to detect an abnormal cardiac rhythm (arrhythmia) quickly and to allow prompt, appropriate action, should cardiac arrest recur*
- during cardiac arrest, *to establish the underlying rhythm and provide appropriate treatment*
- any procedure involving sedation or anaesthesia, *to detect complications promptly and to allow prompt, appropriate action.*

While any of the situations above may also be an indication for 12-lead ECG recording, other factors that would alert you to the need for this include:
- cardiovascular or conduction abnormalities, such as electrolyte or metabolic imbalance, or drug overdose, *to detect an abnormal cardiac rhythm (arrhythmia) quickly and to allow prompt, appropriate action, should cardiac arrest occur* (Jevon 2009)
- a history of life-threatening cardiac arrhythmias, *to detect a deterioration or complications promptly and to allow prompt, appropriate action*
- during and following any invasive cardiac procedure, *to detect complications and to allow prompt, appropriate action*
- acute coronary syndromes, *to detect an arrhythmia quickly and to allow prompt, appropriate action;* a 12-lead ECG will help to establish the area of the heart affected and the associated culprit artery.

EQUIPMENT

- Skin preparation equipment:
  - cleansing agent
  - scissors/razor
- Disposable single-use adhesive electrodes (compatible with the cardiac monitor and ECG machine)
- Cardiac monitor and ECG machine with associated wires
- Electrical supply

OUTLINE OF THE PROCEDURE

Preparing the Patient

While cardiac monitoring is a relatively straightforward procedure, problems can be experienced as a result of poor technique relating to preparation of the skin or attachment of the electrode leads. Careful attachment of the electrodes to the skin is the most important step in obtaining a good-quality ECG tracing (Oster 2014).

The skin, muscle, bone and tissues of the body provide a natural resistance (impedance) to any electrical signals. The outermost layer of the skin (stratum corneum) contains many layers (Waugh & Grant 2014), which can cause a high impedance to the signals being sent to the ECG monitor (Oster 2014). Removal of the stratum corneum at the site where the adhesive electrodes will be placed will significantly reduce this impedance and improve the quality of the signal being received by the monitor (Oster 2014).

Unless there is good contact between the skin and the electrode pad, distortions (artefacts) may appear in the tracing, making analysis of the rhythm more difficult. Artefact may also be caused by interference: for example, from mobile telephones, or from siting the leads over large areas of muscle.

GUIDELINES AND RATIONALE FOR THIS NURSING PRACTICE

Continuous Cardiac Monitoring

- Explain the nursing practice to the patient *to obtain consent and cooperation.* Patients should be encouraged to be active partners in their care.
- Wash your hands *to prevent cross-infection between patients* (World Health Organization 2018).
- Observe the patient throughout this activity for any signs of discomfort or distress. Do this *to allow the nurse to intervene immediately in the event of an adverse reaction.*

- Assess the patient's chest to establish the optimal site for electrode placement. This should be over bone, as opposed to fatty areas and major muscles. Do this *to help reduce motion-related artefact and optimize the ECG signal strength* (Resuscitation Council (UK) 2016).
- If the patient is hirsute (hairy) at the proposed site for electrode application, the hair should be trimmed *to augment electrode adhesion and the clarity of the ECG trace* (Oster 2014).
- For **routine** monitoring, clean the skin at the electrode application site using soap and water, and dry with a cloth or gauze *to augment electrode adhesion and the clarity of the ECG trace* (Oster 2014).
- In patients who are sweating excessively (diaphoresis) or who have greasy or oily skin, alcohol swabs can be used as a method of cleansing the skin in preparation for electrode placement (Resuscitation Council (UK) 2016). In such cases, the alcohol must be fully dried prior to application of the electrodes to the skin. Alcohol should not be used routinely, *as it can cause dehydration of the skin and, consequently, further increase skin impedance* (Oster 2014).
- If the ECG monitor has press stud-style lead wires, attach these to the electrode before placing the electrode on the patient *to avoid potential patient discomfort as a result of pressing these on to the electrode, once they have been positioned on the patient* (Oster 2014).
- Most ECG monitor wires are colour-coded red, yellow and green to help with correct placement (Resuscitation Council (UK) 2016). Once the wires are connected to the adhesive electrode, a simple way to remember the correct placement is: place the **r**ed on the **r**ight shoulder joint; the **ye**llow (**le**mon) on the **le**ft shoulder joint, and **g**reen at the **s**pleen (left upper abdomen or lower chest wall) (Fig. 15.1).
- This placement will enable monitoring using modified limb leads I, II or III (Resuscitation Council (UK) 2016). Select lead II on the monitor, *as this normally provides the best view of the P wave and QRS complex.*
- Ensure that the ECG 'gain switch' on the monitor is set correctly. The gain will increase the size of the QRS complex, should it be required to provide a clearer picture (Jevon 2007).

12-Lead ECG

- Explain the nursing practice to the patient *to obtain consent and cooperation.* Patients should be encouraged to be active partners in their care.
- Wash your hands *to prevent cross-infection between patients* (World Health Organization 2018).
- Observe the patient throughout this activity for any signs of discomfort or distress. Do this *to allow the nurse to*

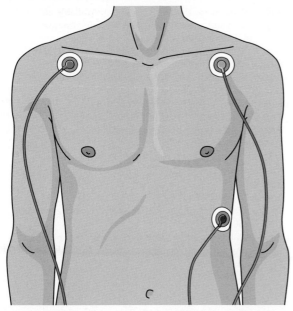

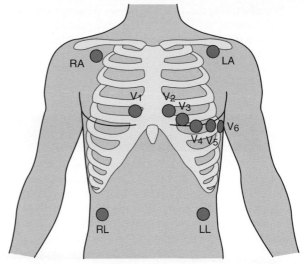

Fig. 15.2 Position of electrodes for 12-lead ECG. *LA,* left arm; *LL,* left leg; *RA,* right arm; *RL,* right leg.

Fig. 15.1 Cardiac monitoring: position of chest leads.

intervene immediately in the event of an adverse reaction.

- Assess the patient's chest to establish the optimal site for electrode placement. This should be over bone, as opposed to fatty areas and major muscles. Do this *to help reduce motion-related artefact and optimize the ECG signal strength* (Resuscitation Council (UK) 2016).
- If the patient is hirsute (hairy) at the proposed site for electrode application, hair should be trimmed *to augment electrode adhesion and the clarity of the ECG trace* (Oster 2014).
- For **routine** monitoring, clean the skin at the electrode application site using soap and water, and dry with a cloth or gauze *to augment electrode adhesion and the clarity of the ECG trace* (Oster 2014).
- In patients who are sweating excessively (diaphoresis) or who have greasy or oily skin, alcohol swabs can be used as a method of cleansing the skin in preparation for electrode placement (Resuscitation Council (UK) 2016). In such cases, the alcohol must be fully dried prior to application of the electrodes to the skin. Alcohol should not be used routinely, *as it can cause dehydration of the skin and, consequently, further increase skin imped-ance* (Oster 2014).
- Apply the electrodes as indicated in Fig. 15.2 (Romano 2015) *to ensure an accurate ECG:*

- Apply the bipolar limb leads to the right arm, left arm and left leg
- Apply the ground electrode to the right leg
- Apply the precordial leads to the chest as follows:
  V_1: the electrode is placed in the fourth intercostal space, on the right sternal border
  V_2: the electrode is placed in the fourth intercostal space, on the left sternal border
  V_3: the electrode is placed midway between V_2 and V_4
  V_4: the electrode is placed in the fifth intercostal space, on the anterior mid-clavicular line
  V_5: the electrode is horizontally aligned with V_4, on the anterior axillary line
  V_6: the electrode is placed on the mid-axillary line and aligned horizontally with V_4.
- Ask the patient to stay as still as possible and press the 'start' or 'run' button to commence the ECG recording.
- Obtain a tracing and ensure that the patient details are correct.

Post-Procedure Care: Continuous Cardiac Monitoring and 12-Lead ECG

- Wash your hands *to prevent cross-infection between patients* (World Health Organization 2018).
- Document your findings appropriately, comparing past recordings, and report any abnormal findings immediately *to enable early intervention to improve the problem.*

- In undertaking this practice, nurses are accountable for their actions, the quality of care delivered and record-keeping in accordance with the Nursing and Midwifery Council (2018).
- Always leave the patient comfortable with their nurse-call system close to hand.

 PATIENT/CARER EDUCATION: KEY POINTS

By its very nature, ECG monitoring can be a cause of anxiety for patients and their carer, particularly when alarms sound (Higgins 2011). It is therefore important to discuss the reasons for ECG monitoring and explain the normal values expected on the monitor, as well as describing the alarm settings to both patient and carer.

It is also important to warn patients that certain activities, such as movement and brushing the teeth, can cause the monitor alarms to sound (Higgins 2011).

REFERENCES

Higgins, D., 2011. ECGs 1: how to carry out monitoring. Nursing Times 107 (27), 12–13.

Jevon, P., 2007. Cardiac monitoring. Part 1–Electrocardiography (ECG). Nursing Times 103 (1), 26.

Jevon, P., 2009. ECGs for Nurses. Blackwell, Oxford.

Nursing and Midwifery Council, 2018. The Code: Professional Standards of Practice and Behaviour for Nurses, Midwives and Nursing Associates. NMC, London. Available at: https://www.nmc.org.uk/globalassets/sitedocuments/nmc-publications/nmc-code.pdf.

Oster, C.D., 2014. Proper skin prep helps ensure ECG trace quality. 3M Health Care, St. Paul, MN.

Resuscitation Council (UK), 2016. Advanced Life Support, seventh ed. RCUK, London.

Romano, M., 2015. The Electrographic Leads. In: Romano, M., Atlas of Practical Electrocardiography. Available from: https://doi-org.gcu.idm.oclc.org/10.1007/978-88-470-5741-8_2.

Waugh, A., Grant, A., 2014. Ross & Wilson Anatomy and Physiology in Health and Illness E-Book. Elsevier Health Sciences.

Woodrow, P., Davies, S., 2009. An introduction to electrocardiogram interpretation: part 1. Nursing Standard 24 (12), 50–57.

World Health Organization, 2018. Five moments for hand hygiene. Available at: http://www.who.int/gpsc/tools/Five_moments/en/.

? SELF-ASSESSMENT

1. What are the indications for continuous cardiac monitoring?
2. What are the indications for performing a 12-lead ECG?
3. How would you prepare the patient for a 12-lead ECG or continuous cardiac monitoring?
4. How would you encourage concordance with ECG monitoring?

16

Enemas and Suppositories: Administration

There are two parts to this chapter:
1. Administration of a suppository
2. Administration of an enema

1. ADMINISTRATION OF A SUPPOSITORY

INDICATIONS AND RATIONALE FOR ADMINISTERING A SUPPOSITORY

A suppository is torpedo-shaped with a pointed end (apex) and a blunt end. It contains a medicinal substance that can be introduced into the rectum; this will eventually dissolve and may be absorbed by the rectal mucosa. The blunt end, which is concave, has a useful indentation for the finger to push against it. This enables patients who are self-administering to insert the suppository without fully inserting their finger.

Indications for suppository use are:
- *to relieve constipation*
- *to evacuate the bowel prior to bowel surgery or certain investigations*
- *to treat haemorrhoids or anal pruritus*
- *to administer medicines*, e.g. antibiotics, bronchodilators or analgesics.

An appropriately trained nurse prescriber has the ability to assess, diagnose and prescribe a suitable suppository to rectify severe constipation. This is a specialized extended role recognized by a registerable qualification with the Nursing and Midwifery Council (NMC). An awareness of the Rome II Criteria for constipation (Box 16.1) offers guidance for the practitioner diagnosing constipation, as does a digital rectal examination (*see* Ch. 34).

Exclusions and Contraindications

Registered nurses should not administer suppositories when there is:
- intestinal obstruction
- an acute abdominal condition
- acute inflammatory bowel disease

BOX 16.1　Rome II Criteria for Constipation (Adults)

A diagnosis of constipation requires two or more of the following symptoms to be present for at least 3 months (not necessarily consecutive) in the preceding 12 months:

1. Straining at defaecation for at least a quarter of bowel movements
2. Lumpy and/or hard stools for at least a quarter of bowel movements
3. A sensation of incomplete evacuation for at least a quarter of bowel movements
4. Less than three bowel movements a week
5. Manual manœuvres to facilitate a quarter of bowel movements (e.g. digital evacuation or support of the pelvic floor)
6. Loose stools not present and insufficient criteria met for irritable bowel syndrome.

From Drossman DA: Rome II: The Functional Gastrointestinal Disorders. McLean, VA, 2000, Degnon Associates.

- severe dehydration
- allergy to components.

Precautions

- History of abuse
- Rectal/anal pain
- Recent anal/rectal surgery
- Recent anal/rectal trauma
- Obvious rectal bleeding
- Spinal injury
- Elderly and debilitated patients

OUTLINE OF THE PROCEDURE

Traditionally, suppositories were inserted pointed end first. However, studies by Abd-El-Maeboud et al. (1991) and Moppett (2000) suggested that suppositories should be inserted blunt end first. These studies assert that it is easier for the suppository to be retained if inserted this way, due to the squeezing action of the anal sphincter against the apex, and that this pushes the suppository into the rectum. A suppository also needs to be placed against the bowel wall, particularly if it is for constipation. The technique for insertion in this case is important, as the patient with constipation is most probably already experiencing discomfort. Several reports on which end of the suppository to insert first have challenged the two earlier studies and the subject remains controversial (Bradshaw & Price 2006; Kyle 2009). The suppository requires body heat for it to dissolve and become effective; if it is not positioned correctly, this leads to ineffective treatment. One argument in favour of insertion blunt end first is that this may be easier for patients who self-administer, and they do not need to insert a finger to push the suppository forward. Bradshaw & Price (2006) and Kyle (2009) therefore advocate a common-sense approach. There is a paucity of research on which end of the suppository should be inserted first; until further studies are available, practitioners should follow manufacturer's guidance and local policy/procedures, and be knowledgeable about the procedure, the rationale for the administration of suppositories and their effects.

Suppositories are of value in emptying the rectum. Glycerine suppositories lubricate hard, dry stools, whereas bisacodyl suppositories will have a mild stimulant effect on the rectum. Delivery of the suppository is relatively painless and the medicine is well absorbed through the rectal mucosa. It is of benefit to those who are unable to swallow medicine, e.g. during a seizure, when experiencing severe nausea and vomiting, if there is a low level of consciousness or if the patient has a needle phobia. Glycerine suppositories should be inserted directly into the faeces and allowed to dissolve, mainly because they have a mild irritant effect but also because they act as a faecal softener (Joint Formulary Committee 2015).

Nurses must also be mindful of the implications of any invasive procedure and demonstrate sensitivity and tact in conducting this procedure. There are potential alerts to consider, such as previous radiotherapy to the area, detection of a previously undiagnosed rectal carcinoma or a past history of sexual abuse.

◎ EQUIPMENT

- Patient's prescription
- Tray on a flat surface
- Non-sterile disposable gloves
- Apron
- Medical wipes/tissue
- Water-soluble lubricant
- Protective covering
- Receptacle for soiled waste
- Prescribed suppository
- Access to toilet facilities/bedpan/commode

GUIDELINES AND RATIONALE FOR THIS NURSING PRACTICE

Prior to Examination

- Check the prescription details ('The Five Rights of Medicine Administration'; *see* Ch. 2).

- Ensure that the suppository has not exceeded the expiry date and the packaging is intact.
- Explain the procedure to the patient.
- Obtain informed consent and document this in the nursing notes.
- Ask the patient if they wish to have a chaperone present.
- Give the patient the opportunity to empty their bladder.
- A medicated suppository should be administered after the patient has emptied their bowels (if possible).
- Ensure that privacy and dignity are maintained at all times.
- A bedpan, commode or toilet should be readily available.
- Ask the patient to remove their clothing from the waist down and offer assistance if required.
- Ask the patient to lie in the left lateral position with the knees flexed (if possible) *to enable easy passage of the suppository into the rectum by following the natural anatomy of the colon.*
- Wash your hands and put on a disposable apron and gloves.
- Place a protective pad under the patient's hips and buttocks.

Procedure

- Explain the nursing practice to the patient *to gain consent and cooperation.*
- Ensure that a toilet or commode is available and accessible.
- Explain to the patient that you will be inserting the suppository.
- Wash your hands and apply disposable gloves.
- Insert one lubricated gloved finger slowly into the patient's rectum and undertake digital rectal examination *to check for the presence of faecal matter and its amount and consistency* (*see* the Bristol stool chart, Ch. 34).
- Slowly withdraw your finger from the patient's rectum to avoid spasm of the anal sphincter.
- Check the prescription chart with a qualified member of staff to ensure that the suppository is the correct one and is being administered to the correct patient *to avoid errors in the administration of medicines.*
- Follow the manufacturer's instructions. Lubricate the suppository: use water with glycerine suppositories, and lubricating jelly with bisacodyl suppositories *to ease insertion and avoid trauma to the anal mucosa* (Joint Formulary Committee 2015).
- Assist the patient into the left lateral position with their buttocks near the edge of the bed *to allow ease of access to the rectal sphincter.*

- Observe the patient throughout the procedure *to monitor for signs of distress or discomfort.*
- Place a protective covering under the patient's buttocks *to avoid soiling by faecal matter.*
- Squeeze some lubricating gel on to a medical wipe or tissue and lubricate the blunt end of the suppository *to ease insertion.*
- Apply disposable gloves and an apron *to protect yourself.*
- Part the patient's buttocks with your non-dominant hand *to allow easier access to the anal sphincter.*
- With your dominant hand, gently insert the blunt end of the suppository into the rectum between the anal wall and stool, advancing it in an upward and slightly backward direction for about 5 cm *to follow the natural line of the rectum* (Galbraith et al. 2007). Repeat this procedure if a second suppository is to be inserted. Withdraw the gloved finger.
- Dry the perianal area of the patient with tissue *to clean any soiling* and place the tissue in a disposal bag.
- Ensure that the patient has access to toilet facilities and is not left on bed to evacuate the bowel. *Gravity, with the patient sitting on a commode or toilet, is more effective for emptying the bowel.*
- Ask the patient to retain the suppository/suppositories for approximately 20 minutes, as per manufacturer's instructions, *to allow the suppository to dissolve and release its active ingredients through the rectal mucosa.*
- Remove the gloves and apron, disposing of them as per the infection prevention and control manual. **Wash your hands** (refer to the local hand hygiene policy).
- Allow the patient to dress in private, unless they require assistance.
- Assess the result of the procedure, discuss it with the patient and record it in the bowel chart.
- Document in the nursing notes all observations, findings and ongoing treatment/management *to ensure safe practice and enable prompt and appropriate medical and nursing interventions to be initiated.* Use the Bristol stool chart to document the type of stool passed (Heaton 2000).
- Registered nurses must only supply and administer medicines in accordance with the processes listed in *Standards for Medicines Management* (Nursing and Midwifery Council 2015) and in accordance with *The Code* (Nursing and Midwifery Council 2018). Treatments should be compatible with any other treatments patients are receiving, including over-the-counter medicines where possible (Nursing and Midwifery Council 2018).

PATIENT/CARER EDUCATION: KEY POINTS

In partnership with the patient/carer, ensure that they are competent to carry out any practices required.

Information should be given on an appropriate point of contact for any concerns that may arise.

The patient should be informed of the reasons for administering the medicine via the rectal route, as this route may be unknown to them. The patient will also require education in the self-administration of suppositories.

If suppositories are being prescribed to relieve constipation, it may be appropriate to discuss lifestyle interventions and behaviour modification for fluids, and for increasing fibre and exercise, as well as other dietary requirements.

Information should be given about bowel training, suggesting that the patient develops the habit of emptying the bowel at the same time every day: on waking is a useful time, whether or not they feel the urge to defaecate. Taking a hot drink prior to the morning habit also helps to stimulate the gastrocolic reflex, which assists in evacuating the bowel. Adopting the correct positioning on the toilet to decrease straining is also helpful.

A full bowel assessment for constipation and the completion of a three-day food journal are useful to resolve the issue of constipation.

2. ADMINISTRATION OF AN ENEMA

INDICATIONS AND RATIONALE FOR ADMINISTERING AN ENEMA

An enema is the introduction of liquid into the rectum by means of a tube. It is used:

- **to relieve severe constipation:** potential complications of unresolved constipation include abdominal pain and distension, confusion, nausea and vomiting, overflow diarrhoea, and abdominal obstruction or perforation
- **to evacuate the bowel prior to surgery, X-ray or another investigation**
- **to administer medicine.**

Enemas are contraindicated in:
- colonic obstruction
- paralytic ileus
- frailty
- situations where administration of large amounts of fluid high into the colon might cause perforation.

An appropriately trained nurse prescriber has the ability to assess, diagnose and prescribe a suitable suppository to rectify severe constipation. This is a specialized extended role recognized by a registerable qualification with the NMC. An awareness of the Rome II Criteria for constipation (see Box 16.1) offers guidance for the practitioner diagnosing constipation, as does a digital rectal examination (see Ch. 34).

 EQUIPMENT

- Flat surface/tray/trolley
- Prescribed enema (warmed to body temperature)
- Protective covering for the bed
- Disposable gloves
- Apron
- Water-soluble lubricant
- Medical wipes/tissues
- Commode/bedpan/access to toilet facilities
- Receptacle for soiled disposable items

TYPES OF ENEMA

There are three main types of enema (Fig. 16.1):
- Medication: enemas containing medication that should be retained as long as possible and should be inserted very slowly over half an hour.
- Evacuant: stimulant enemas that are usually returned, with faecal matter and flatus, within a few minutes. Solutions containing phosphates or sodium citrate are commonly used.
- Retention: enemas that soften and lubricate the faeces, and should be retained for a specified time; they usually contain arachis or olive oil. They may be inserted at bedtime to be retained overnight for maximum efficiency of action. The speed of introduction of the fluid will have an impact on peristalsis: the faster the introduction, the greater the effect. They should therefore be administered slowly.

Micro-enemas are also available, which cause less discomfort to patients when administered. Other enemas can be obtained with long delivery tubes to facilitate self-insertion by patients.

Prior to the administration of any enema, the nurse should check that the patient is not allergic to latex, phosphate or peanuts (arachis oil enemas contains peanut oil).

Large-volume enemas are not for use in patients with a neurogenic bowel or spinal injury as part of their bowel

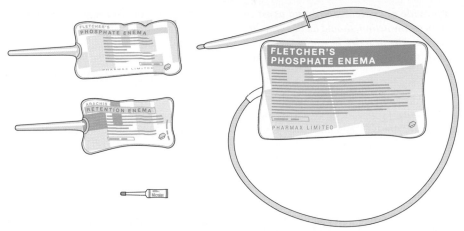

Fig. 16.1 Examples of disposable enemas.

management programme. This is due to the fact these patients cannot retain the volume of the enema for it to be effective, and over-distension of the bowel may stimulate autonomic dysreflexia (Multi-disciplinary Association for Spinal Cord Injury Professionals 2012; Coggrave 2008).

Bowers (2006) states that phosphate can be absorbed systematically and can accumulate; phosphate enemas should therefore be used with caution. They are contraindicated in patients with impaired renal function and should not be given to this patient group. When this type of enema is being used, it is vital for a good fluid intake to be maintained (Dougherty & Lister 2015).

GUIDELINES AND RATIONALE FOR THIS NURSING PRACTICE

- Explain the nursing practice to the patient *to gain consent and cooperation and to check for any previous rectal problems or allergies.*
- Assemble and prepare the equipment *to maintain efficiency of practice.*
- Warm the enema by immersing it in a jug of water (Higgins 2006).
- If necessary, allow the patient to empty the bladder first *to reduce discomfort during the procedure.*
- Ensure the patient's privacy and help the patient into the left lateral position *to allow ease of access to the anal sphincter.*
- Place the protective covering under the patient's buttocks *to contain any soiling or leakage.*
- Put on the disposable gloves and apron.
- The foot of the bed may be elevated to an angle of 45 degrees when a retention enema has been administered, *to facilitate retention.*

- Lubricate the end of the enema tube *to ease entry into the rectum,* and ask the patient to take deep breaths *to encourage relaxation and reduce discomfort on insertion of the enema.* If any persistent resistance is felt or the patient experiences pain, discontinue the procedure immediately and seek assistance. Care should be taken when there are haemorrhoids or anal fissures present and to avoid damaging the rectal mucosa when inserting the tube of the enema into the rectum.
- Squeeze a small amount of fluid down the tube *to expel the air, as air in the rectum will cause discomfort.*
- Insert the tube into the rectum in an upward and slightly backward direction for about 7.5 cm, *to follow the natural line of the rectum.*
- Administer the solution gently and slowly *to minimize any discomfort,* squeezing the bag and rolling it up so that all the contents are administered.
- Observe the patient throughout this activity *to detect any signs of discomfort or distress.*
- **STOP** if there is anal bleeding, if the patients asks you to or if there are signs of autonomic dysreflexia.
- Remove the tube when the prescribed amount has been administered and dry the anal area *to prevent any irritation.*
- The protective covering may be left in place *to help prevent soiling of bed linen by leaking faecal matter.*
- Provide toileting facilities when required. Access to a toilet is preferable *as it reduces the patient's embarrassment.*
- Ensure that the patient is left feeling as comfortable as possible, *to maintain the quality of this nursing practice.*
- Dispose of the equipment safely *to protect others.*
- Document this nursing practice appropriately, monitor the after-effects and report any abnormal findings

immediately *to provide a written record and assist in the implementation of any action, should an abnormality or adverse reaction to the practice be noted.*

- Under the heading of 'Preserve Safety', *The Code* of the NMC states:

You make sure that patient and public safety is protected. You work within the limits of your competence, exercising your professional 'duty of candour' and raising concerns immediately whenever you come across situations that put patients or public safety at risk. You take necessary *action to deal with any concerns where appropriate. Recognise and work within the limits of your competence.* (2018: 13)

ADDITIONAL ISSUES TO CONSIDER

The patient has the right to request a chaperone, as this is an invasive and highly embarrassing procedure. The patient's decision should be documented in the nursing notes. Nurses must be aware of any cultural or religious beliefs or restrictions the patient may have that might prohibit the procedure.

PATIENT/CARER EDUCATION: KEY POINTS

If the enema is being administered to relieve constipation, advice should be given on preventing recurrence. The long-term use of laxatives, opiates, anticholinergics, iron, antidepressants and anti-Parkinsonian medicines has been implicated in increasing the risk of constipation. The nutritional status of the patient, including their diet, meal provider and oral hygiene, should all be covered in a full assessment. It may be appropriate to offer dietary information leaflets to patients and carers to assist them in maintaining both a high-fibre diet and an adequate fluid intake. Patients who have limited mobility have a greater tendency to experience constipation.

If this procedure is performed within the patient's home, it may be appropriate for the nurse to leave prior to the enema achieving its effects. Under these circumstances the nurse should tell the patient how long the enema needs to be retained for maximum effectiveness, and should ensure that further contact is made with the patient to ask whether a satisfactory result was obtained.

It may be appropriate to teach the patient or carer how to (self-)administer an enema if constipation is likely to recur.

Information should be given on an appropriate point of contact for any concerns that may arise.

REFERENCES

Abd-el-Maeboud, K.H., el-Naggar, T., el-Hawi, E.M., et al., 1991. Rectal suppository: common sense and mode of insertion. The Lancet 338 (8770), 798–803.

Bowers, B., 2006. Evaluating the evidence for administering phosphate enemas. British Journal of Nursing 15 (7), 378–381.

Bradshaw, A., Price, L., 2006. Rectal suppository insertion: the reliability of the evidence as a basis for nursing practice. Journal of Community Nursing 16 (1), 98–103.

Coggrave, M., 2008. Neurogenic Continence. Part 3: bowel management strategies. British Journal of Nursing 17 (5), 962–968.

Dougherty, L., Lister, S.E., 2015. The Royal Marsden Hospital Manual of Clinical Nursing Procedures, ninth ed. Wiley Blackwell, London.

Galbraith, A., Bullock, S., Manias, E., et al., 2007. Fundamentals of Pharmacology: An Applied Approach for Nursing and Health, second ed. Prentice Hall, Harlow.

Heaton, K.W., 2000. Bristol Stool Form Scale. University of Bristol, Bristol.

Higgins, D., 2006. How to administer an enema. Nursing Times 102 (20), 24–25.

Joint Formulary Committee, 2015. British National Formulary. BMJ Group and Pharmaceutical Press, London, p. 68.

Kyle, G., 2009. Should a suppository be inserted with the blunt end or the pointed end first, or does it matter? Nursing Times 105 (2), 16.

Moppett, S., 2000. Which way is up for a suppository? Nursing Times 96 (26), 196–197.

Multi-disciplinary Association for Spinal Cord Injury Professionals (MASCIP), Guidelines for Management of Neurogenic Bowel Dysfunction in Individuals with Central Neurological Conditions, 2012. Coloplast, Denmark.

Nursing and Midwifery Council, 2015. Standards for Medicines Management. NMC, London.

Nursing & Midwifery Council, 2018. The Code: Professional Standards of Practice and Behaviour for Nurses, Midwives and Nursing Associates. NMC, London. Available at: https://www.nmc.org.uk/globalassets/sitedocuments/nmc-publications/nmc-code.pdf.

WEBSITES

https://www.bladderandbowel.org/ *Bladder and Bowel Community*

https://improvement.nhs.uk/documents/3074/Patient_Safety_Alert_-_safer_care_for_patients_at_risk_of_AD.pdf *NHS Improvement: Resources to support safer bowel care for patients at risk of autonomic dysreflexia, 2018*

https://www.mascip.co.uk/wp-content/uploads/2015/02/CV653N-Neurogenic-Guidelines-Sept-2012.pdf *Coloplast and the Multidisciplinary Association of Spinal Cord Injured Professionals*

https://rcni.com/hosted-content/rcn/continence/home *Royal College of Nursing: Bowel and Bladder Continence*

https://www.rcn.org.uk/professional-development/publications/pub-003226 *Royal College of Nursing: Management of lower bowel dysfunction, including digital rectal examination and digital removal of faeces*

https://www.spinal.co.uk/wp-content/uploads/2017/05/Autonomic-Dysreflexia.pdf *Spinal Injuries Association: Living with spinal cord injury factsheet: autonomic dysreflexia*

SELF-ASSESSMENT

1. Identify four indications that would lead to a suppository being prescribed.
2. List some common types of suppository and their action.
3. What position should a patient be in before you administer a suppository?
4. Which way should a suppository be inserted?
5. What health education should you give to a patient who has received a suppository to relieve constipation?
6. Discuss the Rome II Criteria for constipation.
7. Describe three types of enema.
8. Describe the optimum length of time each type of enema should remain in situ prior to evacuation.
9. List the equipment required for the administration of an enema.

17

Eye Care and Administration of Eyedrops

There are four parts to this chapter:
1. Eye swabbing
2. Eye irrigation
3. Instillation of eyedrops
4. Instillation of eye ointment

LEARNING OUTCOMES

By the end of this chapter, you should be able to:
- prepare the patient for these four nursing practices
- collect and prepare the equipment
- carry out eye swabbing, eye irrigation, the instillation of eyedrops and the instillation of eye ointment.

BACKGROUND KNOWLEDGE REQUIRED

- Revision of the anatomy and physiology of the eye
- Revision of 'Administration of Medicines' (*see* Ch. 2) and aseptic technique (*see* Ch. 40)

1. EYE SWABBING

INDICATIONS AND RATIONALE FOR EYE SWABBING

Eye swabbing is carried out:
- *to soothe the eye when a patient is suffering from an insensitive or diseased eye*
- *to precede the instillation of an eyedrop or the application of an eye ointment*
- *to remove eye discharge and/or crusts.*

⊚ EQUIPMENT

- Sterile eye dressing pack containing a gallipot, small and other gauze swabs, or gauze swabs and a disposable towel
- Sterile swabbing solution: usually normal saline solution, to soften any crusted discharge
- Good light source
- Trolley or tray for equipment
- Receptacle for soiled disposable items

GUIDELINES AND RATIONALE FOR THIS NURSING PRACTICE

- Explain the practice to the patient *to gain consent and cooperation.*
- Wash your hands *to reduce cross-infection* (World Health Organization 2009).
- Collect and prepare the equipment *to ensure that all the equipment is available and ready for use.*
- Ensure the patient's privacy *to reduce anxiety.*
- Prepare the patient by helping them into a comfortable position, either lying down or seated with the head inclined backwards, *to allow the patient to maintain the position during the practice and permit easy access to the patient's eyes.*
- Observe the patient throughout this activity *to note any signs of distress.*
- Position the light source *to allow maximum observation of the patient's eyes without the beam shining directly into them.*
- Open and arrange the equipment *to prepare for the practice.*
- Wash and dry your hands *to reduce the risk of cross-infection* (World Health Organization 2009).

- Place the disposable towel around the patient's neck *to catch any spillages and protect the patient's clothing.*
- Lightly moisten the gauze swab in the prescribed solution. *Excess moisture will cause the patient's face to be soaked with the cleansing solution.*
- Ask the patient to close their eyes *to reduce the risk of corneal damage* (Shaw 2016).
- Gently swab from the inner canthus to the outer canthus of the eye, using each swab only once *to decrease the risk of cross-infection from one eye to the other or infection of the lacrimal punctum.* (If both eyes are being swabbed, the healthy eye should be treated first, as this also reduces the risk of cross-infection.)
- Gently dry the patient's eyelids *to remove excess moisture.*
- Ensure that the patient is left feeling as comfortable as possible *to maintain the quality of this nursing practice.*
- Dispose of the equipment safely *to reduce any health hazard.*
- Document the nursing practice appropriately, monitor the after-effects and report any abnormal findings immediately, *to provide a written record and assist in the implementation of any action, should an abnormality or adverse reaction to the practice be noted.*
- In undertaking this practice, nurses are accountable for their actions, the quality of care delivered and record-keeping according to *The Code* of the Nursing and Midwifery Council (2018), which includes record-keeping.

2. EYE IRRIGATION

INDICATIONS AND RATIONALE FOR EYE IRRIGATION

Irrigation involves the continuous washing of the eye surface with fluid. It is performed *to aid the removal of a corrosive substance from the eye.*

◉ EQUIPMENT

- Waterproof sheet
- Cotton towel
- Sterile eye dressings pack containing a gallipot, small and other gauze swabs, and a disposable towel
- Irrigation fluid: e.g. sterile water or sterile normal saline
- Lotion thermometer
- Irrigating utensil: e.g. undine or intravenous giving set
- Receiver for the irrigating fluid
- Trolley or adequate surface for equipment
- Receptacle for soiled disposable items

GUIDELINES AND RATIONALE FOR THIS NURSING PRACTICE

- Explain the nursing practice to the patient *to gain consent and cooperation.*
- Wash the hands *to reduce cross-infection* (World Health Organization 2009).
- Collect and prepare the equipment *to ensure that all the equipment is available and ready for use.*
- Ensure the patient's privacy *to reduce anxiety.*
- Observe the patient throughout this activity *to note any signs of distress.*
- Warm the irrigating fluid to 37.8°C and check with the thermometer, *to ensure the comfort of the patient when the irrigating fluid is applied.*
- Help the patient into a suitable position, either sitting or lying with the head and neck well supported, *to allow the patient to maintain the position throughout the practice and permit easy access to the eyes.*
- Apply the waterproof sheet and towel around the patient's neck *to absorb any spillage.*
- Help the patient to turn their head to the side of the affected eye *to prevent any (or further) damage to the other eye by the corrosive substance when irrigation is commenced.*
- Wash and dry your hands *to reduce cross-infection* (World Health Organization 2009).
- Position the receiver below the affected eye, against the patient's cheek, *to collect the used irrigating fluid.*
- Remove any discharge from the eye with a gauze swab *to prevent contamination of the eye when the irrigation commences.*
- Explain to the patient that the flow of fluid is about to begin, *allowing the patient to prepare for the introduction of the fluid.*
- Hold the eyelids apart with your first and second fingers *as the natural defence mechanism of closing the eyes when an object approaches closely will interfere with the practice.*
- Direct the flow from the irrigator on to the patient's cheek *to check that the temperature is comfortable for the patient.*
- Hold the irrigator 2.5 cm above the eye *to allow the easy direction of the flow of fluid over the eye and prevent further damage to the eye.*
- Direct a steady flow of irrigating fluid from the inner canthus to the outer canthus of the eye, *allowing the fluid to cover the whole of the eye surface.*
- Ask the patient to move the eye up, down and all around *to ensure that the whole eye is irrigated.*

- Remove the equipment from the patient and ensure that the patient is left feeling as comfortable as possible, *to maintain the quality of this practice.*
- Dispose of the equipment safely *to reduce any health hazard.*
- Document the nursing practice appropriately, monitor the after-effects and report any abnormal findings immediately, *to provide a written record and assist in the implementation of any action, should an abnormality or adverse reaction to the practice be noted.*
- In undertaking this practice, nurses are accountable for their actions, the quality of care delivered and record-keeping according to *The Code* of the Nursing and Midwifery Council (2018), which includes record-keeping.

3. INSTILLATION OF EYEDROPS

INDICATIONS AND RATIONALE FOR INSTILLATION OF EYEDROPS

Instillation involves the introduction of a liquid into a cavity drop by drop. In certain disease conditions and following injury, eyedrops are prescribed:

- *to apply a local anaesthetic topically prior to diagnostic investigations,* e.g. tonometry, the removal of a foreign body or minor surgery
- *to apply an antibiotic or anti-inflammatory medicine topically*
- *to apply a muscle constrictor or dilator to the eye topically*
- *to apply an artificial lubricant for the eye topically.*

> ### ⊚ EQUIPMENT
>
> - Sterile eye dressings pack containing a gallipot, small and other gauze swabs, and a disposable towel
> - Sterile solution: usually normal saline, for swabbing settings
> - Eyedrops to be administered
> - Automatic dropper for self-administration
> - Light source
> - Trolley or tray for equipment
> - Patient's prescription
> - Receptacle for soiled disposable items

GUIDELINES AND RATIONALE FOR THIS NURSING PRACTICE

- Explain the nursing practice to the patient *to gain consent and cooperation.*
- Wash your hands *to reduce cross-infection* (World Health Organization 2009).
- Collect and prepare the equipment *to ensure that all the equipment is available and ready for use.*
- Ensure the patient's privacy *to reduce anxiety.*
- Observe the patient throughout this activity *to note any signs of distress.*
- Help the patient into a comfortable position *to allow easy access to the patient's eye and permit the patient to maintain the position throughout the practice.*
- Position the light source *to provide good visualization of the eye.*
- Check the medicine prescription against the label on the eyedrops *to ensure that the correct medication will be administered* (Shaw 2016).
- Check the expiry date on the bottle of eyedrops, *to ensure the administration of stable medication.*
- Verify which eye should receive the drops *to ensure that the correct eye receives the medication.*
- Wash and dry the hands *to reduce cross-infection* (World Health Organization 2009).
- Swab the eye clean if a discharge is present *to remove contaminated debris.*
- Hold a swab in your non-dominant hand under the lower lid margin *to remove excess moisture after instillation of the drops.*
- Ask the patient to look up and evert the lower lid, *to prevent the patient being aware of the approaching dropper.*
- Hold the dropper in the dominant hand *to provide controlled application*, about 2 cm above the eye, and allow one drop to fall into the lower conjunctival sac (Fig. 17.1)
- Ask the patient to close the eye *to remove excess moisture.*
- Ensure that the patient is left feeling as comfortable as possible, *to maintain the quality of this practice.*
- Dispose of the equipment safely *to reduce any health hazard.*
- Document the nursing practice appropriately, monitor the after-effects and report any abnormal findings immediately, *to provide a written record and assist in the implementation of any action, should an abnormality or adverse reaction to the practice be noted.*
- In undertaking this practice, nurses are accountable for their actions, the quality of care delivered and record-keeping according to *The Code* of the Nursing and Midwifery Council (2018), which includes record-keeping.

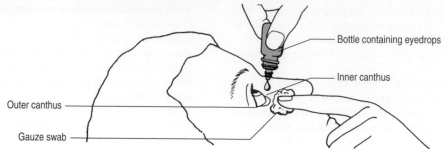

Outer canthus

Gauze swab

Bottle containing eyedrops

Inner canthus

Fig. 17.1 Installation of eyedrops: the lower lid is pulled gently downwards to create a pouch into which the drop is placed.

4. INSTILLATION OF EYE OINTMENT

INDICATIONS AND RATIONALE FOR INSTILLATION OF EYE OINTMENT

In certain disease conditions, and following injury, eye ointment is prescribed:
- *to instil a medicine topically in place of eyedrops when a prolonged action of the medicine is required*
- *to form a protective film over the corneal surface of the eye*
- *to act as a soothing agent for the patient suffering from an inflamed eye or lid margin.*

EQUIPMENT

- Sterile eye dressings pack containing a gallipot, small and other gauze swabs, and a disposable towel
- Sterile solution: usually normal saline, for swabbing settings
- Eye ointment to be administered
- Trolley or tray for equipment
- Light source
- Receptacle for soiled disposable items

GUIDELINES AND RATIONALE FOR THIS NURSING PRACTICE

- Explain the nursing practice to the patient *to gain consent and cooperation.*
- Wash your hands *to reduce cross-infection* (World Health Organization 2009).
- Collect and prepare the equipment *to ensure that all the equipment is available and ready for use.*

- Ensure the patient's privacy *to reduce anxiety.*
- Observe the patient throughout this activity *to note any signs of distress.*
- Help the patient into a comfortable position *to allow easy access to the patient's eye and permit the patient to maintain the position throughout the practice.*
- Position the light source *to provide good visualization of the eye.*
- Check the medicine prescription against the label on the tube of eye ointment *to ensure that the correct medication will be administered.*
- Check the expiry date on the tube of ointment *to ensure the administration of stable medication.*
- Verify which eye should receive the ointment, *ensuring that the ointment is inserted into the correct eye.*
- Wash and dry your hands *to reduce cross-infection* (World Health Organization 2009).
- Swab the eye clean *to remove all traces of the previously instilled ointment and/or discharge.*
- Hold a swab in your non-dominant hand under the lower lid margin *to remove excess ointment after instillation.*
- Ask the patient to look up and evert the lower lid *to prevent the patient seeing the approaching nozzle, which may cause the eyelid to close.*
- Hold the tube of ointment in your dominant hand *to permit good control over insertion of the ointment.*
- With the nozzle of the tube 2.5 cm above the lower lid, squeeze the tube *to allow a ribbon of ointment to run into the lower conjunctival sac from the inner to the outer canthus* (Fig. 17.2).
- Ask the patient to close the eye *to remove excess ointment.*
- Inform the patient that they may experience blurred vision for a few minutes following the instillation of the ointment *until the oily/greasy base disperses over the eye.*

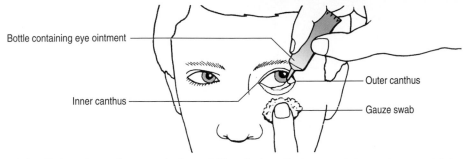

Fig. 17.2 Instillation of eye ointment: the lower lid is pulled gently downwards to create a pouch into which the ointment is placed.

- Ensure that the patient is left feeling as comfortable as possible, *to maintain the quality of this practice.*
- Dispose of the equipment safely *to reduce any health hazard.*
- Document the nursing practice appropriately, monitor the after-effects and report any abnormal findings immediately, *to provide a written record and assist in the implementation of any action, should an abnormality or adverse reaction to the practice be noted.*
- In undertaking this practice, nurses are accountable for their actions, the quality of care delivered and record-keeping according to *The Code* of the Nursing and Midwifery Council (2018), which includes record-keeping.

PATIENT/CARER EDUCATION: KEY POINTS

In partnership with the patient and/or carer, ensure that they are competent to carry out any practices required. Information should be given on an appropriate point of contact for any concerns that may arise.

The patient/carer may need to be taught one or all parts of this nursing practice. A patient who needs to use an automatic dropper will require adequate information and practice to ensure skilled use of the equipment.

The nurse should ensure that the patient at home stores the medication safely and correctly.

The nurse has a responsibility to provide and encourage the education of the general population in the first aid measures needed following contamination of the eye by a corrosive substance.

REFERENCES

Nursing and Midwifery Council, 2018. The Code: Professional Standards of Practice and Behaviour for Nurses, Midwives and Nursing Associates. NMC, London. Available at: https://www.nmc.org.uk/globalassets/sitedocuments/nmc-publications/nmc-code.pdf.

Shaw, M., 2016. How to administer eye drops and eye ointment. Nursing Standard (Royal College of Nursing (Great Britain): 1987). 30(39), pp. 34.

World Health Organization, 2009. WHO Guidelines on Hand Hygiene in Health Care. World Health Organization. Available at: http://apps.who.int/iris/bitstream/handle/10665/44102/9789241597906_eng.pdf;jsessionid=CED4477EC4770D98BE1DCF80F4B3DCAF?sequence=1.

WEBSITES

https://www.nmc.org.uk *Nursing and Midwifery Council*

SELF-ASSESSMENT

1. In what circumstances should eyes be swabbed?
2. What equipment is required for eye swabbing/
3. Why is eye irrigation carried out?
4. In what direction should fluid flow during eye irrigation?
5. Why is it necessary to observe the patient during any of the procedures described in this chapter?

18

First Aid: Physical

LEARNING OUTCOMES

By the end of this chapter, you should be able to:
- understand the basic principles of first aid
- perform first aid in a safe, effective and person-centred manner
- provide life-saving assistance to an ill or injured person until definitive medical treatment can be accessed.

BACKGROUND KNOWLEDGE REQUIRED

- Revision of the contents of a first aid bag or kit (if available)
- Revision of the Nursing and Midwifery Council (NMC) information on responding to unexpected incidents or emergencies (Nursing and Midwifery Council 2017)
- Revision of the recovery position
- Revision of the use of the DR.ABC principles to identify any life-threatening problems and communicate your findings to an operator or medical personnel

INDICATIONS AND RATIONALE FOR FIRST AID

First aid comprises a series of simple, potentially life-saving steps that an individual can perform with minimal equipment. Although it is not a legal requirement to respond to an emergency situation outside of work, nurses have a professional duty to respond and provide care within the limits of their competency. First aid may be required on occasions that you find yourself involved in an unexpected incident or emergency away from your normal place of work, where people may require care, e.g. someone who is having a heart attack, has a strain or sprain, or is bleeding heavily.

OUTLINE OF THE PROCEDURE

The principles of first aid are to preserve life and limit patient deterioration. First aid is the help given to someone who is injured or ill, to keep them safe until they can be given more advanced medical treatment by seeing a doctor or health professional or by going to hospital. The role of a first aider is to give someone this help, while making sure that they and anyone else involved are safe and do not make the situation worse.

The first aider must utilize their knowledge to carry out a primary assessment to deal with any potentially life-threatening conditions in order of priority. This means following the 'DR.ABC': Danger, Response, Airway, Breathing and Circulation (St John Ambulance 2015). After the primary assessment, you can then move on to the secondary assessment to question the casualty about what has happened and to see if they have any other illnesses or conditions. As a first aider, you may also need to decide whether they need an ambulance.

Up-to-date and safe knowledge of first aid training is an essential aspect of professional practice for nurses and midwives (Johnson 2013).

EQUIPMENT

If a first aid bag or kit is available, it may contain the following (this list is not exhaustive and will vary):
- Triangular bandage
- Non-adherent simple dressing
- Surgical tape
- Burn dressing
- Conforming bandage
- Non-sterile gloves
- Foil blanket

If no equipment is available, the nurse should improvise with materials at the scene. For example, a scarf can be used as a sling, and Clingfilm can be used as a temporary dressing for burns.

GUIDELINES AND RATIONALE FOR THIS NURSING PRACTICE

Principles

Nurses should only perform interventions in which they are competent and should act according to their professional code (Nursing and Midwifery Council 2018).

- There is no expectation that you should put your own safety at risk. *The Code* **(2018) makes it clear that nurses and midwives must take account of their own safety, the safety of others and the availability of other care options (this may include paramedics, ambulance crews or military personnel at the scene of an incident or emergency).** You may be able to help or assist in this type of situation, but you should always follow the advice of the emergency services at the scene of an incident or emergency and find a place of safety if told to do so.
- If you are near or at your place of work, you should always follow your employer's emergency and major incident planning policies (Nursing and Midwifery Council 2017).
- Only move on to a secondary assessment once the primary assessment is completed and you have succeeded in dealing with any life-threatening conditions (St John Ambulance 2015).
- The primary assessment by the first aider should include the following line of investigation, using the DR.ABC principles.

Primary Assessment

The primary assessment is a quick way to find out if someone has any injuries or conditions that are life-threatening. By following each step methodically, you can identify each life-threatening condition and deal with it in order of priority (St John Ambulance 2015).

- It is essential to assess the environment and first ensure that it is safe. If it is not, you should move to a place of safety and then ensure that the emergency services have been contacted by you or someone close to you. Only then should you consider providing care if it is safe to do so (Nursing and Midwifery Council 2017). Check that the area and surroundings are safe for you to respond. Check for environmental hazards, such as toxic substances if a spillage has occurred, pets in a home or personal safety in a quiet street if it is dark. If the person to be treated presents with signs of body fluids or is bleeding, use gloves, if available, to protect yourself before performing first aid. Plastic bags could be used when gloves are not available.

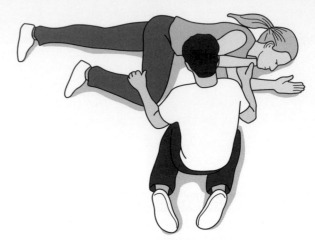

Fig. 18.1 The recovery position.

- Use the DR.ABC principles (danger, response, airway, breathing and circulation; see later for details) *to identify any life-threatening problems.* **If you require medical assistance, call 999/112, state that you are a nurse and use the ABC principles to communicate your findings to the operator** (St John Ambulance 2015).
- If the person appears to be unconscious, i.e. looks as if they are asleep but is unable to respond to noise or body contact, it is likely that they are unresponsive. **Check for breathing by using 'look, listen and feel' for normal breathing: chest movement, and sounds and breaths on your cheeks. Do this for no more than 10 seconds.** If the person is breathing and shows signs of life, place them in the recovery position (Fig. 18.1), unless they appear to have injuries that prevent you from moving them. However, the person's airway must be clear and this takes priority over concerns regarding moving the individual. Ensure that the airway is clear and maintain this until help arrives.
- If there are no signs of life, follow the basic life support guidelines produced by the Resuscitation Council (UK) (2015).
- Only move on to the secondary assessment if you have already done the primary assessment and have succeeded in dealing with any life-threatening conditions.
- Then you can start questioning the casualty about what has happened and carefully check for any other injuries or illnesses. If you can, jot down everything you find out and give all this information to the emergency services or whoever takes responsibility for the casualty.

DR.ABC

Danger

If someone needs help, before you go up to them check – is it safe?

- *No:* If you can see or hear any danger nearby, for you or the casualty, such as broken glass or oncoming traffic, then make the situation safe before you go any closer.
- *Yes:* If you cannot see or hear any danger, then it is safe to approach.

Response

Do they respond when you ask them 'Are you alright?' or if you say 'Open your eyes!'?

- *No:* If they do not respond, pinch their ear lobe or gently shake their shoulders; with a child, tap their shoulder; with a baby, tap their foot. If they still do not respond, you can presume that they are unresponsive and move on to the next stage: airway. Someone who is unresponsive should always take priority, so you should treat them first and as quickly as possible.
- *Yes:* If the person responds by making eye contact with you or making some gesture, then you know that they are responsive and you can move on to the next stage: airway.

Airway

Is their airway open and clear?

- *No – responsive:* If they are responsive, treat them for conditions that may be blocking their airway, such as choking. Only move on to the next stage – breathing – once the airway is open and clear.
- *No – unresponsive:* If they are unresponsive, tilt their head and lift their chin to open their airway. Only move on to the next stage – breathing – once the airway is open and clear.
- *Yes:* If the airway is open and clear, move on to the next stage – breathing.

Breathing

Are they breathing normally? You need to look, listen and feel to check that they are breathing.

- *No – responsive:* If they are responsive, treat them for whatever is stopping them breathing, e.g. an obstructed airway. Then go to the next stage – circulation.
- *No – unresponsive:* If they are unresponsive and not breathing, call 999/112 for an ambulance, or ask someone else to call if possible. Start giving chest compressions and rescue breaths: cardiopulmonary resuscitation (CPR; *see* Ch. 8). If this happens, you probably will not move on to the next stage, as the casualty needs resuscitation.
- *Yes:* If they are breathing normally, move on to the next stage – circulation.

Circulation

Are there any signs of severe bleeding?

- *Yes:* If they are bleeding severely, control the bleeding with your gloved fingers, dressing or clothing, call 999/112 for an ambulance and treat them to reduce the risk of them going into shock.
- *No:* If they are not bleeding and you are sure you have dealt with any life-threatening conditions, then you can move on to the secondary assessment, to check for any other injuries or illnesses.

Secondary Assessment

The secondary assessment involves questioning the casualty about what has happened and carefully checking for any other injuries or illnesses.

The secondary assessment will involve the first aider taking a history from the patient or from bystanders who may have key information. What symptoms does the casualty have and are there any signs to be concerned about? A head-to-toe check of the casualty can help determine this (St John Ambulance 2015).

Event History

- Ask the casualty to describe exactly what happened in the lead-up to them feeling unwell or injuring themselves.
- You can ask other people near the scene too and also look for clues. For example, if a car accident is involved, the impact on the car will help you work out what type of injury the casualty could have.

Medical History

- Then, ask them to tell you their medical history. Use the word **AMPLE** to remember all the things you need to ask them:
  - **Allergy** – do they have any allergies?
  - **Medication** – are they taking any regular or prescribed medication?
  - **Previous medical history** – did they already have any conditions?
  - **Last meal** – when did they last eat something?
  - **Event history** – what happened?

Symptoms

- Ask the casualty to give you as much detail as possible about how they feel. Listen carefully to what they say and make notes, if possible. Here are the key questions:
  - Can they feel any pain?
  - Can they describe the pain, e.g. is it constant or irregular, sharp or dull?

- What makes the pain better or worse?
- When did the pain start?

Signs

- Check the casualty over from head to toe, using all your senses – look, listen, feel and smell.
- You may have to loosen, open, cut away or remove clothing. Ask permission to do this and make sure you are sensitive and discreet.
- Make a note of any minor injuries as you go. Return to these only when you have finished checking the whole body, to make sure you do not miss any more serious injuries.

Head-to-Toe Examination

- *Breathing and pulse:* How fast and strong is the breathing and pulse?
- *Bleeding:* Check the body from head to toe for any bleeding.
- *Head and neck:* Is there any bleeding, swelling, sensitivity or a dent in the bone, which could mean a fracture?
- *Ear:* Do they respond when you talk to them? Is there any blood or clear fluid coming from either ear? If so, this could mean a serious head injury.
- *Eyes:* Are they open? What size are the pupils? If they are different sizes, this could mean a head injury.
- *Nose:* Is there any blood or clear fluid coming from the nostrils? This could mean a serious head injury.
- *Mouth:* Check the mouth for anything that could block the airway. Look for mouth injuries or burns and anything unusual in the line of the teeth.
- *Skin:* Note the colour and temperature of the skin. Pale, cold, clammy skin suggests shock. A flushed, hot face suggests fever or heatstroke. A blue tinge suggests lack of oxygen from an obstructed airway, poor circulation or asthma.
- *Neck:* Loosen any clothing around the neck to look for signs such as a medical warning medallion or a hole in the windpipe. Run your fingers down the spine without moving it to check for any swelling, sensitivity or deformity.
- *Chest:* Check if the chest rises easily and evenly on each side as the casualty breathes. Feel the ribcage to check for any deformity or sensitivity. Note if breathing is difficult or painful in any way.
- *Collarbone, arms and fingers:* Feel all the way along the collarbones to the fingers for any swelling, sensitivity or deformity. Check the casualty can move their elbows, wrists and fingers.
- *Arms and fingers:* Check they do not have any unusual feeling in their arms or fingers. If their fingertips are pale or greyish-blue, this could suggest that the blood is not circulating properly. Also look for any needle marks on the forearms, which suggest drug use. See if there is a medical warning bracelet.
- *Spine:* Check whether they have lost any movement or sensation in their legs or arms. Do not move them to check their spine, as they may have a spinal injury. Otherwise, gently put your hand under their back and check for any swelling or soreness.
- *Abdomen:* Gently feel the abdomen to check for any signs of internal bleeding, like stiffness or soreness, on each side.
- *Hips and pelvis:* Feel both hips and the pelvis for signs of a fracture. Check the clothing for any signs of incontinence, which may suggest a spinal or bladder injury, or bleeding from body openings, which may suggest a pelvic fracture.
- *Legs:* Check the legs for any bleeding, swelling, deformity or soreness. Ask them to raise one leg and then the other, and to move their ankles and knees.
- *Toes:* Check movement and feeling in their toes. Compare both feet and note the colour of the skin: greyish-blue skin could suggest a problem with the circulation or an injury due to cold, like hypothermia.

When to Call an Ambulance

- Before you call for an ambulance, you need to assess the casualty. To do this, follow the steps of the primary assessment, to see if they have any life-threatening or other serious conditions.
- If the area is not safe for you to assess the casualty, then call an ambulance straight away.
- If someone's condition is life-threatening or very serious, then call 999/112 for medical help.
- If someone's condition is not serious, then you need to decide if they need treatment or not, and what options there are: e.g. driving them to hospital or calling their doctor's surgery for medical advice.

PATIENT/CARER EDUCATION: KEY POINTS

When delivering any type of first aid care, it is important for carers/healthcare professionals to act only within the limits of their knowledge and competence. It is acknowledged that not all healthcare professionals are qualified first aiders, but they may be able to support other members of the emergency services or those injured or distressed in other ways.

Working in emergency situations can be highly traumatic for bystanders and healthcare professionals, and appropriate debriefing may have to be considered after the events.

REFERENCES

Johnson, P., 2013. First aid training in pre-registration nurse education. Nursing Standard 22 (51), 42–46.

Nursing and Midwifery Council, 2018. The Code: Professional Standards of Practice and Behaviour for Nurses, Midwives and Nursing Associates. NMC, London. Available at: https://www.nmc.org.uk/globalassets/sitedocuments/nmc-publications/nmc-code.pdf.

Nursing and Midwifery Council, 2017. Information for Nurses and Midwives on Responding to Unexpected Incidents or Emergencies. London.

Resuscitation Council (UK), 2015. Adult Basic Life Support and Automated External Defibrillation. RCUK, London.

St John Ambulance (2015) First Aid Tips, Information & Advice. Available at: http://www.sja.org.uk/sja/first-aid-advice.aspx.

St John Ambulance, St Andrew's First Aid, British Red Cross, 2014. First Aid Manual, tenth ed. Dorling Kindersley, London.

SELF-ASSESSMENT

Reflective Activity: Providing Emergency Assistance

Consider the following scenario. A person collapses with chest pain and subsequently loses consciousness. Breathing is compromised and the individual appears to be in shock. Describe the actions you would take if this occurs in:

- the clinical setting
- a supermarket.

You might think about the following:

- Assessing the situation: check for risks and dangers from the incident itself and from the immediate environment.
- Obtaining help: this may necessitate using public telephones or sending bystanders to convey messages.
- Finding out what is wrong with the person: if there is more than one casualty involved, what are your priorities?
- Providing emergency assistance: this may entail performing basic life support until the arrival of medical assistance.
- Offering support: reassure and manage relatives or bystanders once you have declared yourself to be a nurse or health professional; this immediately raises certain expectations.

(Adapted from St John Ambulance et al. 2014.)

19

Fundamental Care

There are three parts to this chapter:
1. Bed bath, immersion bath and showering
2. Facial shave
3. Hair washing.

Due to the volume of material on personal hygiene, guidelines for mouth care and skin care are given in separate chapters (*see* Ch. 21 and Ch. 27).

LEARNING OUTCOMES

By the end of this chapter, you should be able to:
• prepare the patient for these nursing practices
• collect the equipment
• carry out a bed bath
• help the patient with an immersion bath or shower
• carry out a facial shave
• wash the hair of a bed-fast or ambulant patient.

BACKGROUND KNOWLEDGE REQUIRED

• Revision of the anatomy and physiology of the skin tissue
• Revision of 'Integrity of the Skin' (*see* Ch. 21) and 'Oral Hygiene' (*see* Ch. 27)
• Review of local policy on pre- and postoperative skin care
• Revision of infection control policy in respect of skin care, hair infestation and cleaning of equipment
• Review of local policy on moving and handling
• Review of local policy on these practices

INDICATIONS AND RATIONALE FOR PERSONAL HYGIENE

A patient may require personal hygiene care:
• to clean the skin prior to surgery
• postoperatively, following major surgery when mobility is restricted

• following an acute illness, e.g. myocardial infarction
• while in an unconscious state
• following trauma, e.g. a patient in traction
• when extremely weak and debilitated as a result of the prolonged effects of a disease, trauma or a treatment being administered.

For infection control purposes, personal hygiene equipment should be for the use of a single patient or should be cleaned according to local policy. The nurse should cleanse their hands before and after each practice, according to local policy, and wear a disposable plastic apron.

1. BED BATH, IMMERSION BATH AND SHOWERING

EQUIPMENT

• Soap or prescribed antibacterial preparation/aqueous cream/emulsifying lotion
• Patient's toiletries, such as deodorant
• Bath towels
• Two face cloths/sponges or disposable wipes: disposable wipes are preferred, as pathogenic organisms can multiply on face cloths/sponges
• Disposable paper towel or similar
• Patient's brush and comb
• Nail scissors and nail file, if required
• Clean nightdress, pyjamas or clothing
• Clean bed linen
• Plastic apron and disposable gloves
• Continence products if required
• Equipment for catheter care (*see* Ch. 11), if required
• Equipment for skin care (*see* Ch. 21)
• Equipment for mouth care (*see* Ch. 27)
• Receptacle for the patient's soiled clothing
• Receptacle for soiled bed linen
• Receptacle for soiled disposable items

Continued

Additional Equipment
- Two basins with warm water (35–40°C) (bed bath)
- Trolley or adequate surface (bed bath)
- Bath thermometer (immersion bath)
- Chair or shower stool (immersion bath and shower)
- Bathing/showering equipment aids as appropriate (immersion bath and shower)

GUIDELINES AND RATIONALE FOR THIS NURSING PRACTICE

Bed Bath

- Explain the nursing practice to the patient *to gain consent and cooperation.*
- Collect and prepare the equipment *to ensure that all equipment is available and ready for use, and to minimize interruptions during the procedure.*
- Wash and dry your hands and put on a clean disposable apron *to prevent cross-contamination.*
- Ensure the patient's privacy *to reduce anxiety and promote dignity.*
- Observe and communicate with the patient throughout this activity *to note any signs of distress, pain or discomfort, and to establish and maintain a therapeutic relationship.*
- Check that the bed brakes are in use *to prevent the patient or nurse sustaining an injury from a sudden, uncontrolled movement of the bed.*
- Adjust the bed height *to ensure safe moving and handling practice.*
- Help the patient into a comfortable position *to permit the nurse easy and comfortable access to the patient.*
- Arrange the furniture around the patient's bed space *to allow easy access to equipment on the trolley or surface.*
- Remove any excess bed linen and bed appliances if in use, *to allow easy access to the patient,* but leaving the patient covered with a bed sheet *to maintain modesty.*
- Help the patient to remove their pyjamas or gown and anti-embolic stockings, if required, *to reduce exertion, as this can be a strenuous activity for a person who is in a weakened state.*
- Check the temperature of the basin of water or encourage the patient to do so if possible, to *ensure that the water is warm but not hot, to avoid skin damage.*
- Check with the patient whether they use soap or an alternative product on their face *to provide person-centred,*

individualized care. Alternative soap substitutes and emollients are recommended *to maintain skin health.*
- Wash, rinse and dry the patient's face, ears and neck; when possible, assist patients to do this for themselves *to encourage independence.*
- If a face cloth is used, the second face cloth should be used to wash the rest of the body; the use of disposable wipes is preferred *to reduce the risk of cross-infection.* Nevertheless, the patient's preferences should be considered, *to provide person-centred, individualized care.*
- Expose only the part of the patient's body being washed *to maintain the patient's modesty, dignity and self-esteem.*
- Wash, rinse and thoroughly dry the patient's body in an appropriate order, such as the upper limbs, chest and abdomen, genitalia, lower limbs, back and sacrum, *to prevent excessive exertion on the part of the patient.*
- When washing the patient's limbs, first wash the limb furthest away from you *to allow the assistant to dry that limb as the other limb is being washed, thus reducing the time during which the patient's body is exposed to the cooling effect of the environment.*
- Where possible, assist the patient to immerse the feet and hands in the basin of water (Fig. 19.1).
- As each part of the patient's body is washed, observe the skin for any blemishes, redness, discoloration, dryness

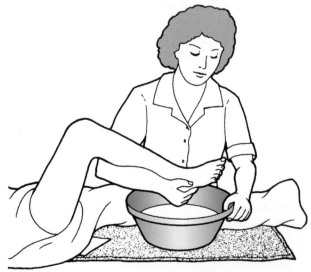

Fig. 19.1 Foot immersion: the patient's foot and leg should be supported. The upper limbs can be supported in a similar way.

or excessive moisture, *to alert the nurse to the potential problem of pressure sore development and/or skin disease* (*see* 'Integrity of the Skin', Ch. 21).

- Put on disposable gloves and assist the patient to wash, rinse and dry the genitalia using disposable wipes, washing from the front of the perineal area to the back in females *to prevent cross-infection from the anal region;* in uncircumcised male patients, draw the foreskin back for cleaning and replace it *to prevent paraphimosis.*
- Carry out catheter care (*see* Ch. 11) or use appropriate continence products if required.
- Remove the gloves and decontaminate your hands *to prevent cross-contamination.*
- Change the water as it cools or becomes dirty, and immediately after washing the patient's genitalia, *to prevent the cooling of the patient and reduce the risk of cross-infection,* respectively.
- When the patient is turned on to their side and their back has been washed, put on disposable gloves and wash, rinse and dry the sacrum using disposable wipes, *to prevent cross-infection from the anal region.*
- Change the water immediately after washing the sacrum or leave this action until last, *to reduce the risk of cross-infection from the normal skin flora of the perineal region to the rest of the skin.*
- Remove the gloves and decontaminate your hands *to prevent cross-contamination.*
- If the patient's bottom sheet is to be changed, this should be done when the patient is turned on to their side to have their back washed, *to minimize exertion for the patient.*
- Apply body deodorants and/or other toiletries as desired by the patient, *to ensure person-centred, individualized care.*
- Help the patient to dress in clean pyjamas or gown and replace anti-embolic stockings, if required, *to promote dignity and to reduce exertion on the part of the patient.*
- Assist the patient to cut and clean the fingernails and toenails, if required and unless otherwise indicated, *to prevent injury, reduce the risk of cross-infection and promote comfort and self-esteem.*
- Remove any soiled or damp bed linen and remake the patient's bed *to promote patient comfort and dignity.*
- Assist the patient with mouth care (*see* Ch. 27) *to promote a positive body image and to minimize the risk of infection.*
- Assist the patient to brush or comb their hair into its usual style, *to promote independence, dignity and self-esteem.*
- Ensure that the patient is left feeling as comfortable as possible *to maintain the quality of this nursing practice.*

- Rearrange the furniture as wished by the patient *to keep any articles needed within easy reach and to give the patient control of the environment.*
- Dispose of the equipment safely *to reduce any health hazard and to prevent cross-infection.*
- Wash and dry your hands *to prevent cross-infection.*

Immersion Bath

- Discuss the arrangements for the bath with the patient *to gain consent and cooperation and encourage participation in care.* In the community, the patient should have an assessment carried out; this will cover the need for equipment available from occupational therapy and whether help with bathing and showering should be given by social care staff.
- Help the patient to collect and prepare the equipment *to have everything ready for use and to minimize disruptions.*
- Wash and dry your hands and put on a clean disposable apron *to prevent cross-infection.*
- Help the patient to the bathroom; this may include the use of mechanical lifting aids or mobility aids if the patient has any difficulty with mobilizing.
- Ensure the patient's privacy as far as possible, *to respect individuality and maintain dignity and self-esteem.*
- Prepare the water in the bath, maintaining a safe temperature, and gain the patient's approval, *to ensure person-centred, individualized care.*
- Help the patient to undress if they need help, *to encourage the patient to be as independent as possible.*
- Observe and communicate with the patient throughout this activity *to observe for any signs of distress, pain or discomfort, and to establish and maintain a therapeutic relationship.*
- Help the patient into the bath. For some patients, mechanical aids may be used as appropriate, according to the manufacturer's instructions.
- Help the patient to wash, commencing with the face and neck *to use clean water first on these areas.*
- Help to wash the patient's hair if required (see later in this chapter).
- Help the patient out of the bath. The patient may sit on a chair that is protected with a towel *to promote comfort and minimize the risk of falling.*
- Help the patient to dry as required *to encourage independence.*
- Apply body deodorants and/or other toiletries as desired by the patient, *to ensure person-centred, individualized care.*
- Help the patient to dress as required, *to promote the patient's self-esteem and independence;* the patient should choose what they want to wear.

- Allow the patient time to clean their teeth or dentures at the basin, *to promote oral hygiene and health,* giving help as required.
- Help to brush or comb the patient's hair *to maintain dignity and self-esteem.*
- Help the patient to a chair or bed as is chosen, or as the condition allows, for a period of rest after the exercise of bathing.
- Ensure that the patient is left feeling as comfortable as possible *to promote relaxation.*
- Clean the bath according to local policy *to promote a safe environment.*
- Dispose of equipment safely *to prevent any transmission of infection.*
- Wash and dry your hands *to prevent cross-infection*.

Showering

Many clinical areas have open shower units where patients can be assisted to a fixed seat (Fig. 19.2) or can be transferred in a mobile shower chair.

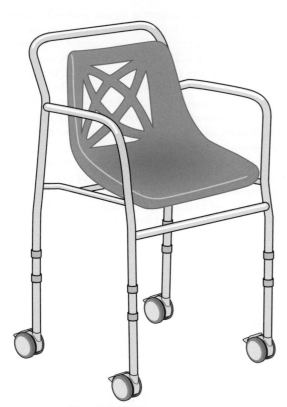

Fig. 19.2 Mobile shower chair.

- Discuss the arrangements for the shower with the patient *to gain consent and cooperation.*
- Help to collect and prepare the equipment *to have everything ready for use.*
- Wash and dry your hands *to prevent cross-infection.*
- Help the patient to the shower room. This may include the use of mechanical lifting aids or mobility aids if the patient has difficulty with mobilizing.
- Help the patient to undress as required, *to maintain privacy and dignity, and to respect individuality.*
- Help the patient to sit on the shower chair or stool *to minimize the risk of falls.*
- Adjust the flow of water from the shower *to maintain a safe water temperature.*
- Help the patient to wash while showering, as required, *to provide an enjoyable body wash.*
- Help the patient to wash their hair if required (see later in this chapter) *to promote self-esteem.*
- Help the patient to dry.
- Proceed as for 'Immersion Bath' in the previous section.

For All these Practices

- Document the nursing practice appropriately, monitor any after-effects and report abnormal findings immediately, *to provide a written record and assist in the implementation of any action, should an abnormality or adverse reaction to the practice be noted.* Do this *to facilitate communication with other team members.*
- In undertaking these practices, nurses are personally and professionally accountable for their actions, and for the safety, quality, assessment, evaluation and documentation of care delivered (Nursing and Midwifery Council 2018a; Nursing and Midwifery Council 2018b).

2. FACIAL SHAVE

⊚ EQUIPMENT

- Bowl of hand-hot water
- Patient's own razor, disposable safety razor or electric shaver for single-patient use
- Shaving soap and brush or shaving foam/gel
- Face cloth or disposable wipe
- Towel
- Receptacles for used razor and soiled disposable items
- Aftershave (if used by patient)
- Plastic apron

GUIDELINES AND RATIONALE FOR THIS PRACTICE

Facial Wet Shave

- Explain the nursing practice to the patient *to gain consent and cooperation.*
- Collect and prepare the equipment *to ensure that all equipment is available and ready for use and to minimize interruptions during the procedure.*
- Wash and dry your hands and put on a clean disposable apron *to prevent cross-contamination.*
- Ensure the patient's privacy *to reduce anxiety and promote dignity.*
- Observe and communicate with the patient throughout this activity *to note any signs of distress, pain or discomfort, to establish and maintain a therapeutic relationship, and to ascertain patient's preferences, e.g. sideburns.*
- Protect the patient's upper body with a towel *to avoid the patient's clothing becoming damp.*
- Note any skin blemishes *to avoid tissue damage during shaving.*
- Wet the patient's face with warm water and use the shaving brush to produce a good lather from the shaving soap, or use shaving foam/gel as per manufacturer's instructions. Apply over the face and neck *to ease the shaving procedure and prevent unnecessary skin trauma.*
- Hold the skin taut with your non-dominant hand, and with your dominant hand use short strokes on the skin, moving the razor in the direction of the hair growth and holding the razor at a 45-degree angle to the skin *to ensure a close shave.*
- Start with the cheeks and neck, then shave the chin and above the lip (Mackie 2013) *to ensure a methodical, thorough shave.*
- After each stroke, rinse the razor in warm water *to prevent blockage of the blades with hair.*
- When you are shaving the neck, it may be helpful for the patient to flex his neck *to ensure a close shave.*
- On completion, rinse the skin and pat it dry with a clean towel *to remove all traces of soap/foam/gel and dry the face.*
- Apply aftershave if requested by the patient and provide a mirror if required.
- Dispose of all equipment in line with local infection control policies.

Facial Dry Shave

This is often the preferred method, especially if the patient is on anticoagulant therapy that will increase the risk of bleeding if the skin is cut with a razor. Electric shavers should

not be shared among patients, as this presents a cross-infection risk.

- Ensure the skin is clean and dry.
- Hold the skin taut with one hand. With the other hand, place the shaver head against the skin and use short, circular movements to remove hair growth.
- Apply aftershave if requested by the patient.
- On completion, clean the shaver as per manufacturer's instructions.

For Wet and Dry Shaves

- Document the nursing practice appropriately, monitor any after-effects and report abnormal findings immediately, *to provide a written record and assist in the implementation of any action, should an abnormality or adverse reaction to the practice be noted.* Do this *to facilitate communication with other team members.*
- In undertaking these practices, nurses are personally and professionally accountable for their actions, and for the safety, quality, assessment, evaluation and documentation of care delivered (Nursing and Midwifery Council 2018a; Nursing and Midwifery Council 2018b).

3. HAIR WASHING

EQUIPMENT

- Small jug or hair spray tap attachment or showerhead
- Towels
- Plastic sheeting
- Absorbent pad
- Earplugs
- Patient's shampoo/conditioner
- Patient's own brush and/or comb
- Face cloth or disposable cloth
- Plastic apron
- Hairdryer
- Trolley or adequate surface for equipment
- Receptacle for soiled disposable items

Additional Equipment for a Bed-Fast Patient
- Basin
- Large container of warm water
- Container for used water or a bed-fast rinser

GUIDELINES AND RATIONALE FOR THIS PRACTICE

If hair is being treated for a hair infestation, then local guidelines should be followed, according to current effective treatments. Infection control policies should be adhered to in order to prevent spread to family members, other patients and staff.

Washing the Hair of a Bed-Fast Patient

- Explain the nursing practice to the patient *to gain consent and cooperation.*
- Collect and prepare the equipment *to ensure that all equipment is available and ready for use and to minimize interruptions during the procedure.*
- Wash and dry your hands and put on a clean disposable apron *to prevent cross-contamination.*
- Ensure the patient's privacy *to reduce anxiety and promote dignity.*
- Observe and communicate with the patient throughout this activity *to note any signs of distress, pain or discomfort, to establish and maintain a therapeutic relationship, and to establish the patient's preferences.*
- Move the bed away from the wall and remove or fold down the headboard of the bed *to facilitate access.*
- Fold bedding and clothing down and cover the patient's chest with a towel. Use the plastic sheeting *to protect the top part of the sheet underneath the patient.*
- Place a towel around the patient's shoulders. Put a towel on the table, then put the bed-fast rinser, if available, on top. The spout should be situated over an empty bowl on the floor to collect the water from the bed-fast rinser. An absorbent pad should be placed under the bowl *to absorb any water spillage.*
- Help the patient to position themselves so that their head is on the bed-fast rinser.
- If a bed-fast rinser is not available, one person should support the patient's neck and head over a basin during this practice *to minimize discomfort.*
- If the patient is unable to lie flat, they can sit upright, supported by pillows with the head bent forward over a basin on the bed trolley, *to promote comfort and allow the patient to maintain the position during the practice.*
- Protect the patient's eyes with the face cloth or disposable cloth, or, if the patient prefers, they may keep their eyes closed *to prevent irritation from the shampoo.*
- Earplugs may also be used, unless contraindicated, *to prevent water and shampoo from entering the ear canal* (Peate & Lane 2015).
- Using the basin to catch the water, wet the patient's hair and apply the shampoo *to commence washing the patient's hair.*
- Rinse off the lather *to remove the shampoo and leave the patient's hair clean.* Repeat if the patient wishes.

- Apply the patient's hair conditioner, if used, and leave for the manufacturer's recommended time or according to the patient's preferences before rinsing *to help detangle the hair and improve the hair's appearance.*
- Towel the hair dry *to remove excess moisture.*
- Replace the headboard and ensure the patient is comfortable, *to minimize discomfort.*
- Assist the patient to comb their hair into its usual style and dry using the hairdryer *to promote dignity and allow a positive body image to be maintained.*
- Ensure that the patient is left feeling as comfortable as possible, *to confirm the quality of care delivered.*
- Dispose of the equipment safely *to reduce any health hazard.*
- Wash and dry your hands *to prevent cross-infection.*

Washing the Hair of an Ambulant Patient

This procedure can be carried out at the washbasin, or as part of a shower or immersion bath using a hair spray tap attachment or showerhead.

- Help the patient to the bathroom and ensure that they are sitting comfortably, *to promote comfort and allow the patient to maintain the position during the practice.*
- If the patient is having their hair washed at the basin, then protect their clothing using plastic sheeting to reduce water penetration and drape a towel around the shoulders *to absorb any water spillage.*
- Protect the patient's eyes with the face cloth or disposable cloth *to prevent irritation from the shampoo.*
- Using the small jug or the hair spray tap attachment, wet the hair and apply the shampoo *to commence washing the patient's hair.*
- Rinse off the lather *to remove the shampoo and leave the patient's hair clean.*
- Repeat if the patient wishes.
- Apply the patient's hair conditioner, if used, and leave for the manufacturer's recommended time, or according to the patient's preferences, before rinsing, *to help to detangle the hair and improve the hair's appearance.*
- Towel the hair dry *to remove excess moisture.*
- Assist the patient to comb their hair into its usual style and dry using the hairdryer, *to promote dignity and allow a positive body image to be reinstated.*
- Ensure that the patient is left feeling as comfortable as possible *to confirm the quality of care delivered.*
- Wash and dry your hands *to prevent cross-infection.*

For All Patients

- Document the nursing practice appropriately, monitor any after-effects and report abnormal findings immediately, *to provide a written record and assist in the implementation of any action, should an abnormality or adverse reaction to the practice be noted.* Do this *to facilitate communication with other team members.*

- In undertaking these practices, nurses are personally and professionally accountable for their actions, and for the safety, quality, assessment, evaluation and documentation of care delivered (Nursing and Midwifery Council 2018a; Nursing and Midwifery Council 2018b).

ADDITIONAL INFORMATION

In many societies, feeling fresh and clean is known to create a positive body image and maintain dignity and self-esteem. The nurse should be sensitive to the beliefs of different cultures regarding the practice of bathing and personal care. Cultural, ethnic and religious preferences should therefore be observed in respect of personal hygiene (Downey & Lloyd 2008).

It is necessary to wash the skin at regular intervals to keep the natural flora of microorganisms within manageable limits. When a patient is confined to bed, a bed bath is one of the nursing practices used to reduce the potential problem of cross-infection or self-infection during the period of vulnerability caused by illness (Downey & Lloyd 2008).

All equipment used should be clean or disposable, and all precautions must be taken to prevent cross-infection. Equipment should be cleaned and dried thoroughly, according to local policy. Both at home and in hospital, it is preferable for the patient to have a personal washbasin during the period of confinement to bed.

In general, bathing at home is no longer the responsibility of the community nursing service but has become the task of social care workers. However, it is important for guidance to be provided by nurses with regard to skin products, especially for patients with urinary or faecal incontinence (*see* later). If the bed bath is part of an overall package of care, such as for a terminally ill patient, the community nurse will be involved in the management of the delivery of care.

The patient should be offered the facilities to empty their bladder prior to commencing a bed bath, immersion bath or shower.

Skin is easily damaged through contact with urine and faeces. The patient with incontinence is at risk of developing incontinence-associated dermatitis (Voegeli 2016). Voegeli (2016) advises the following:

- full assessment and management of the incontinence
- optimization of nutritional and fluid intake, and use of appropriate continence products and toileting techniques

- provision of a structured skin care regime involving the use of skin cleanser and a protectant, rather than washing with soap and water
- restriction of these products to single-patient use to prevent cross-infection
- care taken in the selection of cleansers and barrier creams because some include chemicals that can further irritate the skin.

Patient movement during a bed bath should be kept to a minimum, especially when a patient suffers from dyspnoea; changing the bottom sheet should, for example, be planned to minimize movement and effort if the patient is acutely ill. When oxygen therapy is being administered, the mask or cannula can be removed for facial cleansing, hair care and mouth care at separate times during the bed bath.

The nurse and patient should talk to each other during personal hygiene care but this may have to be kept to a minimum when the patient is acutely ill. Nurses should take care not to 'talk over' the patient during personal hygiene activities, as this is likely to make the experience feel less personal and dignified for the patient. For all patients, but especially those who are acutely ill or unconscious, non-verbal cues can be used as a method of communication, and touch may be particularly important.

The nurse should check that the patient who is suffering pain has had recent pain relief before starting personal hygiene activities, as movement during bathing and hair washing may exacerbate pain.

A patient who does not wash on a regular basis may require some assistance and education from the nurse on the benefit of this practice during their period of incapacity. Assisting a patient who has a pyrexia with personal hygiene can be comforting in terms of removing excess perspiration and providing clean, fresh clothing.

In hospital, it is usual to have disposable toiletries available in ward areas for patients who may have been admitted as an emergency, until their own personal equipment is brought from home. When possible, patients should be dressed in their own bed clothing for their comfort and to help maintain their individuality.

A patient who has the power, movement or sensation of a limb altered either temporarily or permanently, such as by the position of an intravenous infusion or following a cerebrovascular accident, will require some assistance and education on how to dress and undress during a bed bath. The weak or affected limb is undressed last and dressed first.

Soap and detergents should be avoided, as they can increase the pH of the skin, which can result in a breakdown of the skin's natural barrier and may contribute to skin irritation (Cowdell 2011; Voegeli 2016). A patient who has dry skin may have an aqueous cream or emollient prescribed, and some products can be added to the water for washing. It must be remembered that all skin-cleansing products have the potential to cause irritation and, when used, their effects must be carefully evaluated. If soap is used, the skin must be rinsed well and thoroughly dried, using a blotting motion rather than rubbing, to reduce the potential for skin irritation. The nurse should carry out skin care (*see* Ch. 21) during personal hygiene.

Patients should be assisted to keep their fingernails and toenails clean and manicured. A podiatry service may not be available for all patients but should be used when special care has to be taken of a patient's nails, e.g. a patient with diabetes or peripheral vascular disease, to prevent injury to the nail or nailbed. The nurse may assist the patient to apply nail polish, if clinically appropriate and desired.

When patients are confined to bed, the friction between their heads and the pillow can cause their hair to become tangled and matted. A patient's hair should therefore be brushed and combed into its usual style during personal hygiene and at regular intervals throughout the day to prevent tangling and discomfort to the patient.

The patient can have their hair washed while in bed to maintain its cleanliness (*see* earlier). Should a patient be confined to bed over a prolonged period, a hairdresser or barber may be required to cut and style the hair to improve morale.

Before starting personal hygiene care, the nurse should check that the environment around the patient's bed space is at a comfortable temperature and that no draughts are evident. During the procedure, the nurse should ensure that the patient is kept warm, as an excessive loss of body heat can lead to hypothermia.

A patient confined to bed not only will feel more comfortable but also will benefit psychologically from assisted personal care. The provision of privacy during this nursing practice is very important in the maintenance of the patient's dignity, self-esteem and individuality.

When possible, help patients to maintain their dignity, individuality and independence by allowing them to wash and dry any part of their body they wish, such as their face, hands and pubic area. Allow patients to make decisions as to which clothing they wish to wear. The use of body deodorant, perfume and make-up is determined by personal preference, and the nurse should be guided by patients in their application.

An alternative to the traditional bed-bath procedure is a commercial pack that provides disposable single-use products. A small study by Nøddeskou et al. (2014) identified the fact that disposable commercial bed-bath packs were as popular with elderly patients as traditional bed baths, and more popular with nursing staff, and compared favourably to the traditional methods in terms of cost. Gillis et al. (2016) studied skin hydration in nursing home residents using disposable bed baths and found no adverse effect from using them. The use of these products should be considered where appropriate, taking into account availability and patient preferences.

Before and after bathing and showering, a chair should be available so that the patient can sit to dry or dress themselves with minimal danger of falling.

The water temperature of an immersion bath should be checked to ensure that there is no danger of scalding; the maximum temperature should be 43°C. The ability to judge temperature may be impaired in elderly patients or those with diabetic neuropathy, so the water temperature should always be checked by a nurse or other responsible adult. The use of a bath thermometer will help with this.

The bath, shower area and all equipment used should be cleaned in accordance with local policies and manufacturer's instructions after each use. If the nurse is not confident that this has been done, the bath should be cleaned before preparing it for the patient in order to prevent any cross-infection.

Mechanical lifting aids should be used appropriately, according to the manufacturer's instructions, to help the patient in and out of the bath or shower. In the community, this will be in accordance with the individualized community bathing assessment. The maximum recommended weight limits for any mechanical lifting aid must be checked and adhered to, with specialist bariatric equipment sourced if required.

The patient's manual handling plan should be followed in order to prevent injury to the patient and the staff. For safety, it is advised that a frail, disabled or elderly person should always enter and leave a bath while sitting rather than by climbing over the side of the bath. Variable height or adjustable baths may be used.

To prevent the patient or staff slipping, the spillage of water on to the floor should be avoided; any spills that do occur should be dried immediately.

PATIENT/CARER EDUCATION: KEY POINTS

In partnership with the patient and/or carer, ensure that they are competent to carry out any practices required. Information should be given on an appropriate point of contact for any concerns that may arise.

The carer may be taught how to perform this nursing practice. Preventing infection by maintaining personal hygiene should be explained to the patient and carers.

👥 PATIENT/CARER EDUCATION: KEY POINTS—cont'd

Advice on the direction of washing from the anal region to the rest of the perineal area to reduce the risk of cross-infection should also be given.

The importance of a safe water temperature for bathing and showering should be explained, and the height of the controls or taps may need to be adapted for safe use.

The use of aids, both simple and mechanical, should be explained to the patient. This helps to maintain a safe environment by preventing accidental falls and also ensures safe moving and handling techniques for nurses and carers. Advice and teaching on the availability of aids and the adaptation of the patient's home should be part of the responsibilities of the community nursing team and the occupational therapist.

The patient should understand the importance of reporting any redness, swelling or breakdown of the skin to the nurse or medical practitioner so that any further deterioration in skin condition can be prevented.

It is important for carers to understand how to protect skin from damage caused by urine and faeces. Incontinence-associated dermatitis is commonly observed in patients who are incontinent (Voegeli 2016). Carers need to be advised on how to avoid this. Voegeli (2016) recommends avoiding the use of soap and water in favour of less alkaline skin cleansers and the use of appropriate barrier products.

REFERENCES

Cowdell, F., 2011. Older people, personal hygiene and skin care. Medsurg Nursing 20 (5), 235–240.

Downey, L., Lloyd, H., 2008. Bed bathing patients in hospital. Nursing Standard 22 (34), 35–40.

Gillis, K., Tency, I., Roelant, E., et al., 2016. Skin hydration in nursing home residents using disposable bed baths. Geriatric Nursing 37, 175–179.

Mackie, S., 2013. Renal nursing basics: nail care and facial shaving. Journal of Renal Nursing 1 (3), 127–129.

Nøddeskou, L., Hemmingsen, L., Hordam, B., 2014. Elderly patients' and nurses' assessment of traditional bed bath compared to prepacked single units – randomized control trial. Scandinavian Journal of Caring Sciences 29, 347–352.

Nursing and Midwifery Council, 2018a. The Code: Professional Standards of Practice and Behaviour for Nurses, Midwives and Nursing Associates. NMC, London. Available at: https://www.nmc.org.uk/globalassets/sitedocuments/nmc-publications/nmc-code.pdf.

Nursing and Midwifery Council, 2018b. Future Nurse: Standards of Proficiency for Registered Nurses. NMC, London. Available at: https://www.nmc.org.uk/globalassets/sitedocuments/education-standards/future-nurse-proficiencies.pdf.

Peate, I., Lane, J., 2015. Washing a patient's hair in bed: a care fundamental. British Journal of Healthcare Assistants 9 (3), 114–118.

Voegeli, D., 2016. Incontinence-associated dermatitis: new insights into an old problem. The British Journal of Nursing 25 (5), 256–262.

❓ SELF-ASSESSMENT

1. Under what circumstances would a patient require help with personal hygiene?
2. How can the skin be protected from urine and faecal damage?
3. What precautions should be taken to ensure the patient is not at risk during this practice?
4. What alternative products could be used instead of soap?

Infection Prevention and Management

The application of effective infection control precautions (IPCs) reduces the risk to patients and staff of acquiring healthcare-associated infection (HAI). For effective application, staff must have the capability to apply these principles and this involves knowledge and understanding of the actions required and identification of appropriate opportunities to apply them (Atkins 2018).

Patient/client safety is often not about finding new knowledge but about taking what is already known and putting it into practice (Woodward 2018). This chapter covers standard and transmission-based precautions; consideration must be given to how to take responsibility for applying the IPC knowledge gained from this chapter to everyday practices.

INDICATIONS AND RATIONALE FOR INFECTION PREVENTION AND CONTROL

The European Centre for Disease Prevention and Control undertook a survey of HAI from 2011 to 2012 across 33 countries, including the United Kingdom. The reported HAI rate was between 4.8% and 7.2%, with acute hospitals standing at 5.7%. This figure represents 81,089 patients on any given day. The most frequently reported types of HAI were pneumonia and lower respiratory tract infection, surgical site infection and urinary tract infection (European Centre for Disease Prevention and Control 2012). Acquiring an infection while in hospital can lead to delayed discharge, further courses of treatment such as antibiotics, and possible surgery. Patients with acute and chronic conditions may also face serious complications that can lead to the need for intensive care and/or an increased risk of death.

The majority of HAIs are avoidable. Standard infection control precautions (SICPs) are a practical way to prevent HAI in patients/clients, health and social care staff, and visitors. The best outcomes are achieved when everyone at each level of the care system is involved (World Health Organization 2016).

There are 10 SICPs and these form the skills for preventing and controlling infection. They reflect the duty of care that nurses and midwives have to follow the code of practice published by the Nursing and Midwifery Council (2018). *The Code* sets the standards of practice and behaviour for which all nurses are accountable. It prioritizes the patient/client and ensures that nurses have the knowledge and skills required to deliver safe, effective practice. Infection control is therefore a key element of the skills required to be an effective practitioner.

SICP 1 GENERAL PRINCIPLES OF HAND HYGIENE

Hand hygiene is the single most effective SICP in the prevention of HAI. It requires planning to ensure that staff can undertake hand hygiene at the right time, using the correct hand hygiene products and technique.

Preparing for Hand Hygiene

To maximize the effectiveness of hand hygiene the following principles must be adhered to:

- Ensure that nails are short.
- Avoid false nails, nail extensions, gels and varnish.
- Roll up sleeves.
- Remove all jewellery (including wristwatch).

Products for Hand Hygiene

Choose the product most appropriate for the task or procedure:

- plain liquid soap and running water
- alcohol-based hand rub (ABHR)
- surgical hand scrub (liquid soap containing a skin disinfectant)
- surgical hand rub (alcohol-based solution).

Key Factors in Routine Hand Hygiene

- ABHRs are recommended for routine hand hygiene on visibly clean hands (World Health Organization 2009).
- Manufacturer's instructions should be followed on the quantity of ABHR to be used, ensuring that all areas of the hands are covered and rubbing continuously until the alcohol has completely evaporated.
- Since alcohol is not a cleansing agent, hand-washing with plain soap and water is required on visibly soiled hands (or when the patient/client has a vomiting and/or diarrhoeal illness).
- If soap and water are chosen, fresh running water should be used and plain liquid soap.
- Hot water can damage skin, therefore should be avoided.
- It is important to avoid skin irritation by drying hands thoroughly, with a patting technique rather than rubbing, using a clean/disposable towel and applying hand moisturizer.

Technique for the Skill of Routine Hand Hygiene (World Health Organization 2009)

1. Wet hands with fresh running water.
2. Apply plain liquid soap (enough to cover hands).
3. Rub hands together palm to palm.
4. Right palm over left dorsum (back of second hand) with interlaced fingers, and vice versa.
5. Palm to palm with fingers interlaced.
6. Backs of fingers to opposing palms with fingers interlocked.
7. Rotational rubbing of left thumb clasped in right palm, and vice versa.
8. Rotational rubbing, backwards and forwards with clasped fingers of right hand in left palm, and vice versa.
9. Rinse hands with water.
10. Dry hands thoroughly with a disposable paper towel using a patting technique rather than rubbing.
11. If the tap does not have a hands-free mechanism, use the paper towel to turn it off.

When to Undertake the Skill of Routine Hand Hygiene

The World Health Organization (2009) has highlighted critical points at which hand hygiene should be undertaken, based on the care situation. These include:

- before touching the patient/client
- before clean and aseptic procedures
- after body fluid exposure risk
- after touching the patient/client
- after touching the patient's/client's immediate surroundings.

Technique for the Skill of Surgical Hand Scrub/Rub

Both surgical scrub and rub are undertaken before all surgical and some invasive procedures. Preparation is the same as for routine hand hygiene. Nail picks, rather than nailbrushes, should be used to remove dirt from nails. WHO (2009) recommends particular steps for both scrub and rub.

Technique for Effective Surgical Hand Scrub

1. Wash hands with non-antimicrobial liquid soap and running water, using the normal steps for hand-washing (if hands are visibly soiled) immediately prior to beginning the surgical hand antisepsis.
2. Start timing. Wet hands and forearms. Scrub each side of each finger, between the fingers, and the back and front of the right hand for 2 minutes (using an antimicrobial soap).
3. Scrub the right arm, keeping the hand higher than the arm at all times to prevent recontamination of the hands by water from the elbows, and to stop bacteria-laden soap and water contaminating the hands.
4. Wash each side of the arm from the wrist to the elbow for 1 minute.
5. Repeat the process on the other hand and arm, keeping hands above elbows at all times. (If the hand touches anything at any time, the scrub must be lengthened by 1 minute for the area that has been contaminated.)
6. Rinse hands and arms by passing them through the water in one direction only, from fingertips to elbow. Do not move the arm back and forth through the water.

7. Hold hands above elbows.
8. Hands and arms should be dried using a sterile towel and aseptic technique before putting on gown and gloves.

Technique for Effective Surgical Rub

1. Wash hands with plain liquid soap.
2. Put approximately 5 mL (three doses) of ABHR (or as per manufacturer's instructions) in the palm of your left hand, using the elbow of your other arm to operate the dispenser.
3. Dip the fingertips of your right hand in the hand rub to decontaminate under the nails (5 seconds).
4. Smear the hand rub on the right forearm up to the elbow. Ensure that the whole skin area is covered by using circular movements around the forearm until the hand rub has fully evaporated (10–15 seconds).
5. Repeat steps 1–4 for the left hand and forearm.
6. Put approximately 5 mL (three doses) of ABHR in the palm of your left hand, covering the whole surface of the hands up to the wrist with ABHR, rubbing palm against palm with a rotating movement.
7. Rub the back of the left hand, including the wrist, moving the right palm back and forth, and vice versa.
8. Rub palm against palm back and forth with fingers interlinked.
9. Rub the back of the fingers by holding them in the palm of the other hand with a sideways back-and-forth movement.
10. Rub the thumb of the left hand by rotating it in the clasped palm of the right hand, and vice versa.
11. When the hands are dry, sterile surgical clothing and gloves can be put on.

SICP 2 PERSONAL PROTECTIVE EQUIPMENT

Personal protective equipment (PPE) is recommended for use in health and social care where there is a recognized need to protect staff from the risks associated with specific tasks. It is a legal requirement for employers to provide appropriate PPE and also instruction and training on when and how to use all PPE provided (Health and Safety Executive 2013). For IPC, PPE can include gloves, gowns, aprons, masks and eye protection. Most are for single use, with the exception of some eye protection and respiratory hoods, which may have reusable components depending on make. All PPE should be readily accessible for those who are required to wear it, and employees have a responsibility to select the appropriate PPE and to wear it correctly.

Gloves

Gloves are single-use disposable items that should be chosen for fit and purpose, and are either sterile or non-sterile. Sterile gloves are generally worn during surgical procedures or for clean invasive procedures where local protocol requires them to be worn. Non-sterile gloves are recommended where protection against blood and body fluid contamination is anticipated. On removal, gloves should be discarded as clinical waste (or as domestic waste if in the home setting) and hand hygiene performed after disposal.

Fluid-Resistant Surgical Masks

Fluid-resistant surgical masks are recommended for use by staff when there is a risk of blood or body fluid splashing on to the mouth and respiratory mucosa. The mask should be changed when there is moisture build-up from extended use or following gross contamination with blood/body fluids. Respiratory protective equipment is covered under 'Transmission-based Precautions' later in this chapter.

Eye Protection

Eye protection must be worn when the risk of blood or body fluid splashing on to the eyes is likely. Normal glasses are not a substitute. If the eye protection is not single-use, then nurses should be familiar with the process for decontamination of all reusable parts after use and undertake this immediately on removal.

Aprons/Gowns

Disposable plastic aprons are generally worn to protect the uniform or personal clothing when contamination with blood or body fluids is anticipated. On completion of a task, the apron must be removed immediately and discarded as clinical waste (or as domestic waste if in the home setting).

Sterile gowns are generally worn in the operating theatre, where there is a greater risk of blood or body fluid contamination, and also for certain aseptic procedures when local protocol dictates they must be worn. See the relevant local protocol for further guidance.

SICP 3 CLEAN ENVIRONMENT (INCLUDING SICP 4 MANAGEMENT OF BLOOD AND BODY FLUID SPILLAGE)

In 2017, the Scottish Government Health Department published the Health and Social Care Standards (2017), which state that when care is delivered in a building owned by an organization, the care environment will be clean, tidy and well maintained. Pathogens that cause HAI are often found on hospital surfaces such as curtains, bed rails and care equipment (Han et al. 2015). Cleaning is important in all care settings to reduce the risks to staff, patients/clients and visitors from contact with blood and body fluids and from infectious materials.

The public expects that the environment in which they receive care, and the equipment used during the delivery of that care, will be visibly clean and will cause them no harm.

A clean environment is one that is free from dust, dirt and debris. To achieve this, cleaning schedules that include method, frequency and monitoring must be in place. Routine cleaning is achieved with detergent and water.

- All areas that require cleaning should be accessible to staff.
- Debris and dirt should first be removed.
- A fresh solution of detergent and warm water should be applied with a clean cloth or mop.
- Disinfectants should not be used routinely other than for sanitary fittings and for blood spillage.

SICP 5 CLEAN CARE EQUIPMENT

Equipment used on a patient/client can become contaminated with blood and body fluids and act as a vehicle to transmit pathogens from one person to another. Outbreaks have been linked to reusable equipment that has not been cleaned satisfactorily before being reused.

Equipment used in the delivery of care can be divided into four categories:

- single use (use once and discard)
- single patient use (decontaminate between uses on the same patient)
- reusable invasive device (clean and sterilize between uses on multiple patients)
- reusable non-invasive device (clean, or clean and disinfect, between uses on multiple patients).

Manufacturer's instructions on cleaning and decontamination must be sourced and followed to ensure safe and effective equipment use.

Routine Cleaning

Routine cleaning can be undertaken with a solution of water and disposable cloth, or with commercially available detergent wipes. Once clean, equipment should be thoroughly dried before being stored in a clean, dry environment.

Disinfection

Reusable non-invasive equipment that has come into contact with mucous membranes, non-intact skin, blood/body fluids or infectious agents should be cleaned and then disinfected. The choice of disinfectant will be stipulated by the manufacturer and by local infection control policy.

Sterilization

Although sterilization is not addressed as part of this chapter, it is important to note that reusable invasive equipment, such as surgical instruments, must be cleaned and then sterilized between each use.

SICP 6 DISPOSAL OF HEALTH AND SOCIAL CARE WASTE

Providers of healthcare have a legal duty of care to have systems in place to ensure that all waste generated is segregated, labelled, stored and disposed of in appropriate waste streams. Compliance with health waste regulations will result in cost savings to the health service and direct environmental benefits (Department of Health 2013). Healthcare waste is classified according to whether it is deemed hazardous (medicinal, chemical or infectious) or non-hazardous.

In the healthcare environment, waste that may pose a risk of infection is known as clinical waste and can include swabs, bandages, dressings and so on. All healthcare workers have a duty of care to align their practice with the policies and procedures commensurate with their current healthcare employer.

Healthcare organizations must use an approved (UN 3291) colour coding system for segregation of waste, as laid out in Table 20.1.

SICP 7 REPROCESSING OF LAUNDRY

Reusable healthcare laundry must be managed so that it does not pose a risk to staff and patients. Health Protection Scotland (2018b) recommends categorizing laundry into used, infected and heat-labile to ensure appropriate handling and reprocessing. Current recommendations for reprocessing are:

TABLE 20.1   Colour Coding for Waste Segregation

Type of Waste	Waste Container/ Colour	Contents
Clinical waste	Orange bags	Dressings, swabs
	Yellow bags	Ethical (e.g. body parts) and highly infectious waste
	Yellow rigid containers	Sharps (e.g. needles, blades)
Domestic/ household waste	Clear or black bags Rigid containers	Cardboard, plastics, paper, glass

From Health Protection Scotland: *National Infection Prevention and Control Manual*, 2018. Available at: https://www.nipcm.hps.scot.nhs.uk

- 65°C temperature hold for a minimum of 10 minutes within the wash cycle *or*
- 71°C for not less than 3 minutes.

When handling used laundry, healthcare workers should consider the use of PPE (a disposable plastic apron and gloves) to prevent contamination of uniform/clothing and hands. It is good practice to bring a used laundry receptacle to the bedside for immediate removal. On removal of PPE, hand hygiene should be performed.

Healthcare organizations will have a procedure in place to segregate, store and remove used laundry safely to be washed in an approved laundry that meets required standards for reprocessing.

SICP 8 MANAGEMENT OF OCCUPATIONAL EXPOSURE AND SHARPS INJURY

Employers have a legal responsibility for the management of sharps and other injuries under the Health and Safety (Sharps Instruments in Healthcare) Regulations 2013, to ensure that risks to employees from sharps injury are assessed and controls are in place to mitigate any risk. Assessment includes avoiding the use of sharps where possible and also using alternative non-sharp devices as far as is practical. Staff must receive training that covers:

- safe use and disposal of sharps, including safety devices (sharps users)
- immediate action to be taken if a sharps injury occurs.

SICP 9 RESPIRATORY HYGIENE

The Centres for Disease Control (2012) advocates the use of respiratory hygiene/cough etiquette for patients and staff who have a respiratory infection, to reduce the spread of respiratory secretions. These include:

- encouraging the use of a tissue to cover the mouth and nose during coughing and sneezing
- placing the tissue in the nearest waste bin immediately after use
- performing hand hygiene.

For respiratory hygiene to be effective, tissues, waste bins and hand hygiene facilities must be provided and within reach of patients.

SICP 10 PATIENT/CLIENT ASSESSMENT AND ACCOMMODATION

Patients should be assessed on admission to an acute hospital setting and throughout their stay until discharge. The assessment is required to identify potential infection risks that can be transmitted to other patients, staff and visitors. Signs and symptoms of infection, such as fever, rash, cough or vomiting and diarrhoea, should trigger further investigation to rule out infection. In addition, questions about hospitalization outside the UK, travel and previous colonization/infection with resistant organisms (e.g. meticillin-resistant *Staphylococcus aureus* (MRSA), carbapenemase-producing Enterobacteriaceae (CPE)) are now mandatory in UK hospitals to ensure that patients are accommodated appropriately. This might be:

- a single room with en-suite facilities
- a single room with mechanical ventilation that prevents the flow of air out of the room into the ward
- a cohort area for multiple patients with the same infection
- a specialist centre in the UK equipped with facilities that have controlled ventilation for infections that are life-threatening, such as viral haemorrhagic fever.

Patients/clients in care homes should, as far as possible, be facilitated to stay in their bedroom to limit contact with other patient/clients while they are infectious.

Patients/clients attending outpatient clinics should be encouraged to rearrange their appointment if possible when they have symptoms of an infectious disease. This could be at the end of a clinic, to allow for cleaning and for reduced contact with others in the waiting area.

Early and ongoing assessment ensures that appropriate precautions are instigated so that the risk is minimized as soon as possible.

TRANSMISSION-BASED PRECAUTIONS

Where a patient is considered to have an infection that can be transmitted to others, additional precautions should be considered as well as SICPs, including patient accommodation, respiratory protective equipment, and enhanced cleaning of the environment, care equipment and laundry.

Microorganisms can spread in one or more of the following ways: by contact, by droplet or by being airborne.

Contact

This is the most common route of spread and can take place:

- directly, from person to person, skin to skin, body fluids and blood
- indirectly, on contaminated hands or equipment, or in the environment.

Droplet

Spread is via respiratory secretions of more than 5 μm in size, which travel up to 1 metre during coughing and sneezing, landing on the mucous membranes of the eyes, nose or mouth. This route requires close contact.

Airborne

Spread is via respiratory secretions of 5 μm or less in size, which become airborne and, when inhaled, reach the alveoli of the lungs. Airborne spread does not require close contact; merely being in the same room is enough, as particles are transported much further due to their size.

RESPIRATORY PROTECTIVE EQUIPMENT

All employers in the UK have a legal responsibility to provide staff with the correct PPE to control substances hazardous to health in the workplace (Health and Safety Executive 2013). Whichever type of respiratory protective equipment (RPE) is chosen, it must comply with the Personal Protective Equipment Regulations (Health and Safety Executive 1992).

Respiratory protection is recommended for staff when:
- they are caring for a patient/client with an infectious disease transmitted by the airborne route
- they are undertaking aerosol-generating procedures on a patient with an infectious disease transmitted by the airborne or droplet route.

The RPE can take the form of either a mask with inbuilt filter, which relies on the user to draw in air through normal breathing, or a powered hood with battery pack, which mechanically circulates air within the hood. It is recommended that filtering face piece masks (FFP3), which filter pathogens such as viruses, bacteria and fungal spores, and meet Standard EN149:2001, are provided for staff where this level of protection is required (Health Protection Scotland 2018a). Before using an FFP3 mask, the wearer must be tested to ensure that a good fit can be created around the face. In the UK, FFP3 masks are available from more than one manufacturer and it is therefore important for the wearer to be fit-tested for the specific mask that will be available for their use. Respiratory hoods do not need fit-testing before use but do require training on their use and decontamination. It is important to note that a fluid-resistant surgical mask should not be used as a substitute for RPE.

Staff should familiarize themselves with local policies on the RPE available, including training opportunities. They should also consider which procedures they undertake that might be considered aerosol-generating. Health Protection Scotland (2018a), in the *National Infection Prevention and Control Manual*, lists the following as having the potential for aerosol generation:
- intubation and extubation
- manual ventilation
- open suctioning
- cardiopulmonary resuscitation

- bronchoscopy
- surgery and post-mortem procedures involving high-speed devices
- some dental procedures (e.g. drilling)
- non-invasive ventilation (NIV), e.g. bi-level positive airway pressure (BiPAP) and continuous positive airway pressure (CPAP) ventilation
- high-frequency oscillating ventilation (HFOV)
- induction of sputum.

The wearing of any PPE should be considered as part of a risk assessment of the infectious nature of the patient and the mode of transmission of the infectious agent.

PATIENT/CARER EDUCATION: KEY POINTS

- demonstrate hand hygiene to patients and carers. Explain how they can help to reduce the risk of infection by undertaking hand hygiene themselves
- encourage patients to report symptoms such as diarrhoea and/or vomiting, fever, rash immediately so that appropriate patient placement can be reviewed
- provide information to patients / carers on their infection status and explain how they can help to reduce the risk of transmission
- explain to patients / carers why staff may wear personal protective clothing such as disposable apron, gloves and masks
- encourage carers not to visit if they themselves have an infection

---

REFERENCES

Atkins, L., 2018. Using the Behaviour Change wheel in infection prevention and control practice. Journal of Infection Prevention 17 (2), 74–78.

Centers for Disease Control, 2012. Respiratory Hygiene/Cough Etiquette in Healthcare Settings. Available at: https://www.cdc.gov/flu/professionals/infectioncontrol/resphygiene.htm.

Department of Health, 2013. Environment and sustainability Health Technical Memorandum 07-01: Safe management of healthcare waste. Available at: https://www.gov.uk/government/publications/guidance-on-the-safe-management-of-healthcare-waste.

European Centre for Disease Prevention and Control, 2012. Point prevalence survey of healthcare-associated infections and antimicrobial use in European acute care hospitals. Available at: https://ecdc.europa.eu/sites/portal/files/media/en/publications/Publications/healthcare-associated-infections-antimicrobial-use-PPS.pdf.

Han, J.H., Sullivan, N., Leas, B.F., et al., 2015. Cleaning Hospital room surfaces to prevent health Care-Associated infections. Annals of Internal Medicine 163 (8), 598–607.

Health Protection Scotland, 2018a. National Infection Prevention and Control Manual. Available at: https://www.nipcm.hps.scot.nhs.uk.

Health Protection Scotland, 2018b. National Guidance for Safe Management of Linen in NHSScotland. Available at: https://www.hps.scot.nhs.uk/resourcedocument.aspx?id=6613.

Health and Safety Executive, 1992. Personal protective equipment at work: Personal Protective Equipment at Work Regulations 1992. Guidance on Regulations L25, third ed. Available at: http://www.hse.gov.uk/pUbns/priced/l25.pdf.

Health and Safety Executive, 2013. Personal protective equipment (PPE) at work. A brief guide. Available at: https://www.hse.gov.uk/toolbox/ppe.htm.

Nursing and Midwifery Council, 2018. The Code: Professional Standards of Practice and Behaviour for Nurses, Midwives and Nursing Associates. NMC, London. Available at: https://www.nmc.org.uk/globalassets/sitedocuments/nmc-publications/nmc-code.pdf.

Scottish Government Health Department, 2017. Health and Social Care Standards: My Support, My Life. Available at: https://hub.careinspectorate.com/.

Woodward, S., 2018. Implementing change: lessons from the patient safety movement. Journal of Infection Prevention 17 (2), 79–82.

World Health Organization, 2009. WHO guidelines on hand hygiene in health care. First global patient safety challenge: clean care is safer care. Available at: https://apps.who.int/iris/bitstream/handle/10665/44102/9789241597906_eng.pdf?sequence=1.

World Health Organization, 2016. Health care without avoidable infections: The critical role of infection prevention and control. Available at: http://apps.who.int/iris/bitstream/handle/10665/246235/WHO-HIS-SDS-2016.10-eng.pdf;jsessionid=ECBB926FE972BB021BCD8AFDBC0FE0B2?sequence=1.

? SELF-ASSESSMENT

1. Familiarize yourself with your local IPC policies and protocols, and consider how they affect you and your colleagues.
2. Choose three care scenarios that you are likely to undertake with a patient/client:
   - Consider the most appropriate time to carry out hand hygiene and how this will be achieved.
   - Discuss which items of PPE you should wear and why. Consider what might prevent you from achieving this and how this problem can be overcome.
   - How would you explain to your patient/client why you are taking these precautions?
3. Describe how you might assess your patient/client for signs of infection.
4. Identify three pieces of care equipment that you use with your patient/client. Think about how you clean each one after use. If any is single-use, how will you dispose of each piece?
5. Read your local policies and protocols on:
   - disposal of waste
   - processing of laundry
   - reporting of sharps injury and occupational exposure to blood and body fluids.

Integrity of the Skin

INDICATIONS AND RATIONALE FOR SKIN CARE

This care involves the maintenance of a patient's skin viability by ensuring skin cleanliness, relieving skin capillary pressure, ensuring adequate nutritional status and monitoring potential problems. Skin care is indicated for every patient, but specific circumstances increase the need for care when:
* the patient is incontinent
* the patient's mobility is temporarily or permanently impaired, e.g. a bed-fast, paralysed or unconscious patient
* the patient has a poor nutritional status
* the patient has impaired peripheral circulation.

GUIDELINES AND RATIONALE FOR THIS NURSING PRACTICE

* Explain the nursing practice to the patient *to gain consent and cooperation.*

* Ensure the patient's privacy *to reduce anxiety and promote dignity.*
* Wash the hands *to reduce the risk of cross-infection* (Loveday et al. 2014).
* Observe and communicate with the patient throughout this activity *to note any signs of distress or discomfort and to promote dignity and independence.*
* Assess the patient's risk factors for developing a pressure ulcer, utilizing one of the risk assessment scales, *to permit preventive care to be implemented*. This should be performed as part of the initial assessment process within 6 hours of admission to hospital, or at the first face-to-face visit by community nursing services, after any interventional procedure, and at regular intervals throughout care when the patient's condition changes (National Institute for Health and Care Excellence 2014; National Institute for Health and Care Excellence 2015).
* Assess the patient using a malnutrition screening tool, such as the Malnutrition Universal Screening Tool (MUST) (BAPEN 2003), *to ascertain the patient's nutritional status, as malnutrition increases the risk of skin breakdown.*
* Identify individual problem areas, such as a patient with peripheral vascular disease or peripheral neuropathy whose affected limb may be at greater risk than the rest of their body, as there will be increased risk of the

TABLE 21.1   Adapted Waterlow Pressure Area Risk Assessment Chart

Risk	Score
Sex	
Male	1
Female	2
Age	
14–49	1
50–64	2
65–74	3
75–80	4
81+	5
Build/Weight for Height (Body Mass Index (BMI) = Weight in kg/Height in m^2)	
Average: BMI 20–24.9	0
Above average: BMI 25–29.9	1
Obese: BMI >30	2
Below average: BMI <20	3
Continence	
Complete/catheterized	0
Incontinent urine	1
Incontinent faeces	2
Doubly incontinent (urine and faeces)	3
Skin Type: Visual Risks Area	
Healthy	0
Tissue paper (thin/fragile)	1
Dry (appears flaky)	1
Oedematous (puffy)	1
Clammy (moist to touch)/pyrexia	1
Discoloured (bruising/mottled)	2
Broken (established ulcer)	3
Mobility	
Fully mobile	0
Restless/fidgety	1
Apathetic (sedated/depressed/reluctant to move)	2
Restricted (restricted by severe pain or disease)	3
Bedbound (unconscious/unable to change position/traction)	4
Chairbound (unable to leave chair without assistance)	5
Nutritional Element	
Unplanned weight loss in past 3–6 months:	
<5%	0
5–10%	1
>10%	2

TABLE 21.1 Adapted Waterlow Pressure Area Risk Assessment Chart—cont'd

Risk	Score
BMI:	
>20	0
18.5–20	1
<18.5	2
Patient/client acutely ill or no nutritional intake >5 days	2
Special Risks: Tissue Malnutrition	
Multiple organ failure/terminal cachexia	8
Single organ failure, e.g. cardiac, renal, respiratory	5
Peripheral vascular disease	5
Anaemia = Haemoglobin <8 g/dL	2
Smoking	1
Special Risks: Neurological Deficit	
Diabetes/multiple sclerosis/cerebrovascular accident/motor/sensory/paraplegia: max. 6	4–6
Special Risks: Surgery/Trauma	
On table >6 hours	8
Orthopaedic/below waist/spinal (up to 48 hours post op)	5
On table >2 hours (up to 48 hours post op)	5
Special Risks: Medication	
Cytotoxic, anti-inflammatory, long-term/high-dose steroid: max. 4	4
Total Score	
Date	
Initials	
Time	

More than one score/category can be used: 10+ = 'at risk'; 15+ = 'high risk'; 20+ = 'very high risk'. Undertake and document the risk assessment within 6 hours of admission or on first home visit. Reassess if there is a change in the individual's condition and repeat regularly, according to local protocol. Ensure that the plan of care is implemented/reviewed for all identified areas of concern. Write, imprint or attach a label, stating surname, forenames, date of birth, location, CHI number (in Scotland) and sex.
Adapted from Healthcare Improvement Scotland/National Association of Tissue Viability Nurse Specialists (Scotland) 2014. Risk Assessment Chart Waterlow v2 30th October 2014 www.healthcareimprovementscotland.org/our_work/patient_safety/tissue_viability.aspx

development of a pressure ulcer due to vascular insufficiency and altered sensation, respectively.

- Devise and document a bespoke care plan for people who are assessed as at high risk of developing a pressure ulcer (National Institute for Health and Care Excellence 2014). In doing so, consideration should be given to the risk and skin assessment, the need for additional pressure relief, the ability to self-mobilize, individual preferences and any pre-existing comorbidities, *to reduce the risk of development of a pressure ulcer.*

- Relieve the pressure exerted on the skin surface by regularly changing the patient's body position (National Institute for Health and Care Excellence 2014) and using pressure-relieving devices (National Institute for Health and Care Excellence 2014) *to prevent or reduce devitalization of healthy tissue.*

- Support the patient's body and limbs in natural positions *to promote comfort and prevent damage,* and maintain joint and muscle movement with passive and active exercises.

- A patient who is assessed as having a high risk factor will require frequent, e.g. 2–4-hourly, changes of position *to relieve the pressure of the soft tissues against bone* and frequent reassessment (National Institute for Health and Care Excellence 2014). For some patients, a high-specification foam mattress may be required. A turning chart may be used to record the time, position of the patient and signature of the nurse or carer.
- Reduce the pressure, friction and shearing forces on the skin with the use of any of the recommended aids available, such as a high-specification foam mattress or a pressure-redistributing surface (National Institute for Health and Care Excellence 2014), *to reduce the factors contributing to pressure ulcer development.*
- Cleanse the skin of an incontinent patient or a patient who is perspiring profusely, *to reduce the number of microorganisms on the skin, which will be greatly increased*. Avoid the use of soap, *to prevent the alkaline content drying the skin and depleting it of its natural oils* (Voegeli 2016).
- Dry the skin thoroughly by patting it gently *to minimize the proliferation of microorganisms on the skin surface, thereby diminishing the risk of infections.*
- Consider the use of barrier creams to prevent skin damage in adults at risk of developing incontinence-associated dermatitis (Voegeli 2016) *to minimize the risk of developing lesions associated with incontinence.*
- Examine and classify (Box 21.1) the patient's skin during this nursing practice, checking for skin integrity, discoloration and disparities in heat, and turgor and moisture, which may be indicative of the development of a pressure ulcer (Whiteing 2009; National Institute for Health and Care Excellence 2014).

BOX 21.1   Pressure Injury Stages

Pressure Injury

A pressure injury is localized damage to the skin and underlying soft tissue, usually over a bony prominence or related to a medical or other device. The injury can present as intact skin or an open ulcer, and may be painful. The injury occurs as a result of intense and/or prolonged pressure or pressure in combination with shear. The tolerance of soft tissue for pressure and shear may also be affected by microclimate, nutrition, perfusion, comorbidities and condition of the soft tissue.

Stage 1 Pressure Injury: Non-Blanchable Erythema of Intact Skin

Intact skin with a localized area of non-blanchable erythema, which may appear differently in darkly pigmented skin. Presence of blanchable erythema or changes in sensation, temperature or firmness may precede visual changes. Colour changes do not include purple or maroon discoloration: these may indicate deep tissue pressure injury.

Stage 2 Pressure Injury: Partial-Thickness Skin Loss With Exposed Dermis

The wound bed is viable, pink or red, and moist, and may also present as an intact or ruptured serum-filled blister. Adipose (fat) and deeper tissues are not visible. Granulation tissue, slough and eschar are not present. These injuries commonly result from adverse microclimate and shear in the skin over the pelvis and shear in the heel. This stage should not be used to describe moisture-associated skin damage (MASD), including incontinence-associated dermatitis (IAD), intertriginous dermatitis (ITD), medical adhesive-related skin injury (MARSI) or traumatic wounds (skin tears, burns, abrasions).

Stage 3 Pressure Injury: Full-Thickness Skin Loss

Adipose tissue (fat) is visible in the ulcer, and granulation tissue and epibole (rolled wound edges) are often present. Slough and/or eschar may be visible. The depth of tissue damage varies by anatomical location; areas of significant adiposity can develop deep wounds. Undermining and tunnelling may occur. Fascia, muscle, tendon, ligament, cartilage and/or bone are not exposed. If slough or eschar obscures the extent of tissue loss, this is an unstageable pressure injury.

Stage 4 Pressure Injury: Full-Thickness Skin and Tissue Loss

Full-thickness skin and tissue loss with exposed or directly palpable fascia, muscle, tendon, ligament, cartilage or bone in the ulcer. Slough and/or eschar may be visible. Epibole (rolled edges), undermining and/or tunnelling often occur. Depth varies by anatomical location. If slough or eschar obscures the extent of tissue loss, this is an unstageable pressure injury.

Obscured Full-Thickness Skin and Tissue Loss

Full-thickness skin and tissue loss, in which the extent of tissue damage within the ulcer cannot be confirmed because it is obscured by slough or eschar. If slough or eschar is removed, a stage 3 or stage 4 pressure injury will be revealed. Stable eschar (i.e. dry, adherent, intact

BOX 21.1   Pressure Injury Stages—cont'd

without erythema or fluctuance) on the heel or ischaemic limb should not be softened or removed.

Deep Tissue Pressure Injury (DTPI): Persistent, Non-Blanchable, Deep Red, Maroon or Purple Discoloration

Intact or non-intact skin with a localized area of persistent, non-blanchable, deep red, maroon or purple discoloration, or epidermal separation revealing a dark wound bed or blood-filled blister. Pain and temperature change often precede skin colour changes. Discoloration may appear differently in darkly pigmented skin. This injury results from intense and/or prolonged pressure and shear forces at the bone–muscle interface. The wound may evolve rapidly to reveal the actual extent of tissue injury or may resolve without tissue loss. If necrotic tissue, subcutaneous tissue, granulation tissue, fascia, muscle or other underlying structures are visible, this indicates a full-thickness pressure injury (unstageable, stage 3 or stage 4). Do not use DTPI to describe vascular, traumatic, neuropathic or dermatological conditions.

Additional Pressure Injury Definitions
Medical Device-Related Pressure Injury

This describes an aetiology. Medical device-related pressure injuries result from the use of devices designed and applied for diagnostic or therapeutic purposes. The resultant pressure injury generally conforms to the pattern or shape of the device. The injury should be staged using the staging system.

Mucosal Membrane Pressure Injury

Mucosal membrane pressure injury is found on mucous membranes with a history of a medical device in use at the location of the injury. Due to the anatomy of the tissue, these ulcers cannot be staged.

From National Pressure Ulcer Advisory Panel (2016), http://www.npuap.org/resources/educational-and-clinical-resources/pressure-injury-staging-illustrations/. Used with permission of the National Pressure Ulcer Advisory Panel 2019.

- Use a skilled moving and handling technique when repositioning the patient, and proper positioning to prevent them sliding down in the bed or chair *to reduce the shearing and friction forces exerted on a patient's skin.*
- Maintain, or improve when appropriate, the patient's nutritional status, using the services of a dietitian if necessary, *to prevent poor nutritional and hydration status, which greatly increases the risk of pressure ulcer development.*
- Educate the patient and carers about preventive care for pressure ulcer development when the patient's condition permits: e.g. a patient in traction can assist with pressure relief measures. Patient cooperation and care are vital *to prevent the overall development of pressure ulcers and also facilitate patient empowerment.*
- After giving any of the forms of care above, ensure that the patient is as comfortable as possible *to ensure quality of patient care;* consideration should be given to pain relief strategies before and during and subsequent to any care delivery.
- Dispose of used equipment safely *to reduce any health hazard.*
- Document the nursing practice appropriately, monitor the after-effects and report any abnormal findings immediately, *to provide a written record and assist in the implementation of any action, should an abnormality or adverse reaction to the practice be noted.*

- In undertaking this practice, nurses are accountable for their actions, the quality of care delivered and record-keeping (Nursing and Midwifery Council 2018a; Nursing and Midwifery Council 2018b).

 PATIENT/CARER EDUCATION: KEY POINTS

When a person is assessed as being at significant risk of developing a pressure ulcer, bespoke information about the causes, early indications, implications and methods of prevention should be provided to them and their carers/families (National Institute for Health and Care Excellence 2014). Information should be given on an appropriate point of contact for any concerns that may arise.

A patient who is permanently at risk of pressure ulcer development should be encouraged to take an active role in preventive care. This may involve the nurse teaching the patient how to inspect the skin tissue regularly, e.g. using a mirror to assess skin areas that are difficult to access.

When prolonged or permanent use of pressure-relieving aids is required, the patient and carers should be given information on the safe, continued care of the equipment and on appropriate action, should a fault occur.

REFERENCES

BAPEN, 2003. Malnutrition Universal Screening Tool BAPEN. Available at: https://www.bapen.org.uk/pdfs/must/must-full.pdf.

Loveday, H.P., Wilson, J.A., Pratt, R.J., et al., 2014. Epic3: national evidence-based guidelines for preventing healthcare-associated infections in NHS hospitals in England. The Journal of Hospital Infection 86 (Suppl. 1), S1–S70.

National Institute for Health and Care Excellence, 2014. Pressure ulcers: prevention and management [CG179]. NICE, London. Available at: https://www.nice.org.uk/guidance/cg179/chapter/1-Recommendations.

National Institute for Health and Care Excellence, 2015. Pressure Ulcers Quality Standard [QS89]. NICE, London. Available at: https://www.nice.org.uk/guidance/qs89/chapter/Quality-statement-4-Skin-assessment.

National Pressure Ulcer Advisory Panel, 2016. NPUAP Pressure Injury Stages. Available at: https://www.npuap.org/resources/educational-and-clinical-resources/npuap-pressure-injury-stages/.

National Pressure Ulcer Advisory Panel/European Pressure Ulcer Advisory Panel/Pan Pacific Pressure Injury Alliance, 2014. Prevention and Treatment of Pressure Ulcers: Quick Reference Guide Cambridge Media: Australia. Available at: https://www.npuap.org/wp-content/uploads/2014/08/Quick-Reference-Guide-DIGITAL-NPUAP-EPUAP-PPPIA-Jan2016.pdf.

Nursing and Midwifery Council, 2018a. The Code: Professional Standards of Practice and Behaviour for Nurses, Midwives and Nursing Associates. NMC, London. Available at: https://www.nmc.org.uk/globalassets/sitedocuments/nmc-publications/nmc-code.pdf.

Nursing and Midwifery Council, 2018b. Future Nurse: Standards of Proficiency for Registered Nurses. NMC, London. Available at: https://www.nmc.org.uk/globalassets/sitedocuments/education-standards/future-nurse-proficiencies.pdf.

O'Tuathail, C., Taqi, R., 2011. Evaluation of three commonly used pressure ulcer risk assessment scales. British Journal of Nursing (Tissue Viability Supplement) 20 (6), S27–S34.

Voegeli, D., 2016. Incontinence-associated dermatitis: new insights into an old problem. British Journal of Nursing 25 (5), 256–262.

Whiteing, N.L., 2009. Skin assessment of patients at risk of pressure ulcers. Nursing Standard 24 (10), 40–44.

WEBSITES

https://www.nmc-uk.org *Nursing and Midwifery Council*
https://www.rcn.org.uk *Royal College of Nursing*

SELF-ASSESSMENT

1. Under what circumstances would a nurse be required to provide increased levels of skin care?
2. What are the risk factors associated with pressure ulcer development?
3. What assessment tools are available for nurses to use to assess patients?
4. What actions can be taken by the nurse to minimize the risk of pressure ulcer development?
5. What role can the patient play in pressure ulcer prevention?

Intravenous Therapy

There are three parts to this chapter:
1. Commencing an intravenous infusion
2. Priming the equipment for intravenous infusion
3. Maintaining the infusion for a period of time

LEARNING OUTCOMES

By the end of this chapter, you should be able to:
- prepare and support the patient for these nursing practices
- collect and prepare the equipment
- assist the medical practitioner/nurse with the safe insertion of an intravenous cannula or catheter
- prepare, commence and maintain an intravenous infusion, as prescribed.

BACKGROUND KNOWLEDGE REQUIRED

- Revision of the anatomy and physiology of the cardiovascular system, with special reference to the circulation of the blood and to body fluids
- Revision of aseptic technique (*see* Ch. 40)
- Review of local policy in relation to intravenous therapy

INDICATIONS AND RATIONALE FOR INTRAVENOUS INFUSION

An intravenous infusion is the introduction of prescribed sterile fluid into the blood circulation via a vein. It may be indicated for the following reasons:

- *to maintain a normal fluid, nutrient and electrolyte balance when the patient is unable to maintain adequate intake by mouth and nasogastric feeding is inappropriate,* e.g.:

- a patient during the preoperative, intraoperative and postoperative periods
- a patient who has had surgery involving the gastrointestinal tract
- a patient who has malabsorption problems
- *to replace severe fluid loss in emergency situations,* e.g.:
  - a patient who has severe haemorrhage and/or hypovolaemic shock
  - a patient who has severe burns
  - a patient who is dehydrated by vomiting or diarrhoea usually associated with enteric infection
- *to administer medication when other routes are not appropriate or when there is a need for a rapid onset of action or precise titration of the dose,* e.g.:
  - analgesic medication for rapid pain relief
  - chemotherapy for the treatment of cancers.

1. COMMENCING AN INTRAVENOUS INFUSION

OUTLINE OF THE PROCEDURE

Intravenous therapy is prescribed by the medical practitioner. Peripheral intravenous cannulation is performed by a doctor, or by a nurse or other healthcare practitioner who has undertaken specialist training and is deemed competent to carry out this procedure. The nurse may be required to help with the procedure, to maintain the infusion safely for a period of time and to undertake removal of the cannula.

Using a strict aseptic technique, the practitioner selects a suitable peripheral vein. The insertion site is decontaminated with a single-use application of 2% chlorhexidine gluconate in 70% isopropyl alcohol and allowed to dry before the cannula is inserted (Loveday et al. 2014). A topical preparation of local anaesthetic, e.g. Emla cream, can be applied to the skin surface at least 1 hour prior to the procedure; Ametop may be applied 45 minutes before the procedure (BNF 2018).

A sterile peripheral venous cannula is inserted into the vein so that the prescribed infusion fluid can enter the patient's blood circulation. The infusion fluid flows into the cannula through an administration set that will have been primed ready for use. The cannula is secured in position and covered by a sterile, transparent, semi-permeable dressing (Health Protection Scotland 2014) (Fig. 22.1). The flow of infusion fluid is maintained, and the containers of fluid replaced as prescribed, until the intravenous infusion is discontinued.

Sites Chosen for Intravenous Cannulation

The metacarpal veins and the dorsal venous arch at the back of the hand or the superficial veins of the wrist or lower arm, such as the cephalic or basilic veins, are ideal. The vein should feel soft and bouncy, and refill when depressed (Witt 2011). The veins of the lower limbs are rarely used because of the increased risk of thrombosis as a result of a slower venous flow. The non-dominant limb should be used if possible to minimize the patient's discomfort and promote independence.

◎ EQUIPMENT

- Trolley or tray
- Patient's prescription and fluid balance charts
- Sterile peripheral venous catheters in sizes 16–22 Ch (or Fg), depending on the fluids to be infused
- Single-use tourniquet
- Non-sterile gloves/apron
- Single-use application of 2% chlorhexidine gluconate in 70% isopropyl alcohol to decontaminate the skin, as per local policy
- Sterile, transparent, semi-permeable cannula dressing
- Sterile intravenous administration set

- Prescribed intravenous infusion fluid
- Infusion stand
- Sharps disposal bin
- Receptacle for soiled disposable items

Additional Equipment, if required
- Local anaesthetic and equipment for its administration
- Electronic flow control device (pump) with the appropriate administration set/syringe
- Needle-free cap or extension set

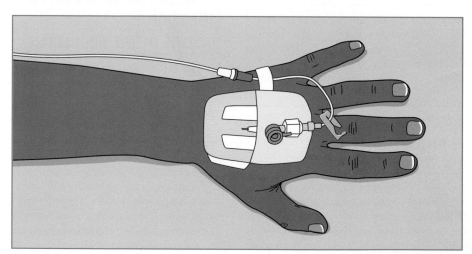

Fig. 22.1 Peripheral intravenous cannula and giving set secured in place with a sterile, transparent, semipermeable dressing.

INFUSION FLUIDS

The commonly prescribed intravenous fluids are (Smith 2017):

- crystalloids:
  - compound sodium lactate, e.g. Ringer's lactate/ Hartmann's solution
  - sodium chloride 0.9%
- colloids:
  - gelofusine
  - hetastarch
- blood (*see* 'Blood Transfusion', Ch. 6)
- parenteral nutrients, via a central venous catheter (*see* 'Parenteral nutrition', Ch. 26).

Intravenous fluids are commercially prepared in sterile containers, which are labelled 'FOR INTRAVENOUS INFUSION'. They may also be prepared by the hospital pharmacy. The containers used for these preparations are frequently soft plastic bags protected by an outer covering (*see* the manufacturer's instructions), although semi-rigid plastic containers continue to be used, mainly for medications.

PERIPHERAL INTRAVENOUS CATHETERS (CANNULAS)

A wide range of intravenous catheters (cannulas) is available (Fig. 22.2). They differ in relation to their size, possession of an injection port and inclusion of a needle-stick protection system. The selection of a suitable catheter should be based on the quantity and nature of intravenous fluid that is to be infused through it and also by the local trust policy. The smallest catheter possible should be selected, ***to prevent damage to the vein*** (Brooks 2016) (Table 22.1).

ADMINISTRATION SETS

Administration sets are commercially prepared in sterile packs. The set contains specialized sterile tubing with a rigid spike at one end, protected by a sterile cover. At the other end is a similarly protected Luer Lock connector. Towards the spike end, the tubing widens into a drip chamber. An adjustable roller clamp surrounds the tubing below the drip chamber, which allows the flow of fluid to be manually regulated at the prescribed flow rate. Blood administration sets include a filter and should be changed when the transfusion episode is complete or every 12

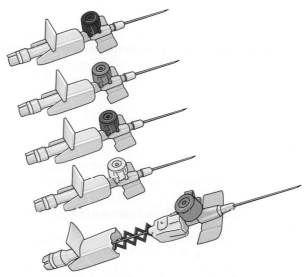

Fig. 22.2 A selection of intravenous catheters.

TABLE 22.1	**Peripheral Intravenous Catheters**		
Gauge (Ch/Fg)	**Typical Manufacturer Colour**	**Approximate Flow Rate (mL/min)***	**Common Uses**
22 Ch	Blue	42	Small, fragile veins, short-term access
20 Ch	Pink	67	Routine infusions, bolus drug administration
18 Ch	Green	103	Rapid infusions, surgical patients
16 Ch	Grey	236	Major trauma or surgery, massive fluid replacement, blood transfusion
14 Ch	Orange	270	Emergency situations

*Flow rates from BD Venflon Pro Safety Shielded IV Catheter.

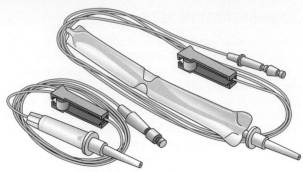

Fig. 22.3 Administration sets.

hours, whichever is sooner (Loveday et al. 2014). Simple administration sets are available without a filter, for the infusion of clear intravenous fluids. Some contain a covered air vent, to avoid the need for an air inlet needle when using glass or rigid plastic fluid containers. Simple administration sets (Fig. 22.3) should be changed every 96 hours (Loveday et al. 2014).

ELECTRONIC FLOW CONTROL DEVICES (PUMPS)

A wide variety of electronic control devices, such as volumetric or syringe pumps, is available. They provide an accurate flow of fluid over a prescribed period of time and may contain additional safety features, such as audible alarms, anti-free-flow protection, air embolism prevention and inline pressure monitoring. The choice of pump is dependent on the required volume of fluid to be infused and the speed of the infusion. The Medicines and Healthcare Products Regulatory Agency (2013) has produced extensive guidance relating to all aspects of the use of such infusion devices. The manufacturer's guidelines must be followed and only the specific administration set for each device should be used. The nurse is responsible for the monitoring of the patient and accountable for use of these devices (Nursing and Midwifery Council 2018).

GUIDELINES AND RATIONALE FOR THIS NURSING PRACTICE

- Help to explain the nursing practice to the patient *to gain consent and cooperation, and to encourage participation in care.*
- Ensure the patient's privacy, *to respect their individuality.*
- Help to collect and prepare the equipment. Wash hands *to reduce the risk of cross-infection* and put on non-sterile gloves *to prevent contamination with body fluids* (Health Protection Scotland 2012).

- Check the prescribed infusion fluid with a registered nurse or medical practitioner, in line with the local policy. This is a legal requirement and part of professional practice.
- Maintaining asepsis, prime the administration set with the infusion fluid, ensuring that all the air is expelled from the system, *to prevent any danger of air embolus.*
- Place the infusion fluid on the stand beside the patient and label it with the date and time.
- Help the patient into as comfortable a position as possible and provide an explanation and reassurance *to minimize their distress during the cannulation procedure.*
- Observe the patient throughout this activity *to monitor any adverse effects.*
- Expose and support the area for cannulation *to facilitate access.*
- Help to prepare the sterile equipment as required, *to maintain a safe environment.*
- Apply pressure around the limb above the cannulation site as directed, with a single-use tourniquet. This will fill the veins with additional blood and so help *to facilitate cannulation.*
- Once the cannula has been successfully inserted, release the pressure, as directed.
- Help to secure the cannula in place with a sterile, transparent, semi-permeable cannula dressing, including a label with the date (Loveday et al. 2014). If a needle-free injection cap is to be used, it should be primed and connected to the cannula at this time.
- Before connecting the intravenous fluid, check the patient's name band, the prescription chart and the infusion fluid, in line with the local policy.
- Using an aseptic non-touch technique, remove the protective caps from the primed administration set and the cannula and connect them together, securing the Luer Lock fitting with a firm twisting action.
- Slowly open the clamp on the administration set, *to commence the flow of fluid to the veins.*
- Regulate the flow rate as prescribed *to maintain the prescribed fluid intake.*
- Ensure that the patient is left feeling as comfortable as possible *to help them continue to tolerate the intravenous therapy.* Comfort helps to reduce stress levels and promotes healing.
- Dispose of equipment safely *to prevent the transmission of infection.*
- Document this nursing practice by filling in the prescription and fluid balance charts and documenting the insertion of the cannula in line with local health authority and trust policy. This will include the date and time of insertion, the location and the type and size of cannula

inserted (Royal College of Nursing 2016). An intravenous cannulation care plan may be used for this process.

* Monitor the after-effects and report any abnormal findings immediately, *to ensure safe practice and enable prompt, appropriate medical and nursing intervention to be initiated as soon as possible.*
* Maintain the infusion at the prescribed flow rate *to continue the treatment.*
* The cannula insertion site and the immediate surrounding tissues must be observed and monitored at least once every shift (Royal College of Nursing 2016), *to identify and respond to signs of complications* (McCallum & Higgins 2012). The use of a recognized assessment scale, such as a Visual Infusion Phlebitis (VIP) score, can be used *to guide the management of the cannula* (Loveday et al. 2014).
* All the equipment connections should be inspected for disconnections, flaws or leakage *to prevent contamination or an air embolus.* The tubing should be inspected *to check there are no air bubbles.*
* Fluid balance charts should be accurately maintained *to enable accurate assessment of the patient's state of hydration.*
* In undertaking this practice, nurses are accountable for their actions, the quality of care delivered and record-keeping in accordance with *The Code* of the Nursing and Midwifery Council (2018).

2. PRIMING THE EQUIPMENT FOR INTRAVENOUS INFUSION

This involves the preparation of the prescribed infusion fluid by running it through the administration set. Asepsis should be maintained during this part of the practice *to prevent any internal or exposed areas being contaminated.*

⊚ EQUIPMENT

* Prescribed intravenous infusion fluid
* Patient's prescription chart
* Sterile administration set
* Receptacle for soiled disposable items
* Infusion stand

GUIDELINES AND RATIONALE FOR THIS NURSING PRACTICE

* Check the infusion fluid, which is prescribed by the medical practitioner. Each container of fluid is checked by either one registered nurse/medical practitioner or two people, one of whom must be a registered nurse or a medical practitioner (*see* 'Administration of Medicines', Ch. 2), depending on the local health authority and trust policy.
* Check the following details against the patient's own prescription documentation, the patient's identification band and the label on the infusion fluid *to make sure that the correct prescribed infusion is given:*
  * the patient's name and unit number
  * the date of the prescription
  * the type of infusion prescribed
  * the amount of infusion prescribed
  * the container labelled 'FOR INTRAVENOUS INFUSION'
  * the expiry date of the infusion fluid
  * the time prescribed for commencement of the infusion
  * the time to be taken for completion of the infusion
  * the signature of the medical practitioner.
* Check the fluid for cloudiness, sediment or discoloration. The container should be inspected for flaws, leaks or evidence of contamination. Any suspect fluid or containers must be discarded immediately, according to the healthcare provider's policy, *to prevent the introduction of infection or contamination, and to maintain a safe environment.*
* Document the signature of the nurse or medical practitioner checking the infusion prescription and record the batch number of the fluid in the documentation. Do this *to allow the particular infusion fluid administered to be identified, should the patient suffer any adverse effects.*

When Using a Soft Plastic Container (Bag)

* Perform the appropriate hand-washing technique and wear non-sterile gloves *to prevent infection* (Health Protection Scotland 2012).
* Remove the outer plastic packaging of the container *to prepare it for use.*
* Remove the administration set from its package *to prepare it for use.*
* Close the flow control clamp *to prevent any uncontrolled flow of fluid.*
* Using a non-touch technique, remove the protective covers from the inlet port on the fluid container and the administration set spike, *to maintain asepsis.*
* Insert the administration set spike firmly through the seal of the inlet port *to make the fluid flow into the first part of the administration set.*
* Hang the infusion fluid on the infusion stand, *so that gravity will aid the flow.*

- Gently squeeze the drip chamber of the administration set *to allow it to half-fill.*
- Slowly open the flow control clamp *to allow the fluid to fill the rest of the tubing slowly.* Once the fluid reaches the end of the tubing, close the flow control clamp. Ensure that no bubbles remain in the tubing, *to prevent any danger of air embolus.*
- Place the free end of the tubing in the notch provided on the flow control clamp *to protect the administration set from contamination.*
- Place the primed equipment on the infusion stand beside the patient's bed *to make it ready for connection to the intravenous cannula.*

The equipment should only be primed immediately prior to the infusion to minimize the risk of infection. If contamination occurs or the container is punctured while the equipment is being primed, the infusion and the administration set are discarded and the procedure recommenced.

When Using a Rigid or Semi-Rigid Plastic Container

- Maintain an aseptic non-touch technique as before.
- Using an administration set with an air vent, prepare it as before.
- Peel off the protective cover of the entry bung on the container.
- Insert the spike of the administration set into the entry bung on the container and twist firmly until the spike is completely inserted.
- Hang the container on the infusion stand *for gravity to aid the flow.*
- Open the air vent and proceed to prime the equipment as before.

3. MAINTAINING THE INFUSION FOR A PERIOD OF TIME

The number of drops per minute required for each particular infusion has to be accurately calculated *to maintain the flow of infusion at the prescribed rate.* Volumetric pumps are now used frequently.

GUIDELINES AND RATIONALE FOR THIS NURSING PRACTICE

Calculating the Flow Rate of Infusion Fluids

All administration sets include details of the number of drops delivered per millilitre for that particular set, this being known as the drop factor. This information is written on the packaging and can be used to calculate the flow rate needed.

The formula used for calculation is as follows:

$$\frac{\text{Total volume of infusion fluid}}{\text{Total time of infusion in minutes}} \times \text{Drops per mL (drop factor)} = \text{drops per minute}$$

Here is an example:
Total volume of fluid = 500 mL
Time for completion = 4 hours, i.e. 240 minutes (4 × 60)
Drop factor = 15
$\frac{500}{240} \times 15 = 31.25$ drops (approximately)

Thus the number of drops required to maintain the infusion at the required rate is 31 per minute when the drop factor is 15 drops per mL.

The position of the cannula in the vein and the movement of the patient's limbs may have an effect on the flow rate. **It is therefore important to assess visually the rate of fall of fluid in the infusion container, as well as to regulate the number of drops required per minute.** For example, when the time for completion is 4 hours, one-quarter of the fluid should have been infused after 1 hour and half the fluid after 2 hours.

Changing the Infusion Container

Within 24 hours, the empty container can be replaced with a full container of prescribed infusion fluid without changing the administration set, depending on the duration of infusion. The containers should be exchanged before the level of fluid drops below the point of the trocar in the neck of the container. Preparation for changing a container should begin while a small amount of fluid remains in the infusion container *to prevent the formation of air bubbles in the system and the danger of air embolus.*

- Explain the nursing practice to the patient *to gain consent and cooperation.*
- Perform hand-washing and maintain asepsis during this practice as before.
- Check the prescribed infusion fluid.
- Prepare the new container of infusion fluid as for priming the equipment.
- Temporarily turn off the infusion by closing the roller clamp.
- Remove the trocar of the administration set from the empty container and insert it into the new infusion fluid, maintaining asepsis.
- Recommence the infusion as soon as possible at the prescribed flow rate.
- Maintain observations as before.
- Dispose of the used container safely *to prevent the transmission of infection.*

- Document the nursing practice appropriately, monitor the after-effects and report any abnormal findings immediately *to ensure safe practice and enable prompt appropriate medical and nursing intervention to be initiated as soon as possible.*
- In undertaking this practice, nurses are accountable for their actions, the quality of care delivered and record-keeping in accordance with *The Code* of the Nursing and Midwifery Council (2018).

Removal of the Intravenous Cannula

This is performed using an aseptic technique when intravenous infusion is discontinued or when a new site for access is needed to continue an infusion. Routine resiting of cannulas is not recommended; they should be removed when complications occur or when they are no longer required (Loveday et al. 2014).

- Explain the procedure to the patient *to obtain consent and cooperation.*
- Ensure the patient's privacy, *respecting their individuality.*
- Close the flow clamp *to discontinue infusion of the fluid.*
- Prepare a trolley and sterile dressings as required, *to maintain a safe environment.*
- Apply non-sterile gloves *to protect against blood-borne infection.*
- Expose the site of insertion of the cannula, *maintaining asepsis.*
- Hold a sterile swab lightly over the entry site using the non-dominant hand and slowly withdraw the cannula with the dominant hand, applying pressure once it has been removed *to reduce the amount of bleeding.*
- Retain pressure on the puncture site as required *until the bleeding stops, maintaining asepsis.*
- Cover the site with a small sterile dressing, *to prevent infection.*
- Dispose of equipment safely *to prevent the transmission of infection.*
- Resume observation of the site as appropriate, *to monitor the healing process.*
- Document the time, date and reason for removal in the appropriate manner, monitor the after-effects and report any abnormal findings immediately, *to ensure safe practice.*
- In undertaking this practice, nurses are accountable for their actions, the quality of care delivered and record-keeping in accordance with *The Code* of the Nursing and Midwifery Council (2018).
- The tip of the cannula is occasionally sent to the laboratory for microbiological investigation. If this is ordered, the tip must be cut off with sterile scissors, put into an appropriately labelled sterile specimen container, maintaining asepsis, and sent to the appropriate laboratory with the completed laboratory form (*see* 'Diagnostic Investigations', Ch. 14).

PATIENT/CARER EDUCATION: KEY POINTS

In partnership with the patient and/or carer, ensure that they are competent to carry out any required practices. Information should be given on an appropriate point of contact for any concerns that may arise.

Explain the reason for the intravenous infusion to the patient. Emphasize the importance of not dislodging the intravenous cannula or dressing, and the dangers of disconnecting the giving set. They can reduce the likelihood of this occurring by keeping the cannulated limb as still as possible.

Advise the patient to notify you if they:

- experience any redness, swelling or pain at the cannulation site, which may be a sign of local infection or of dislodgement of the cannula
- observe that the intravenous infusion fluid container is empty
- hear an audible alarm sounding, if an electronic infusion device (pump) is being used
- require assistance in dressing or mobilization and are hampered in undertaking this because of the intravenous infusion.

REFERENCES

British National Formulary, 2018. https://bnf.nice.org.uk/.

Brooks, N., 2016. Intravenous cannula site management. Nursing Standard 30 (52), 53–62.

Health Protection Scotland, 2012. National Infection Prevention and Control Manual. Available from: https://www.nipcm.hps.scot.nhs.uk/.

Health Protection Scotland, 2014. Preventing infections when inserting and maintaining a peripheral vascular catheter (PVC). Available from: https://www.hps.scot.nhs.uk/haiic/ic/resourcedetail.aspx?id=660.

Loveday, H.P., Wilson, J.A., Pratt, R.J., et al., 2014. Epic3: national evidence-based guidelines for preventing healthcare-associated infections in NHS hospitals in England. Journal of Hospital Infection 86 (Suppl. 1), S1–S70.

McCallum, L., Higgins, D., 2012. Care of Peripheral venous cannula sites. Nursing Times 108 (34/35), 12, 14-15.

Medicines and Healthcare Products Regulatory Agency, 2013. Infusion Systems MHRA. London. Available from: https://assets.publishing.service.gov.uk/government/uploads/system/uploads/attachment_data/file/403420/Infusion_systems.pdf.

Nursing and Midwifery Council, 2018. The Code, Professional standards of practice and behaviour for nurses and midwives. NMC, London.

Royal College of Nursing, 2016. Standards for Infusion Therapy, fourth ed. RCN, London.

Smith, L., 2017. Choosing between colloids and crystalloids for IV infusion. Nursing Times 113 (12), 20.

Witt, B., 2011. Vein selection. In: Philips, S., Collins, M., Dougherty, L. (Eds.), Venepuncture and Cannulation. Wiley-Blackwell, Oxford.

SELF-ASSESSMENT

1. You are asked to assist the competent practitioner in the insertion of an intravenous cannula. List the equipment that will be required and outline the procedure as it should be undertaken.
2. Determine the differences between the various types of administration set and provide examples of the fluids that would be administered via each.
3. Outline the procedure for priming, connecting and administering an intravenous infusion of 1 L of 0.9% sodium chloride over 8 hours.
4. Describe how would you remove a peripheral intravenous cannula.

Lumbar Puncture

INDICATIONS AND RATIONALE FOR LUMBAR PUNCTURE

Lumbar puncture is the insertion of a specialized needle into the lumbar subarachnoid space to gain access to the CSF. This may be required:

- *to obtain a sample of CSF for investigative and diagnostic purposes*, e.g.:
  - a key investigation when diagnosing Alzheimer's disease (Engelborghs et al. 2017)
  - bacteriological investigation in patients suspected of having meningitis or encephalitis
  - cytological investigation in patients suspected of having a malignant tumour
- *to identify the presence of blood in the CSF* following trauma or a suspected subarachnoid haemorrhage
- *to introduce radio-opaque fluid into the subarachnoid space* for radiographic investigation
- *to identify raised intraspinal/intracranial pressure and provide relief*, if appropriate, by removing some of the CSF

- *to introduce intrathecal medication* such as cytotoxic agents or antibiotics.

The procedure may be performed on people who are inpatients or day patients, according to their clinical status. A lumbar puncture should not be performed if raised intracranial pressure is suspected, as the raised pressure might cause the brainstem tissue to herniate through the foramen magnum. This is known as 'coning' and could be fatal (Engelborghs et al. 2017).

OUTLINE OF THE PROCEDURE

A lumbar puncture is performed by a medical practitioner using an aseptic technique. The patient is helped into the correct position. An area of skin above the third, fourth and fifth lumbar vertebrae is prepared and cleansed with alcohol-based antiseptic solution prior to the administration of local anaesthesia. Once the local anaesthetic has taken effect, a special lumbar puncture needle is inserted between the third and fourth, or fourth and fifth, lumbar vertebrae in order to gain access to the subarachnoid space below the spinal cord in the region of the cauda equina (Fig. 23.1). The needle is hollow with a stilette to ease introduction to the subarachnoid space. Once in position, the stilette of the needle is removed. A disposable manometer is attached to the end of the needle via a two-way tap, and the CSF is allowed to flow into the manometer to record the intraspinal pressure. A normal CSF pressure is 60–150 mm H_2O. The pressure will fluctuate with respiration and heartbeat. Coughing will cause the pressure to rise.

When the pressure recording has been completed, the manometer is occluded and 2–3 mL of CSF is allowed to flow into each of the three separate sterile specimen containers as required, while still maintaining asepsis. The specimen containers should be pre-labelled as numbers 1, 2 and 3, as the first specimen may contain blood as a result of the needle being introduced. The containers should collect the specimens sequentially to avoid misinterpretation of results. The medical practitioner will note the colour, consistency and opacity of the CSF, as well as observing the presence or

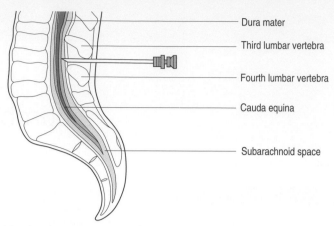

Fig. 23.1 Lumbar puncture: position of the needle in relation to the vertebrae.

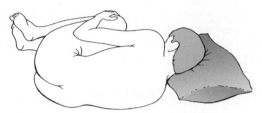

Fig. 23.2 Lumbar puncture: position of the patient. Reproduced with permission from Lindsay KW, Bone I: *Neurology and Neurosurgery Illustrated*, ed 4, Edinburgh, 2004, Churchill Livingstone (Elsevier).

absence of blood. On completion of this stage, the needle is removed, and the puncture site is covered by a small, sterile dressing or plastic sealant spray. Following this procedure, according to local policy and the patient's clinical status, appropriate neurological observations, wound site assessment and the monitoring of any localized pain or headache should be performed (Arevalo-Rodriguez et al. 2016).

Position of the Patient

The correct position is important in order to ensure the success and safety of this procedure. Patients should lie on their side on a firm bed with one pillow, stretching their lumbar vertebrae by flexing their head and neck and drawing their knees up to the abdomen, holding them with their hands (Fig. 23.2). The nurse can assist by supporting the patient behind the knees and the neck, and helping to maintain the extension of the lumbar vertebrae, thus widening the intervertebral space. This will help to ensure that the insertion and correct placement of the lumbar puncture needle are safely achieved. Once the needle is in position, the medical practitioner may ask patients to straighten their legs slowly without moving the position of their back. This

will reduce the intra-abdominal pressure, which can cause an abnormal reading of intraspinal pressure.

This procedure is occasionally performed with a patient sitting straddled on a chair and facing the back of the chair with their head resting on folded arms. This may be required for patients who are not comfortable lying on their side due to dyspnoea or obesity; however, there is evidence to support the theory that a sitting position may cause more severe headache during the procedure (Monserrate et al. 2015).

⊚ EQUIPMENT

- Trolley
- Sterile dressings pack
- Sterile drapes
- Sterile surgical gloves for the medical practitioner
- Lumbar puncture needles of appropriate size
- Spinal manometer
- Two-way tap
- Alcohol-based antiseptic lotion for cleansing the skin
- Local anaesthetic and equipment for its administration
- Syringe and needles for administering the local anaesthetic
- Sterile dressing, e.g. Airstrip or plastic sealant spray
- Three sterile specimen containers appropriately labelled and numbered 1, 2 and 3, completed laboratory forms, and a plastic specimen bag for transportation; these may be required for three separate samples of CSF for microbiological, biochemical and cytological investigation
- Receptacle for disposable items
- Sharps disposal container

LUMBAR PUNCTURE NEEDLE

This is a rigid stainless steel needle, available in sizes between 3.8 and 12.7 cm in length, complete with its own sharp-pointed stilette; this helps the passage of the needle into the correct position. Once the stilette has been removed, the blunt end of the needle lies within the subarachnoid space and should cause no damage to the tissues during the procedure. Needles are usually supplied with their own metal two-way tap but a Luer disposable tap may be used. The length and gauge of the needle will be dependent on the height and weight of the patient, the reason for the lumbar puncture and the experience of the medical practitioner undertaking the procedure.

Following a systematic review of the literature, Arevalo-Rodriguez et al. (2017) found that using needles with an atraumatic tip reduced the risk of headache following lumbar puncture. There is no significant evidence to support the theory that a larger or smaller atraumatic needle prevents post-procedure headache.

GUIDELINES AND RATIONALE FOR THIS NURSING PRACTICE

- Help to explain the procedure to the patient *to gain consent and cooperation, and to encourage participation in care.*
- Ensure the patient's privacy *to respect individuality and maintain self-esteem.*
- Help to collect and prepare the equipment *to ensure the procedure is performed efficiently.*
- Help the patient into the appropriate position and remain with them *to maintain that position and maximize safety during the procedure.*
- Help to prepare the sterile field *to maintain asepsis.*
- Observe the patient throughout this activity to monitor any adverse effects.
- Help to expose the lumbar region of the patient's back and assist the medical practitioner, as required, *to maintain asepsis and reassure the patient.*
- Hold the appropriate sterile containers to receive the flow of CSF as directed, *maintaining asepsis.*
- Once the needle has been removed, apply pressure to the site and cover with a sterile dressing or plastic sealant spray *to prevent leakage of the CSF and maintain asepsis.*
- Help the patient into a comfortable position once the procedure has been completed *to promote comfort and recovery from the procedure;* there is no evidence to support keeping the patient on bed rest to reduce the risk of headache (Arevalo-Rodriguez et al. 2017).

- Dispose of the equipment safely *to comply with health and safety issues and prevent transmission of infection.*
- Monitor the patient's conscious level *to observe for signs of possible brainstem herniation.*
- Monitor the patient's vital signs *to observe for abnormalities.*
- Document the procedure appropriately, monitor any after-effects and report abnormal findings immediately, *to ensure safe practice and enable prompt appropriate medical and nursing action to be initiated.*
- Immediately dispatch the labelled CSF specimens, with their completed forms, to the laboratory *to ensure that investigations are initiated and decisions about appropriate treatment made as soon as possible.*
- In undertaking this practice, nurses are accountable for their actions, the quality of care delivered and record-keeping according to The Code of the Nursing and Midwifery Council (2018).

ADDITIONAL INFORMATION

This is an invasive procedure that involves direct access to the spinal and brain tissue via the CSF. Asepsis should therefore be maintained during and after the procedure, and an adequate hand-washing technique should be practised to prevent cross-infection.

The puncture site should be observed for evidence of localized infection or leakage; accurate observations of the patient's condition will help to monitor any signs of developing infection.

Urgent medical attention must be sought if CSF leakage occurs.

The patient's general and neurological condition, e.g. disorientation, restlessness, drowsiness and nausea, should be noted. Any evidence of cerebral irritability should be observed. Fitting, twitching, spasticity or weakness of limb movements should be reported immediately and recorded. The patient's level of consciousness and vital observations should be recorded as prescribed, depending on their condition. Any rise in temperature that might indicate a developing infection should be reported. Neurological observations should be maintained according to local policy after this investigation (*see* 'The Patient with Impaired Consciousness', Ch. 37).

The patient may complain of a headache following this procedure. Analgesic medication should be administered as prescribed. The nurse should be observant for any non-verbal communication indicating pain, and anticipate the patient's needs as appropriate. The fact that the patient might experience discomfort should be explained.

A normal diet may be ordered as the patient's condition allows and an adequate fluid intake should be maintained following the procedure. Drinks should be easily accessible to the patient and specialized cups or straws used as appropriate.

The patient should have a short period of rest and then mobilize as directed. Mobilization should commence with the patient sitting up in bed for a period of time before progressing to further activity as the condition allows.

PATIENT/CARER EDUCATION: KEY POINTS

The reason for and the importance of the lumbar puncture for diagnostic or therapeutic purposes should be explained to the patient. This should include the fact that the investigation itself should have no long-term effects. The importance of staying in the correct position should be carefully explained and reinforced.

Following the lumbar puncture, the patient should understand the necessity of reporting a headache or any other adverse effects to the nursing staff. Patients who have the procedure performed as an outpatient should be given written instructions with advice on taking appropriate analgesia for headache, care of the puncture site and a contact telephone number in case of any adverse effects at home.

REFERENCES

Arevalo-Rodriguez, I., Ciapponi, A., Roqué i Figuls, M., et al., 2016. Posture and fluids for preventing post-dural puncture headache. The Cochrane Database of Systematic Reviews (3), CD009199.

Arevalo-Rodriguez, I., Muñoz, L., Godoy-Casasbuenas, N., et al., 2017. Needle gauge and tip designs for preventing post-dural puncture headache (PDPH). The Cochrane Database of Systematic Reviews (4), CD010807.

Engelborghs, S., Niemantsverdriet, E., Struyfs, H., et al., 2017. Consensus guidelines for lumbar puncture in patients with neurological diseases. Alzheimer's & Dementia: Diagnosis, Assessment & Disease Monitoring 8, 111–126.

Monserrate, A.E., Ryman, D.C., Shengmai Ma, M.S., 2015. Factors associated with the onset and persistence of post-lumbar headache. Journal of American Medical Association Neurology 72 (3), 325–332.

Nursing and Midwifery Council, 2018. The Code: Professional Standards of Practice and Behaviour for Nurses, Midwives and Nursing Associates. NMC, London. Available from: https://www.nmc.org.uk/globalassets/sitedocuments/nmc-publications/nmc-code.pdf. (Accessed 21 June 2019).

SELF-ASSESSMENT

1. Describe some of the indications for lumbar puncture.
2. Discuss the nurse's role in preparing the patient for lumbar puncture.
3. Why is it important to have specimen containers ready prior to the procedure?
4. Following the procedure, what observations should be made on the patient?
5. What information would a patient need, being discharged following lumbar puncture?

Mental State Assessment

The nursing process is a key framework for practice and involves four phases: assessing, planning, implementing and evaluating. This framework highlights the importance of assessment within nursing practice and suggests that all interventions should flow from the initial assessment phase. Nurses working in clinical practice regularly have to complete nursing assessments but sometimes feel ill-prepared and/or under-supported when expected to complete a mental state assessment (Giandinoto & Edward 2014). The ability to complete a mental state assessment is an important skill for all nurses, especially given the worldwide prevalence of mental health difficulties. Research examining the worldwide prevalence of mental health difficulties between 1980 and 2013 estimates that almost 18% of those taking part were thought to have had a mental health difficulty within the preceding 12 months, and 29% were thought to have had a mental health difficulty at some point in their lives (Steel et al. 2014). The high prevalence of mental health difficulties reported in this research gives an indication of how common mental health difficulties are in society and how many people/families are affected by mental health difficulties.

Nurses working outside mental health settings also have to be able to assess people's mental state because of the known link between physical health and mental health (van den Brink et al. 2014). People with mental health difficulties are at greater risk of physical health difficulties (Scott et al. 2016), and people living with long-term physical health difficulties are more likely to experience mental health difficulties (Doherty & Gaughran 2014). This link is important because not only do mental health difficulties increase the risk of developing other health difficulties (Scott et al. 2016), but also they are associated with high mortality rates (Walker et al. 2015). These factors highlight the need for all nurses to be able to assess mental state, regardless of their field of practice or nursing specialism. However, regular clinical supervision is required to help nurses develop and maintain competence in this area (Cutcliffe et al. 2018).

INDICATIONS AND RATIONALE FOR COMPLETING A MENTAL STATE ASSESSMENT

The 'mental state assessment' is a framework used in clinical settings to assess current mental health and/or diagnose mental health difficulties (Kareem & Ashby 2000). The mental state assessment can be completed at any stage during a care episode, but is often undertaken at the start of a care episode and used for care planning. A good mental state assessment involves establishing a safe environment, being empathic, promoting recovery, being collaborative and using effective communication skills (Lynch et al. 2012). There are many reasons for undertaking a mental state assessment:
- *to assess someone in the community following a new referral to a service*
- *to assess someone who has been admitted to hospital or presented at the accident and emergency department*

- *to assess someone following a recent change in mental health*
- *to assess someone because they are concerned about their own mental health.*

OUTLINE OF THE PROCEDURE

The mental state assessment involves using both observational and interview methods to gather information about a person's current mental state (Mansel and Bradley-Adams 2017). It usually involves assessing different elements, which are listed in Box 24.1. Some guidance is given here to help explain what each element might involve in practice. Remember that there is much variation in how mental state assessments are completed and that there is no firm agreement about what should be included and how the assessments should be carried out (Coombs et al. 2013). This section provides brief guidance for novice and/or inexperienced nurses undertaking mental state assessments. It is for illustrative purposes and not meant to be prescriptive. Nurses can use this framework when completing mental state assessments but should adapt their mental state assessment to reflect the clinical situation and purpose.

Assessing Appearance

A significant amount of information can be gathered through observing a person's appearance. This could include information about whether someone is able to attend to personal care and/or if they are neglecting themselves.

- Observe the appearance and consider whether they are well groomed and whether their clothing is appropriate (e.g. appropriate for the weather).
- Consider whether there is anything unusual about how they present (e.g. being especially thin might alert the assessor to the possibility of an eating disorder).

BOX 24.1 Mental State Assessment

- Appearance
- Speech
- Behaviour
- Mood
- Cognition
- Orientation
- Hallucinations
- Delusions
- Level of distress

From Coombs T, Crookes P, Curtis J: A comprehensive mental health nursing assessment: variability of content in practice, *Journal of Psychiatric and Mental Health Nursing* 20 (2):150–155, 2013, Table 1.

Assessing Speech

This observation can help determine whether there is anything different about how the person is speaking. Speaking faster than normal (e.g. possible pressure of speech) or slurring words (e.g. possible intoxication) might suggest a change in speech pattern and would provide useful assessment information.

- Observe how the person speaks during the assessment and determine whether the rate, rhythm and tone are normal for the person being assessed.
- Listen to the content of what the person is saying to evaluate whether the speech is coherent and/or appropriate for the situation.

Assessing Behaviour

This observation can give an indication of the level of distress experienced by the person being assessed and whether the person is over- or under-active.

- Observe the person being assessed and look for evidence of restlessness, agitation or tension.
- Observe daily routines and activity levels to determine whether the person is more or less active than usual.

Assessing Mood

The assessment of mood involves making the distinction between affect (how an emotion is expressed) and mood (how an emotion is experienced). Terms used to describe affects include: blunted, appropriate or labile. Mood can be described as depressed, calm or anxious.

- Assess mood/affect regularly to determine the person's current emotional state.
- Ask the person to describe how they currently feel.
- Ask the person to describe how they feel using one word (e.g. anxious, depressed, sad or angry).
- Ask the person to rate the intensity of this feeling using a 0–10 scale (i.e. 0 = mild and 10 = severe).
- Ask about how their mood is generally and whether they experience any severe mood changes.

Assessing Cognition

The cognitive element of the assessment involves evaluating a person's alertness, attention, concentration, memory and insight.

- Assess alertness by observing the person during the assessment.
- Assess attention and concentration by asking whether the person can read the paper and/or watch TV as usual.
- Ask the person whether they have noticed any changes in their attention and concentration.
- An informal assessment of short-term memory could involve asking someone to remember three items (e.g.

pen, watch, clock) and then asking them to recall the items after 5 minutes.
- Another informal short-term memory assessment might involve asking someone what they did earlier in the day.

Assessing Orientation

This involves checking whether the person being assessed is orientated in time, place and person.
- Ask the person to state the day, month and year.
- Ask the person to state where they are (e.g. can you tell me where you are, what room you are in, and what floor of the building?)
- Ask the person to recall the name of the assessor and/or a family member who is with them.

Assessing Hallucinations

Hallucinations and other perceptual disturbance can occur in certain types of mental health difficulty (e.g. psychosis). Hallucinations can affect any of the senses (e.g. sight, sound, smell, taste, touch) and might include hearing voices, seeing things that are not there or smelling unusual smells. When assessing mental health, it is important to ask whether the person being assessed has ever experienced hallucinations and to gather as much detail as possible about the nature and extent of any current hallucinations. It is worth asking when the hallucinations occur (e.g. only at night or when alone), how long they go on for (e.g. constant or intermittent), what form they take (e.g. hearing voices or smelling excrement), what happens (e.g. they get anxious or smoke cannabis), and what the person thinks about the experience (e.g. that they are being controlled by higher power or there are covert forces who are going to harm them).
- Have you ever heard voices or seen things that other people did not?
- What happens?
- Can you tell me about the experience?
- When does this happen?
- What makes it happen?
- Does anything make it better or worse?
- What do you think about this?

Assessing Delusions

A delusion is a false belief held strongly by someone in the face of contradictory evidence, which is not in keeping with their cultural background. Delusional thinking can occur when someone is having difficulty with their mental health and is associated with certain kinds of mental health difficulty (e.g. psychosis). Delusional thinking is sometimes termed either grandiose or persecutory in nature.
- Do you ever believe something sinister is happening?
- Do you worry that people are trying to harm you or others?

- Do you know things other people find hard to understand or believe?
- Do you ever think you are gifted or special in some way?

Assessing Level of Distress

Assessing the level of distress is important to determine whether the mental health difficulties are having a negative impact on the person's life. Not all people will experience the same level of distress, and the level of distress will vary over time. This means that it is important to gauge the current level of distress and consider how this compares to normal for that person. An important element of this section of the mental state assessment is evaluating risk. During the mental state assessment, it is important to consider the risk of self-harm, suicide and harm to others (Coombs et al. 2013). It is important for the nurse to ask explicitly about the risk of self-harm, suicide and harm to others. During the assessment the assessor will need to decide whether to complete a full risk assessment and/or refer to specialist services (Bolster et al. 2015).
- Do you have any thoughts of suicide (or self-harm)?
- Do you have a plan to harm yourself (or others)?
- Do you intend to harm yourself (or others)?
- What do you intend to do?
- What could we do to stop you harming yourself (or others)?

◎ EQUIPMENT

A mental state assessment can be completed using very little equipment. Nurses will sometimes take notes using a pen and paper, but it is important for the note-taking not to get in the way of the mental state assessment. If the nurse focuses too much on taking notes during the mental state assessment, it can be difficult to listen properly to the person being assessed.

GUIDELINES AND RATIONALE FOR THIS NURSING PRACTICE

- Read the referral details *to establish the reason for referral and to ensure that you are assessing the right person* (Luu et al. 2016).
- Find a suitable time and place for the assessment, *to ensure that the venue is safe and comfortable during the assessment.*
- Start well by introducing yourself to the person being assessed and explaining what the assessment will involve (Guest 2016).
- Gain consent and explain confidentiality *to promote professionalism* (Nursing and Midwifery Council 2018).
- Establish a rapport and adopt a collaborative approach (Lynch et al. 2012).

- Use effective interpersonal skills and an empathic approach *to build a therapeutic relationship* (Coombs 2011).
- Complete the assessment interview and observations necessary for the mental state examination (Mansel & Bradley-Adams 2017).
- Include explicit questioning about potential risk to self and others (Bolster et al. 2015).
- Look for strengths and promote recovery (Xie 2013).
- Involve the person being assessed (and their family/carers) by asking their opinion and preferences, and including them in the decision-making process (Nursing and Midwifery Council 2018).
- Decide whether you need further information and consider if a comprehensive mental health assessment is required (Coombs et al. 2013).
- Develop a useful formulation or final assessment *to help guide future interventions* (Coombs et al. 2011).
- Explain what is going to happen after the assessment, *to keep the person informed about their care* (Nursing and Midwifery Council 2018).
- Document the assessment using the SBAR approach (situation, background, assessment and recommendations) (Wacogne & Diwaker 2010).

REFERENCES

Bolster, C., Holliday, C., Oneal, G., Shaw, M., 2015. Suicide assessment and nurses: what does the evidence show? Online Journal of Issues in Nursing 20 (2).

Coombs, T., Crookes, P., Curtis, J., 2013. A comprehensive mental health nursing assessment: variability of content in practice. Journal of Psychiatric and Mental Health Nursing 20 (2), 150–155.

Coombs, T., Curtis, J., Crookes, P., 2011. What is a comprehensive mental health nursing assessment? A review of the literature. International Journal of Mental Health Nursing 20 (5), 364–370.

Cutcliffe, J.R., Sloan, G., Bashaw, M., 2018. A systematic review of clinical supervision evaluation studies in nursing. International Journal of Mental Health Nursing.

Doherty, A.M., Gaughran, F., 2014. The interface of physical and mental health. Social Psychiatry and Psychiatric Epidemiology 49 (5), 673–682.

Giandinoto, J.A., Edward, K.L., 2014. Challenges in acute care of people with co-morbid mental illness. British Journal of Nursing 23 (13), 728–732.

Guest, M., 2016. How to introduce yourself to patients. Nursing Standard 30 (41), 36.

Kareem, O.S., Ashby, C.A., 2000. Mental state examinations by psychiatric trainees in a community NHS trust. The importance of a standardised format. Psychiatric Bulletin 24 (3), 109–110.

Luu, N.P., Pitts, S., Petty, B., et al., 2016. Provider-to-provider communication during transitions of care from outpatient to acute care: a systematic review. Journal of General Internal Medicine 31 (4), 417–425.

Lynch, J.M., Askew, D.A., Mitchell, G.K., Hegarty, K.L., 2012. Beyond symptoms: defining primary care mental health clinical assessment priorities, content and process. Social Science & Medicine 74 (2), 143–149.

Mansel, B., Bradley-Adams, K., 2017. 'I AM A STAR': a mnemonic for undertaking a mental state examination. Mental Health Practice 21 (1), 21.

National Institute for Health and Care Excellence, 2011a. Common mental health problems: identification and pathways to care. Available at: https://www.nice.org.uk/guidance/cg123/ifp/chapter/common-mental-health-problems.

National Institute for Health and Care Excellence, 2011b. Service user experience in adult mental health: improving the experience of care for people using adult NHS mental health services. Available at: https://www.nice.org.uk/guidance/cg136/chapter/Introduction.

Nursing and Midwifery Council, 2018. The Code: Professional Standards of Practice and Behaviour for Nurses, Midwives and Nursing Associates. London: NMC. Available at: https://www.nmc.org.uk/globalassets/sitedocuments/nmc-publications/nmc-code.pdf.

Public Health England, 2018. Wellbeing and mental health: applying all our health. Available at: https://www.gov.uk/government/publications/wellbeing-in-mental-health-applying-all-our-health/wellbeing-in-mental-health-applying-all-our-health.

Scott, K.M., Lim, C., Al-Hamzawi, A., et al., 2016. Association of mental disorders with subsequent chronic physical conditions: world mental health surveys from 17 countries. JAMA Psychiatry 73 (2), 150–158.

Steel, Z., Marnane, C., Iranpour, C., et al., 2014. The global prevalence of common mental disorders: a systematic review and meta-analysis 1980–2013. International Journal of Epidemiology 43 (2), 476–493.

van den Brink, A.M., Gerritsen, D.L., Voshaar, R.C.O., Koopmans, R.T., 2014. Patients with mental–physical multimorbidity: do not let them fall by the wayside. International Psychogeriatrics 26 (10), 1585–1589.

Wacogne, I., Diwakar, V., 2010. Handover and note-keeping: the SBAR approach. Clinical Risk 16 (5), 173–175.

Walker, E.R., McGee, R.E., Druss, B.G., 2015. Mortality in mental disorders and global disease burden implications: a systematic review and meta-analysis. JAMA Psychiatry 72 (4), 334–341.

Xie, H., 2013. Strengths-based approach for mental health recovery. Iranian Journal of Psychiatry and Behavioral Sciences 7 (2), 5.

SELF-ASSESSMENT

1. What is the purpose of a mental state assessment?
2. What are the main elements covered within a mental state assessment?

25

Neurological Assessment and Seizure Management

There are two parts to this chapter:
1. Neurological examination.
2. Management of an adult patient who is having a seizure.

1. NEUROLOGICAL EXAMINATION

INDICATIONS AND RATIONALE FOR NEUROLOGICAL EXAMINATION

A full neurological examination involves assessment of the patient's mental status, i.e. level of consciousness (see Ch. 37), cranial nerves, motor and sensory function, reflexes, pupillary responses, cerebellum and vital signs (including respiratory rate, heart rate, temperature, blood pressure and pain assessment). The purpose of the neurological examination is to gather objective data on the functional state of the patient's neurological system (Hickey 2014). This may be required to:
- aid in the diagnosis of neurological disease
- monitor the effect or progression of neurological disease
- evaluate the effectiveness of treatments and interventions during the course of a neurological disease.

OUTLINE OF THE PROCEDURE

This chapter outlines examination of the cranial nerves, and the motor and sensory function of the patient's trunk and limbs. This procedure is carried out by a medical or skilled nurse practitioner (Hickey 2014).

Assessing the Function of the Cranial Nerves

To assess the olfactory nerve (I), the patient is asked to identify the odours of strong-smelling substances, e.g. lavender oil or peppermint oil (Hickey 2014).

The function of the optic nerve (II) is assessed by testing the patient's visual acuity and visual fields. For the visual field test, the practitioner faces the patient, sitting 1-metre away. Each of the patient's eyes is tested separately. The practitioner covers their own left eye, while the patient, with assistance from a nurse if required, covers their right eye. The practitioner holds a pen at arm's length, outside of the field of vision, while instructing the patient to fix their gaze on the practitioner's eyes. As the practitioner advances the pen slowly from outside of the field of vision into the centre, the patient is asked to verbalize when they first see the pen. Loss of field of vision is indicated if the practitioner notes the pen before the patient does. The four quadrants of peripheral vision are tested. Reliable assessment requires the practitioner to have a normal field of vision (Bowie & Woodward 2011a).

The ophthalmoscope is used to observe the health of the inner structures of the eye (Hickey 2014). The patient's eyeball and eyelid movements are observed to assess the function of the oculomotor (III), trochlear (IV) and abducens (VI) cranial nerves. A pen torch is used to assess unilateral and consensual pupillary reactions.

The sensory function of the trigeminal (V) nerve is examined by touching the skin on both sides of the patient's face. A non-sterile swab is stroked across the skin. Variable pressure is applied using a Neurotip™ to observe the patient's ability to discriminate between blunt and sharp sensations (Bowie & Woodward 2011a).

The sensory function of the facial (VII) nerve is assessed by asking the patient to taste and identify various substances, e.g. salt, sugar, vinegar and lemon juice. To prevent inaccurate results, the patient is asked to use a mouth rinse after each substance is tasted (Bowie & Woodward 2011a).

An auriscope is used to examine the ears, while the function of the vestibulocochlear (VIII) cranial nerve is assessed using a tuning fork.

Assessing the Motor and Sensory Function of the Trunk and Limbs

An assessment of the patient's sensation of pain, light touch and temperature is made using a Neurotip™, a piece of gauze and test tubes containing hot and cold water.

A tendon hammer is used when testing a spinal reflex, such as the knee jerk. Assessment of reflexes also requires the use of the pointed end of the tendon hammer for stroking the lateral aspect of the sole of the patient's foot (Bowie & Woodward 2011b). Testing of the muscle strength of each limb is performed by asking the patient to push against the practitioner and grading the strength of the outcome using the Medical Research Council Muscle Strength Grading System (Fig. 25.1) (Medical Research Council 1976; Bowie & Woodward 2011b).

Grade	Muscle state
0	No contraction
1	Flicker or trace of contraction
2	Active movement with gravity eliminated
3	Active movement against gravity
4	Active movement against gravity and resistance
5	Normal power

Data from the Medical Research Council

Fig. 25.1 Medical Research Council Muscle Strength Grading System, MRC 1976. Reproduced with permission from the Medical Research Council.

EQUIPMENT

- Ophthalmoscope
- Pen
- Pen torch
- Auriscope
- Tuning fork
- Neurotip™ (neurological examination tip)
- Non-sterile swab
- Test tubes (filled with hot and cold water)
- Small containers of various strong-smelling substances, e.g. peppermint and lavender oil
- Tendon hammer
- Small samples of salt, sugar, lemon juice and vinegar
- Glass of water for rinsing the patient's mouth
- Trolley or tray for equipment
- Receptacle for used mouth rinse
- Receptacle for soiled disposable items
- Sharps bin to dispose of the Neurotip
- Personal protective equipment, including examination gloves and disposable aprons

GUIDELINES AND RATIONALE FOR THIS NURSING PRACTICE

- Explain the procedure to the patient *to obtain consent* (Nursing and Midwifery Council 2018). Care should be person-centred, and patients should be encouraged to be active partners in their care (McCormack & McCance 2016).
- Wash your hands *to prevent cross-infection* (World Health Organization 2018; Health Protection Scotland 2016).
- Wear personal protective equipment, as appropriate, *to prevent cross-infection and to break the chain of infection* (NHS Education for Scotland 2017).
- Prepare the equipment *to ensure that all the equipment is available, clean and ready for use.*
- Observe the patient throughout the neurological examination for any signs of discomfort or distress. *The nurse should intervene immediately in the event of an adverse reaction* (Nursing and Midwifery Council 2018).
- Protect the patient's privacy and provide reassurance, *to reduce anxiety.*
- Assist the patient into a comfortable position, *firstly to protect the patient's dignity and comfort, and secondly to assist the practitioner to obtain reliable and accurate results for each part of the examination* (Nursing and Midwifery Council 2018).
- The patient may require assistance with further positional changes as the examination progresses, depending on the patient's level of independence and ability.

- Assist the medical practitioner during the examination *to enhance the overall quality of the procedure and protect patient safety* (Nursing and Midwifery Council 2018).
- At the end of the examination, ensure that the patient is left feeling comfortable, *to maintain the quality of the nursing practice.*
- Decontaminate or dispose of the equipment safely in accordance with local policy *to reduce risks to health and safety.*
- Remove all personal protective equipment and dispose of it safely in accordance with local policy, *to prevent cross-infection* (NHS Education for Scotland 2017).
- During and at the end of the procedure ensure that all practitioners observe the five moments of hand hygiene by decontaminating hands at appropriate intervals, *to break the chain of infection* (World Health Organization 2018).
- After the procedure, document the nursing practice appropriately, continue to monitor the patient and report any abnormal findings immediately, *to provide a written record and assist in the implementation of any action, should an abnormality or adverse reaction to the practice be noted* (Nursing and Midwifery Council 2018).
- Nurses are accountable for their actions and inactions, the quality of care delivered and the standard of record-keeping in accordance with *The Code* (Nursing and Midwifery Council 2018).

PATIENT/CARER EDUCATION: KEY POINTS

In partnership with the patient and/or carer, ensure that they are competent to carry out any practices required. Provide the patient and/or carer with information about an appropriate point of contact, should any concerns arise.

The medical practitioner will explain the procedure to the patient to enable consent to be obtained. The nurse should act as an advocate, ensuring that the patient is provided with enough information to provide consent for the examination (Nursing and Midwifery Council 2018).

The results of the examination should be explained and discussed with the patient, to enable a person-centred plan of care to be developed (McCormack & McCance 2016; Hickey 2014).

2. MANAGEMENT OF AN ADULT PATIENT WHO IS HAVING A SEIZURE

A seizure is *'clinical manifestation of presumed or proved abnormal electrical activity in the brain … rang[ing] from a fleeting subjective experience such as déjà vu or a twitch (myoclonic jerk) through to a tonic–clonic convulsion'* (Angus-Leppan 2014: p. 1).

People with epilepsy experience frequent seizures. Seizures associated with epilepsy have recently been reclassified in the International Classification of Seizure Types by the International League Against Epilepsy (2017) (Fisher et al. 2017), based on three characteristics:
- site of seizure onset
- level of awareness during a seizure
- further features of a seizure.

See Fig. 25.2 for an outline summary of types of seizure.

Establishing the location of seizure onset is important because this can be used to guide treatments like choice of medication or surgery. For example, 'focal seizures' begin in a discrete region of neurons on one side of the brain, while 'generalized seizures' begin on both sides of the brain.

'Level of awareness' replaces the term 'level of consciousness' with reference to seizures because 'awareness' can be assessed with greater ease (Fisher et al. 2017; Falco-Walter et al. 2018). Level of awareness correlates directly with patient safety during a seizure (Fisher et al. 2017). 'Focal-aware' is the term used to describe a seizure that starts in one distinct area of the brain, the patient is aware and can interact throughout the seizure; 'Focal impaired awareness' is the term used when a seizure starts in an area of the brain and the patient's awareness is compromised. For example, they may be able to hear, but loose the ability to understand, respond or react. In 'generalized seizures' awareness is always compromised and patients will have no recollection of the events (Fisher et al. 2017). Other types of seizure include 'focal motor seizures', where there is movement associated with the seizure, e.g. jerking or twitching movements, or automatisms (such as lip-smacking) (Falco-Walter et al. 2018). 'Focal non-motor seizures' refer to seizures in which altered sensations or emotions are involved. 'Auras' are short-lasting, occurring at the beginning of a seizure; they involve sensory or psychic experiences (Angus-Leppan 2014; England & Pluegar 2014).

Generalized seizures can be classified as 'motor' or 'non-motor'. 'Generalized motor seizures' include tonic–clonic seizures (convulsion), which are characterized by three phases: prodromal, tonic–clonic and post-ictal. During the 'prodromal phase' the patient may feel irritable or tense, and may experience an aura, but some patients have no warning prior to loss of awareness (England & Pluegar 2014). During the 'tonic–clonic phase', the patient may elicit an ictal cry, experience loss of muscle tone and drop to the ground (England & Pluegar 2014). The body becomes rigid and tonic (stiffens) with rhythmical (clonic) shaking of all four limbs, the torso and the face. The jaw tightens and the patient may bite their tongue. Apnoea induces cyanosis and

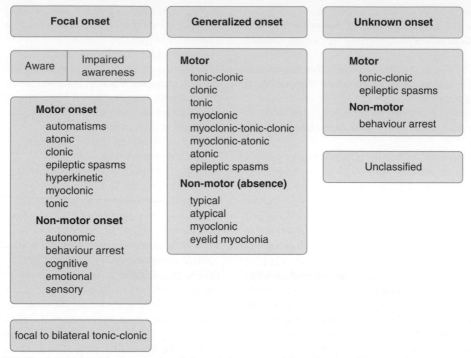

Fig. 25.2 The International League Against Epilepsy's International Classification of Epileptic Seizures, expanded version, 2017. Reproduced with permission from the International League Against Epilepsy (Fisher et al. 2017).

the patient may be incontinent of urine (Angus-Leppan 2014). Tonic–clonic seizures last anything from 1 to 2 minutes. The 'post-ictal phase' spans more than 10 minutes, during which time the patient is drowsy and confused, having an inability to concentrate and a reduced capacity to communicate. Patients can feel fatigued and will forget the event (England & Pluegar 2014).

'Generalized non-motor seizures' refer to 'absences', which last seconds and are associated with disturbances in awareness, activity and possibly deterioration in ability to learn. Absences can occur a few times to several hundred times throughout the day. During an absence attack the patient will not reply when their name is called and they will appear to be staring into space (Angus-Leppan 2014; England & Pluegar 2014).

Aside from epilepsy, seizures can occur at random for a number of other different reasons, including:

• metabolic anomalies, eg hypoglycaemia or hypoxia.
• underlying cardiac or respiratory problems
• drug interactions or toxicities
• alcohol withdrawal
• cerebral infections or space-occupying lesions
• fever (England & Pluegar 2014).

The cause of a seizure must be established and the patient needs to be managed effectively to prevent further seizure

activity (Angus-Leppan 2014). Loss of awareness during seizures carries a risk of other injuries, including falls, head injuries, burns or fractures due to the unpredictable onset of seizure activity (Dickson et al. 2018). Recognizing a seizure is vital to enable first aid to be provided (England & Pluegar 2014).

GUIDELINES AND RATIONALE FOR THIS NURSING PRACTICE

If you observe a patient having a seizure, it is essential to maintain patient safety.

• Remain calm and use the 'DR.ABC' approach (*see* Ch. 18), *to give priority to maintaining the patient's airway, breathing and circulation* (Resuscitation Council UK 2017).
• Avoid placing anything into the patient's mouth during a seizure, *to avoid bite injuries to yourself and to prevent damage to the patient's teeth* (England & Pluegar 2014).
• Stay with the patient for the duration of the seizure, protecting them from physical injury, *to prevent any further physical harm and to observe the progression of the seizure carefully* (England & Pluegar 2014).
• With assistance, once the seizure ends and it is safely possible to do so, position the patient into the recovery

position *to prevent aspiration of oral secretions* (England & Pluegar 2014). This may require the use of additional pillows. Use suction equipment if required and available.

- Carefully note the time of onset and duration of the seizure. Report details of the seizure activity to medical staff and document these on the patient's chart and within their notes (Nursing and Midwifery Council 2018). If this is the patient's first seizure, observers' accounts can assist medical staff with diagnosis (Angus-Leppan 2014; Gloss & Krumholz, 2016). Detail signs that may have preceded the seizure, and note how the patient looked at onset and any changes as the seizure developed. Observe the patient's level of consciousness. Consider if the patient was capable of verbalizing, if their eyes were open, and if there were changes in pupillary size, shape and symmetry. Note whether their eyeballs deviated to the side.
- Support medical staff in caring for the patient by preparing and administering any medications that are prescribed and preparing the patient for any tests or procedures (Nursing and Midwifery Council 2018).
- Within the 'DR.ABC' framework, obtain the patient's vital signs as appropriate (respiratory rate, oxygen saturations, pulse, body temperature and blood pressure; establish their blood glucose level), *to maintain patient safety and to assist medical staff with establishing correctable causes for seizure activity* (Resuscitation Council (UK) 2017).
- Continue to monitor the patient in the post-ictal phase, establishing their recall of events; **if they are confused, disorientated or drowsy, they are at risk of further injury to themselves** (England & Pluegar 2014).
- Assess the severity of any injuries that may have been sustained and seek further medical advice as required.
- Promote the patient's dignity and function as a patient advocate (Nursing and Midwifery Council 2018). Explain the events and any care that is required to the patient *to obtain consent* (Nursing and Midwifery Council 2018). Care should be person-centred, and patients should be encouraged to be active partners in their care (McCormack & McCance 2016).
- Reassure relatives or significant others who are present, *to maintain a calm environment and reduce unnecessary distress for the patient.*
- Continue to observe the patient for further seizure activity and take active measures *to maintain a safe environment for the patient.* Ensure that the patient is further risk-assessed for slips, trips and falls, for pressure ulceration risk and for bed rails; complete the necessary documentation and update the care plan accordingly (Nursing and Midwifery Council 2018).

PATIENT/CARER EDUCATION: KEY POINTS

Self-management is key to stability in the long-term management of seizures associated with epilepsy. Patients, care-givers, friends and work colleagues should be involved in education programmes to support the patient to self-manage. A number of self-help groups and websites are available to help patients and carers to learn about the complexities of managing epilepsy.

The patient and care-giver will need to understand the need to adhere consistently to anti-epileptic drug regimes and engage with therapeutic drug monitoring practices, while learning to identify factors that trigger seizure activity.

Carers will be required to maintain a seizure diary to enable patients to self-regulate their condition. Seizure activity may fluctuate during times of acute illness, as fever can lower the seizure threshold. Various devices are available to detect seizure activity while the patient is sleeping.

Carers will be expected to learn basic life support measures and how to administer seizure-relieving medications, e.g. rectal diazepam (England & Pluegar 2014).

Many adaptations may be required to enable the patient to cope with their activities of daily living. For example, patients may have restrictions placed on their ability to drive or operate machinery, which may have implications for employment; they may also be advised to shower rather than taking baths (Angus-Leppan 2014).

There is evidence to suggest that many patients who experience seizures are admitted to hospital when they could be managed just as effectively at home. A hospital stay can be disruptive and distressing for the patient (Osborne et al. 2015). Carer education is vital to enable the patient to self-manage their condition.

Status epilepticus refers to a seizure lasting longer *'than 5 minutes, or two or more consecutive seizures that occur without complete recovery between them'* (England & Pluegar 2014: p. 661). Status epilepticus is an emergency situation, and the patient requires urgent medical attention structured around the 'DR.ABC' approach (*see* Ch. 18) to manage the airway, arrest the seizure activity, and establish and correct precipitating factors (Manno 2011).

REFERENCES

Angus-Leppan, H., 2014. First seizures in adults: clinical review. British Medical Journal 348, 1–8.

Bowie, I., Woodward, S., 2011a. Assessment, interpretation and management of cranial nerve dysfunction. In: Woodward, S.,

Mestecky, A. (Eds.), Neuroscience Nursing: Evidence-Based Approach. Wiley-Backwell, Oxford.

Bowie, I., Woodward, S., 2011b. Assessment, interpretation and management of altered perceptual motor and sensory function. In: Woodward, S., Mestecky, A. (Eds.), Neuroscience Nursing: Evidence-Based Approach. Wiley-Blackwell, Oxford.

Dickson, J., Asghar, Z., Siriwardena, N., 2018. Pre-hospital ambulance care of patients following a suspected seizure: a cross-sectional study. Seizure: The Journal of the British Epilepsy Association 57, 38–44.

England, K., Plueger, M., 2014. Seizure and epilepsy. In: Hickey, J. (Ed.), The Clinical Practice of Neurological and Neurosurgical Nursing, 7th ed. Lippincott Williams and Wilkins. Philadelphia, PA.

Falco-Walter, J., Scheffer, I., Fisher, R., 2018. The new definition and classification of seizures and epilepsy. Epilepsy Research 139, 73–79.

Fisher, R., Cross, J., French, J., et al., 2017. Operational classification of seizure types by the International League Against Epilepsy: Position Paper of the ILAE Commission for Classification and Terminology. Epilepsia 58 (4), 522–530. doi:10.1111/epi.13670. Available at: https://www.epilepsydiagnosis.org/doc/Fisher_et_al-2017-Seizure_Types-Epilepsia.pdf.

Gloss, D., Krumholz, A., 2016. Managing an unprovoked first seizure in adults. CNS Drugs 30, 179–183.

Health Protection Scotland, 2016. Standard Infection Control Precautions Literature Review: Hand Hygiene. Hand Washing. Available at: https://www.nipcm.hps.scot.nhs.uk/documents/sicp-hand-hygiene-hand-washing-in-the-hospital-setting/.

Hickey, J., 2014. Neurological assessment. In: Hickey, J. (Ed.), The Clinical Practice of Neurological and Neurosurgical Nursing, 7th ed. Lippincott Williams and Wilkins. Philadelphia, PA.

McCormack, B., McCance, T., 2016. Person-Centred Practice in Nursing and Health Care: Theory and Practice, 2nd ed. John Wiley & Sons, Chichester.

Manno, E., 2011. Status epilepticus: current treatment strategies. The Neurohospitalist 1 (1), 23–31.

Medical Research Council, 1976. Aids to examination of the peripheral nervous system. Memorandum no. 45. Her Majesty's Stationery Office, London.

NHS Education for Scotland, 2017. Personal Protective Equipment. Available at: https://www.nes.scot.nhs.uk/education-and-training/by-theme-initiative/healthcare-associated-infections/training-resources/personal-protective-equipment-(ppe).aspx.

Nursing and Midwifery Council, 2018. The Code: Professional Standards of Practice and Behaviour for Nurses, Midwives and Nursing Associates. NMC, London. Available at: https://www.nmc.org.uk/globalassets/sitedocuments/nmc-publications/nmc-code.pdf.

Osborne, A., Taylor, L., Reuber, M., et al., 2015. Prehospital care after a seizure: evidence base and United Kingdom guidelines. Seizure: The Journal of the British Epilepsy Association 24, 82–87.

Resuscitation Council (UK), 2017. Advanced Life Support, 7th ed. Resuscitation Council (UK), London.

World Health Organization, 2018. Five moments for hand hygiene. Available at: https://www.who.int/gpsc/tools/Five_moments/en/.

❓ SELF-ASSESSMENT

1. Which cranial nerves control movement of the eyeballs and eyelids?
2. What techniques are used to assess the patient's responses to touch, pain and temperature?
3. During a neurological examination, how is the muscle strength of a patient's limbs assessed?
4. Discuss the role of the nurse in relation to neurological examination.
5. Outline and discuss the priorities of care for managing a patient who is having a seizure.
6. With reference to relevant underlying anatomy and physiology, provide a rationale for determining the blood glucose level of a patient who is having a seizure.
7. Critically analyse the role of the nurse in supporting self-management in the patient with long-term seizure activity due to epilepsy.

26

Nutrition

There are three parts to this chapter:
1. Feeding a dependent patient
2. Enteral nutrition
3. Parenteral nutrition.

1. FEEDING A DEPENDENT PATIENT

LEARNING OUTCOMES

By the end of this chapter, you should be able to:
- prepare the patient for this nursing practice
- collect and prepare the equipment
- carry out the feeding of a dependent patient.

BACKGROUND KNOWLEDGE REQUIRED

- Revision of the anatomy and physiology of the mouth and oesophagus, with special reference to the physical acts of mastication and swallowing

INDICATIONS AND RATIONALE FOR THE FEEDING OF A DEPENDENT PATIENT

The nurse may be required to feed a dependent patient *to maintain adequate nutrition* in:
- a patient who is unable to use their upper limbs because of paralysis, neuropathy or serious illness
- a patient who has lost upper limb coordination because of physical or mental illness
- a patient who is visually impaired
- a patient who has an oral or facial injury
- a patient who is acutely delirious.

EQUIPMENT

- Feeding utensils: e.g. fork, knife and spoon, drinking cup with a spout or cup with an angled straw; include any items recommended by speech and language therapists or occupational therapists
- Cloth, disposable napkin or paper towel
- Diet, as ordered by the patient, or recommended by the dietitian and/or speech and language therapist
- Trolley or tray for equipment
- Apron
- Receptacle for soiled disposable items

GUIDELINES AND RATIONALE FOR THIS NURSING PRACTICE

In hospital or at home, this practice may be undertaken by the patient's relatives or carers.
- Explain the nursing practice to the patient *to gain consent and cooperation.*
- Collect and prepare the equipment *to ensure that all the equipment is available and ready for use.*
- Help the patient into a comfortable upright position *to allow easy access to the patient and also to allow the patient to maintain their position during the practice.*
- Observe the patient throughout this activity *to note any signs of distress, such as a cough or gurgly voice.*
- Wash your hands and put on an apron *to maintain general hygiene and to reduce the risk of cross-infection.*
- Keep the food not being eaten at a suitable temperature where possible, *to ensure patient satisfaction and enjoyment.*
- Remind the patient of their ordered menu *to permit psychological preparation for the food.*
- When possible, sit down while feeding the patient *to make this an enjoyable social occasion.*

- Ask the patient which food they wish to eat first, *to give the patient some control over the activity.*
- Offer the food to the patient at a rate set by them, *to avoid hurrying them while they are eating, which may induce nausea or vomiting.*
- Place the spoon or fork accurately into the patient's mouth *to prevent gagging or choking.*
- Offer sips of fluid during the meal *to aid in the mastication and swallowing of the food.*
- Discontinue feeding when asked by the patient *to prevent a feeling of distension and excessive fullness.*
- Assist the patient with mouth care following the meal *to promote dental health and possibly reduce the incidence of dental caries.*
- Ensure that the patient is left feeling as comfortable as possible, *to maintain the quality of this nursing practice.*
- Dispose of equipment safely *to reduce any health hazard.*
- Document the nursing practice appropriately, monitor the after-effects and report any abnormal findings immediately, *to provide a written record and assist in the implementation of any action, should an abnormality or adverse reaction to the practice be noted.*
- In undertaking this practice, nurses are accountable for their actions, the quality of care delivered and record-keeping according to *The Code* (Nursing and Midwifery Council 2018).

PATIENT/CARER EDUCATION: KEY POINTS

Advice on a healthy dietary intake and the benefits of such a diet should be given by the registered dietitian to both the patient and the carers. The nurse should reinforce any information and education given by the registered dietitian regarding the constituents of any special diet that is required by the patient.

The involvement of occupational therapists should be considered, as they can assess individuals who have a functional limitation that prevents them from eating independently to maintain their nutritional requirements. Speech and language therapist involvement should be considered for patients with oropharyngeal swallowing difficulties and/or communication problems.

Information regarding the maintenance of oral health should also be given by the nurse. Dental care is important and good oral health is essential for maintaining a satisfactory nutritional status.

2. ENTERAL NUTRITION

LEARNING OUTCOMES

By the end of this chapter, you should be able to:
- prepare the patient for this nursing practice
- collect and prepare the equipment
- describe the principles of enteral feeding
- outline some of the problems of enteral feeding.

BACKGROUND KNOWLEDGE REQUIRED

- Revision of the anatomy and physiology of the gastrointestinal tract
- Revision of the nutritional requirements of the human body

INDICATIONS AND RATIONALE FOR ENTERAL FEEDING

Enteral feeding is the introduction of the daily nutritional requirements, in liquid form, directly into a patient's stomach or small intestine by means of a tube. The tube may be inserted through the nostril and passed down into the stomach, or introduced directly into the stomach or small intestine via a surgical incision made in the abdominal wall.

Enteral feeding may be performed *to maintain adequate nutrition* in the following circumstances:
- obstruction of the oesophagus or gastric outflow, e.g. by a neoplasm
- loss or impairment of the swallowing reflex
- oesophageal or abdominal fistula
- preoperative preparation of malnourished patients
- during radiotherapy or chemotherapy treatment
- postoperatively, after some types of oral, abdominal or oesophageal surgery
- some unconscious or sedated patients
- severe burns.

Enteral feeding can be administered via an enteral feeding pump or by bolus using an enteral feeding syringe. It is given through a fine-bore tube that is attached to an enteral feeding administration set, which is then attached to the prescribed liquid feed. Enteral feeding may also be introduced via a self-retaining tube such as a radiological image-guided gastrostomy (RIG) or percutaneous endoscopic gastrostomy (PEG) tube via a surgical opening in the abdominal wall into the stomach or jejunum. The prescribed liquid feed is available ready-prepared, which can greatly reduce the potential of healthcare-associated infection (National Institute for Health and Care Excellence 2017).

ENTERAL FEEDING VIA A FINE-BORE NASOGASTRIC TUBE AS AN INTERMITTENT BOLUS OR CONTINUOUS PUMP SYSTEM

◎ EQUIPMENT

- Fine-bore nasogastric tube: size 8 or 10 Ch (or Fg) or 10
- Sterile water
- Hypoallergenic tape
- Prescribed liquid enteral feed
- Enteral feeding administration set
- Intravenous infusion stand
- Volumetric feeding pump
- Enteral syringe: 50 mL
- pH indicator strips: to test human gastric aspirate
- Receptacle for soiled disposable items

GUIDELINES AND RATIONALE FOR THIS NURSING PRACTICE

- Explain the nursing practice to the patient *to gain consent and cooperation.*
- Collect and prepare the equipment *to maintain efficiency of practice.*
- Where possible, assist the patient to sit upright with their head well supported and chin tilted downwards *to facilitate tube position.*
- Observe the patient throughout this activity *to detect any signs of discomfort or distress.*
- Insert the fine-bore feeding tube and confirm placement using pH indicator strips. A small amount of stomach contents is aspirated and placed on the pH indicator strip (NHS Improvement 2016). A pH of 5.5 or less indicates that stomach contents have been aspirated and the tube is safe for immediate use. If pH is greater than 5.5 or no gastric aspirate can be aspirated, then an X-ray is required *to confirm the position of the tube.*
- Attach the container of prepared feed to the infusion stand and join the feeding administration set to the container using an aseptic non-touch technique (Rowley et al. 2010).
- Insert the giving set into the feeding pump and prime the set, allowing the feed to run through to the end of the set before it is connected to the feeding tube, *to ensure that minimal air is introduced into the patient's stomach.*

- Ensure that the rate of flow is as prescribed *to avoid the patient's stomach becoming over-distended and producing feelings of nausea.*
- When intermittent bolus feeding is the method of choice, use an enteral syringe to flush the tube with 50 mL of water at the end of the bolus feed *to clear the tube.*
- Ensure that the patient is left feeling as comfortable as possible, *to maintain the quality of this practice.*
- Record appropriately the time of commencement of feeding and the amount and type of feed given, monitor the after-effects and report any abnormal findings immediately, *to provide a written record and assist in the implementation of any action, should an abnormality or adverse reaction to the practice be noted.*
- In undertaking this practice, nurses are accountable for their actions, the quality of care delivered and record-keeping according to *The Code* (Nursing and Midwifery Council 2018).

Single-use fine-bore tubes for continuous enteral feeding are hypoallergenic, and polyurethane- and latex-free; they are available in sizes 8 and 10 Ch (or Fg). They are more comfortable for the patient than wide-bore tubes and less likely to cause ulceration, inflammation, stricture, haemorrhage and erosion of the mucosa (Best 2013; Kurtis 2013). They can remain in place for 90 days before they require renewing.

ENTERAL FEEDING VIA A GASTROSTOMY/ JEJUNOSTOMY TUBE

See Fig. 26.1.

EQUIPMENT

- Sterile water
- Enteral syringe
- Prepared prescribed liquid feed
- Enteral feeding pump, if required
- Enteral feeding administration set, if required
- Intravenous infusion stand, if required
- Receptacle for soiled disposable items

GUIDELINES AND RATIONALE FOR THIS NURSING PRACTICE

- Explain the nursing practice to the patient *to gain consent and cooperation.* Where possible, patients should be encouraged to be active partners in care.
- Assist the patient into a suitable position, e.g. semi-recumbent, *to allow easy access to the gastrostomy site*

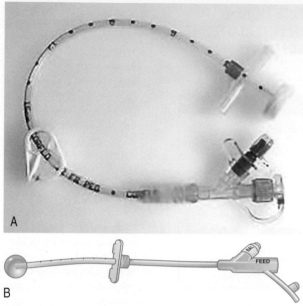

Fig. 26.1 Enteral feeding: examples of gastrostomy tubes. (A) Percutaneous endoscopic gastrostomy (PEG). (B) Radiological image-guided gastrostomy (RIG).

and to lessen the risk of a kink in the tube. Ideally, the patient should not lie flat, as this increases the risk of reflux and aspiration.

- Observe the patient throughout this activity *to detect any signs of discomfort or distress.*
- Collect and prepare the equipment *to maintain efficiency of practice.*
- Insert the administration set into the prescribed feed in an aseptic manner and then attach the pump, if required, *to prevent infection.*
- Prime the set to expel all the air *to prevent unnecessary air being introduced into the stomach, which can cause pain and distension.*
- The plastic cap at the end of the administration set should remain in place at this time *to prevent infection.*
- Flush the tube with about 10–50 mL of sterile water using an enteral feeding syringe *to ensure that the tube is patent.*
- Set the flow to the prescribed rate.
- Disconnect the administration set when all the feed has been delivered.
- Flush the tube using an enteral syringe with sterile water *to clear the tube.*
- Ensure that the patient is left feeling as comfortable as possible, *to maintain the quality of this practice.*

- Dispose of the equipment safely *to reduce any health hazard.*
- Record appropriately the time and amount and type of feed administered, monitor the after-effects and report any abnormal findings immediately, *to provide a written record and assist in the implementation of any action, should an abnormality or adverse reaction to the practice be noted.*
- In undertaking this practice, nurses are accountable for their actions, the quality of care delivered and record-keeping in accordance with *The Code* (Nursing and Midwifery Council 2018).

PATIENT/CARER EDUCATION: KEY POINTS

A clear explanation of the necessity for this form of feeding will help to gain the patient's cooperation.

If the patient is self-administering feeds, the importance of hygiene needs to be stressed (National Institute for Health and Care Excellence 2017).

The feeding pattern recommended by the registered dietitian also needs to be agreed with the patient.

3. PARENTERAL NUTRITION

LEARNING OUTCOMES

By the end of this chapter, you should be able to:
- prepare and support the patient for this nursing practice
- collect and prepare the equipment
- assist the medical practitioner with the insertion of a central venous catheter
- maintain an infusion of parenteral nutrition for a period of time in an acute hospital or community setting.

BACKGROUND KNOWLEDGE REQUIRED

- Revision of the anatomy and physiology of the cardiopulmonary system, with special reference to the circulation of the blood, and the veins of the neck and upper thorax
- Revision of the nutritional needs to maintain health
- Revision of 'Intravenous therapy' (see Ch. 22) and 'Outline of the Procedure' (see later).
- Revision of aseptic technique (see Ch. 40)
- Revision of the 'Infection Prevention and Management' (see Ch. 20)
- Review of local policies regarding parenteral nutrition in both community and institutional care

INDICATIONS AND RATIONALE FOR PARENTERAL NUTRITION

Parenteral nutrition is the intravenous infusion of essential nutrients when the gastrointestinal tract cannot be used (British Association for Enteral and Parenteral Nutrition 2016a). *It may be indicated for anyone who is unable to ingest, digest or absorb sufficient oral or enteral feeding*, e.g.:
- patients who have had surgery involving major resection of the intestine, as they will have a reduced ability to digest food
- patients who have extensive inflammatory disease of the alimentary system, as inflammation of the gut reduces the efficiency of the digestive process
- patients who have gastrointestinal malabsorption problems because, despite a reasonable intake, an inadequate amount of nutrients will be absorbed and available for growth, development and repair of tissues and as a source of energy (Ojo 2017)
- patients who have severe nausea, vomiting and/or mucositis, e.g. following chemotherapy for malignant disease; the intake of adequate food will be compromised

with a resulting increased risk of weight loss, sepsis or bacteraemia (Arends 2018).

'Parenteral nutrition' is the term used when all the patient's nutritional requirements are given by a central venous catheter. However, it has been demonstrated that some parenteral nutrition solutions can be infused for a short time using a peripheral vein access route. Parenteral nutrition may also be given as a supplement to, or as a bridge to, nasogastric or oral feeding.

OUTLINE OF THE PROCEDURE

The procedure for intravenous line insertion is usually performed at the bedside or within the vascular access department. The position of the patient is important during this procedure and depends on the choice of entry site for the intravenous catheter. There are three main access choices:
- Central venous catheter (CVC), non-tunnelled (subclavian or internal jugular veins): the patient lies supine with no pillow, and the neck is extended. The head is rotated away from the site of entry and is well supported in position. The head of the bed is lowered by 10 degrees. This position is important to prevent the development of an air embolus.
- Tunnelled CVC (tCVC) (Hickman line): the patient lies supine with no pillow, and the neck is extended. The head of the bed is lowered by 10 degrees.
- Peripherally inserted central catheter (PICC): the patient lies supine. The chosen arm is extended, with the palm upwards and the elbow supported. PICCs introduced via the cephalic or basilic vein are increasingly being used as technology advances.

The insertion of the intravenous catheter for the infusion of parenteral nutrition is performed by appropriately trained practitioners using an aseptic technique. Personal protective equipment is worn and refers to the following equipment: gloves, apron, eye protection, face shield and face mask (NHS Education for Scotland 2017). Having washed their hands, the practitioner puts on a theatre gown and gloves, and prepares the sterile equipment on the trolley, maintaining asepsis. When the patient is in the correct position (the bed/trolley must have the facility to place the patient in the head-down tilt position, termed the Trendelenburg position), sterile drapes are placed round the area of the access site. A local anaesthetic is usually administered. The skin area of the preferred access site is cleansed prior to the insertion, and following insertion the lumens are flushed with sterile sodium chloride solution. The tube is stitched securely in position and then the access site is covered with a sterile dressing.

A central venous catheter can also be tunnelled subcutaneously so that the entry site to the vein is separated from the skin entry site; this will reduce the risk of infection. This option is chosen when long-term parenteral nutrition is envisaged (Pittiruti et al. 2009).

The concentration of nutrients is an irritant to peripheral vessels and could cause damage to peripheral veins. The infusion fluid enters the circulation, is rapidly diluted by the volume of blood entering the heart and is quickly distributed by the circulation, thus reducing any problems around irritation of the vessels involved.

EQUIPMENT

- As for intravenous infusion (*see* Ch. 22)

Additional Equipment
- Personal protective equipment: sterile surgical gown, gloves, hat, mask and goggle/visor (operator and assistant)
- Sterile drape for trolley, medium drapes and fenestrated drape for patient
- Access to oxygen and suction points
- Patient monitoring equipment
- Near-bedside resuscitation equipment
- Portable ultrasound, sterile probe cover and sterile gel
- 2% chlorhexidine in 70% alcohol for cleansing the skin
- 0.9% sodium chloride vials
- Sterile catheter: appropriate for the site of entry used, e.g. Hickman catheter or triple- or quadruple-lumen catheter
- Sterile needle-free connectors for each lumen and appropriate sutures
- Sterile semi-permeable transparent dressing

PARENTERAL NUTRITION FORMULATION

Parenteral nutrition solutions are supplied by manufacturers complete or as a multi-chamber preparation. Vitamins, trace elements, minerals and water may be added to both regimens; this must be done under controlled aseptic pharmaceutical laboratory conditions (British Association for Parenteral and Enteral Nutrition 2016b). The administrations will be prescribed by the medical practitioner for each 24-hour period according to the patient's nutritional needs and related blood biochemistry.

An adequate supply of micronutrients is essential for patients on parenteral nutrition to prevent deficiencies (British Association for Parenteral and Enteral Nutrition 2016b). Such requirements will vary on an individual patient

basis and will depend on underlying clinical conditions and previous nutritional state:
- carbohydrates, e.g. dextrose
- fats, e.g. Intralipid
- nitrogen, e.g. amino acids such as glutamine.

Many products are available, the choice depending on the patient's needs and the pharmaceutical contractual arrangements within each health board/authority. A number of commercial pharmaceutical companies provide ready-prepared combined parenteral infusion bags for a 24-hour period.

The following may also be added:
- vitamins: some are destroyed by sunlight and so if these are added to a 24-hour parenteral infusion, the container must be covered by a dark bag to exclude light
- electrolytes, e.g. potassium and phosphates
- trace elements, e.g. zinc and magnesium.

TUNNELLED CVC: HICKMAN LINE

A Hickman intravenous catheter may be chosen by the medical practitioner for a parenteral infusion that is needed over the longer term. This radio-opaque silastic catheter has a small, sponge-like Dacron cuff at its distal end. The Hickman line is tunnelled subcutaneously and the cuff helps to retain the line in position as fibrous tissue forms around it. Home parenteral nutrition is required for some patients and they receive extensive training in care and maintenance (British Association for Parenteral and Enteral Nutrition 2016b). It is recommended that parenteral nutrition should be provided only in specialized centres where a coordinated multidisciplinary service is available (British Association for Parenteral and Enteral Nutrition 2016b).

A Hickman line can also be used for the administration of intravenous cytotoxic medications that are prescribed over a long period and which are not suitable for a peripheral infusion because of their irritant properties.

VOLUMETRIC INFUSION DEVICE

Parenteral nutrition should be infused using a continuous volumetric infusion pump. This ensures that the prescribed nutrients are infused at the prescribed rate, suitable for the patient's metabolism. Infusion pumps are primed with a suitable giving set and then attached to an infusion catheter. There are clear manufacturer's instructions for all infusion pumps, which should be followed when setting up infusions.

Infusion pumps can normally be set to give an hourly flow rate of between 1 and 999 mL per hour. All pumps are fitted with a digital readout of details of the infusion and an alarm system that monitors for any occlusion of the lines, air bubbles and completion of the prescribed fluid. New equipment for the controlled administration of intravenous infusion is continually being developed. There are different types of infusion pump available; the choice may depend on the individual health board/authority policy.

GUIDELINES AND RATIONALE FOR THIS NURSING PRACTICE

- Help to explain the procedure to the patient *to gain consent and cooperation, and to encourage participation in care* (British Association for Parenteral and Enteral Nutrition 2016a).
- Ensure the patient's privacy, *to respect individuality and maintain self-esteem.*
- Collect and prepare the equipment *to maintain efficiency of practice.*
- Check the prescribed parenteral nutrition preparation (*see* 'Administration of Medicines', Ch. 2).
- Wash your hands and apply personal protective equipment *to reduce cross-infection* (NHS Education for Scotland 2017).
- Using an aseptic non-touch technique (Rowley 2010), prime the equipment (*see* 'Intravenous Therapy', Ch. 22).

- Help the patient into the appropriate position, depending on the site of entry used for the insertion of the central venous catheter, *to maintain optimum safety for the patient.*
- Observe the patient throughout this activity *to monitor any adverse effects.*
- Commence the infusion of parenteral nutrition at the prescribed rate.
- The infusion is usually covered with a dark bag *to protect any vitamins from light, which may cause their deterioration.*
- Ensure that the patient is left feeling as comfortable as possible *to reduce anxiety and stress.*
- Refer to the infusion device manufacturer's instructions *to maintain the infusion as prescribed.*
- Dispose of the equipment safely *to maintain a safe environment.*
- Document the nursing practice appropriately, monitor the after-effects and report any abnormal findings immediately *to ensure safe practice and enable prompt and appropriate medical and nursing intervention to be initiated.*
- In undertaking this practice, nurses are accountable for their actions, the quality of care delivered and record-keeping according to *The Code* (Nursing and Midwifery Council 2018).

PATIENT/CARER EDUCATION: KEY POINTS

Inpatient parenteral nutrition: explanations about parenteral nutrition, given before, during and after the line has been inserted, as well as the rationale for continuing parenteral nutrition, will help the patient to understand and interpret the condition and its treatment. The nurse should be sensitive to the timing and relevance of the information for each stage of this practice.

Home parenteral nutrition (HPN): in partnership with the patient/parent/carer, an evaluation is made to ensure that they are competent to carry out any practices required, including the principles of asepsis, basic gut and vascular anatomy, the complications of parenteral nutrition and information about their underlying illness. Patients requiring long-term therapy should understand the importance of reporting redness, swelling or pain at the catheter site or any feeling of being generally unwell. Information should be given on an appropriate point of contact for any concerns that may arise.

The HPN team will assess the ability of the patient/parent/carer to perform all aspects of the HPN procedure. This will include teaching the relevant aspects of:

- aseptic technique
- care of the CVC
- observation of the site
- preparation of the intravenous feed
- use of the volumetric infusion pump.

Patient education and all aspects of the discharge planning timeframe will vary greatly and depend on each individual's requirements, underlying medical condition(s) and home circumstances. The nutrition nurse assigned to provide HPN education will organize the discharge and communicate with the community team involved. Written information in the form of a patient information leaflet will be provided, reinforcing the patient/parent/carer's knowledge and confidence.

A relevant contact telephone number to use as a 'helpline' will further improve the patient's confidence and independence.

REFERENCES

Arends, J., 2018. How to feed patients with gastrointestinal Mucositis. Current Opinion in Supportive and Palliative Care 12, 1–6.

Best, C., 2013. Nasogastric tube insertion in adults who require enteral feeding. Nursing Standard 21 (40), 39–43.

British Association for Parenteral and Enteral Nutrition, 2016a. Standards and Guidelines for Nutritional Support of Patients in Hospital. BAPEN, Maidenhead.

British Association for Parenteral and Enteral Nutrition, 2016b. Current perspectives on parenteral nutrition in adults. BAPEN, Maidenhead. Available from: https://www.bapen.org.uk/nutrition-support/parenteral-nutrition.

Kurtis, K., 2013. Caring for adult patients who require nasogastric feeding tubes. Nursing Standard 27 (18), 47–56.

National Institute for Health and Care Excellence, 2017. Nutrition Support for Adults: oral nutrition support, enteral tube feeding and parenteral nutrition, CG32. Available from: https://www.nice.org.uk/Guidance/cg32.

NHS Education for Scotland, 2017. Personal Protective Equipment. Available at: https://www.nes.scot.nhs.uk/education-and-training/by-theme-initiative/healthcare-associated-infections/training-resources/personal-protective-equipment-(ppe).aspx.

NHS Improvement, 2016. Nasogastric Tube Misplacement: Continuing Risk of Death and Severe Harm. NSPA NHS/PSA/RE/2016/006. NHS Improvement, Edinburgh.

Nursing and Midwifery Council, 2018. The Code: Professional Standards of Practice and Behaviour for Nurses, Midwives and Nursing Associates. NMC, London. Available at: https://www.nmc.org.uk/globalassets/sitedocuments/nmc-publications/nmc-code.pdf.

Ojo, O., 2017. The Role of Nutrition and hydration in disease prevention and patient safety. British Journal of Nursing 26 (8), 1020–1022.

Pittiruti, M., Hamilton, H., Biffi, R., et al., 2009. ESPEN Guidelines on Parenteral Nutrition: Central venous Catheters (access, care, diagnosis and therapy of complications). Clinical Nutrition: Official Journal of the European Society of Parenteral and Enteral Nutrition 28, 365–377.

Rowley, S., Clare, S., Macqueen, S., Molyneux, R., 2010. ANTT v2: an updated practice framework for aseptic technique. British Journal of Nursing 19 (5).

WEBSITES

https://www.bapen.org.uk *British Association for Parenteral and Enteral Nutrition*

https://www.nmc-uk.org *Nursing and Midwifery Council*

https://www.rcn.org.uk *Royal College of Nursing*

www.scottishpatientsafetyprogramme.scot.nhs.uk

 SELF-ASSESSMENT

1. When is it necessary to feed a patient?
2. Outline the procedure for feeding a patient.
3. Under what circumstances is it considered necessary to commence enteral feeding?
4. In what ways is enteral feeding administered?
5. When is parenteral nutrition used?

Oral Hygiene

INDICATIONS AND RATIONALE FOR MOUTH CARE

Mouth care is the use of a toothbrush and paste, a mouthwash or other mouth-cleaning preparation to help the patient to maintain the cleanliness of their teeth or dentures and to encourage the flow of saliva to maintain a healthy oropharyngeal mucosa. Good oral health is crucial to meeting fundamental human needs, such as comfort, nutrition, communication and acceptable personal appearance (NHS Quality Improvement Scotland 2004; Best & Hitchings 2015). This nursing practice is also known as oral hygiene and may be required:

- for patients who have not eaten for a period of time or whose diet is restricted, as the reduction in mastication decreases the flow of saliva; this may occur during the preoperative or postoperative period, especially in patients who have undergone oral or abdominal surgery
- for patients who are dehydrated for any reason, as the normal flow of saliva will be reduced
- for patients suffering from nausea or vomiting, as they will be reluctant to eat
- for patients being treated with oxygen therapy, particularly if unhumidified oxygen is being used, as it has a drying effect on the oral mucosa
- for patients who are having radiotherapy or cytotoxic medication for malignant disease, as this may adversely affect the cells of the oral mucosa (NICE 2018)
- for patients with any form of facial paralysis or muscle weakness, as the inability to masticate adequately reduces the flow of saliva and may cause food debris to be retained in the mouth; this may include an unconscious patient or one in the terminal stages of illness
- for patients who have poor manual dexterity or cognitive impairment (Health Education England 2016)
- for patients with an oral infection such as candidiasis.

There is limited research on the frequency of mouth care, which will vary for each individual. The use of an effective oral assessment tool is strongly advised to ensure the early detection of problems within vulnerable patient groups (Bissett & Preshaw 2011). Intensive mouth care may be carried out every 2 hours, whereas mouthwashes may only be required two or three times a day, but frequency should be based on the individual assessment. It is important to note that if some mouthwash products are used inappropriately, they can cause damage to oral mucosa. Products containing chlorhexidine are neutralized by toothpaste and these should not be used together (Health Education England 2016).

◎ EQUIPMENT

- Tray or trolley
- Plastic gloves (non-sterile)
- Pencil torch
- Spatula
- Toothbrush
- Toothpaste
- Container for dentures: for institutional care this should be appropriately labelled
- Beaker
- Bowl or receiver
- Towel or other protective covering
- Mouthwash solution
- Soft tissues for wiping the mouth
- Receptacle for disposable items

Additional Equipment for Specialized Mouth Care as Required
- Mouth-care pack or equivalent equipment
- Foam sticks
- Cotton buds
- Prescribed medication, e.g. an antifungal agent if thrush is diagnosed
- Solution for mouth cleaning
- Lubrication for lips, e.g. Petroleum jelly or lip balm
- Suction equipment

TOOTHBRUSH AND TOOTHPASTE

The patient's own equipment may be used if it is available; otherwise, a soft, small-headed nylon brush and toothpaste can be supplied. This is usually the most appropriate equipment for this nursing practice (Health Education England 2016). Patients should be assisted to brush their teeth if this is possible, using the technique illustrated in Fig. 27.1 to ensure maximum plaque removal and to preserve gum integrity.

FOAM STICKS

Sponge sticks should not be used to clean the patient's teeth or gums, as they do not remove dental plaque. There is also evidence that the sponge head can become detached from the stick and become a choking hazard (Medicines and Healthcare Products Regulatory Agency 2012). Many organizations have banned their use.

SOLUTIONS TO BE USED AS MOUTHWASHES

Various solutions are available, professional knowledge, individual prescription and patient preference influencing the choice. All the solutions used should be clearly labelled and diluted according to their instructions. The procedure

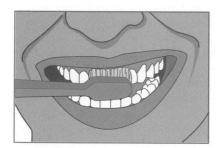
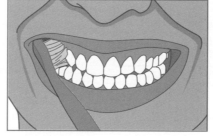
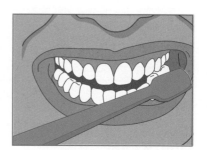
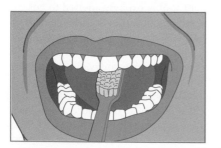
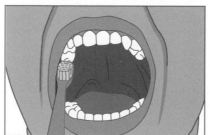
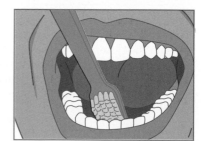

Fig. 27.1 Mouth care: correct method of brushing.

for checking the preparation is as for 'Administration of Medicines' (see Ch. 2).

Saline

This can be made up using common salt: 1 level teaspoon (approximately 4.5 g) in 500 mL of water. It is also available in sterile sachets. Saline is an effective mouthwash for patients who have had oral surgery, especially dental extractions.

Sodium Bicarbonate

This may be made up immediately prior to use: 1 level teaspoon of powder in 500 mL of water. Sodium bicarbonate is a useful mouthwash for dissolving mucus and debris. A stronger solution can be used for soaking dentures before cleaning them.

Chlorhexidine

Chlorhexidine is often used by patients with gum disease or those who have had oral surgery, as it has anti-bacterial properties (Health Education England 2016). It should always be used as directed and in line with medicines management policy.

Water

This may be the most refreshing and appropriate mouthwash to use after brushing the teeth.

OTHER AIDS FOR MOUTH CARE (IF PERMITTED)

Soda Water

This may be appreciated as an alternative mouthwash.

Ice Cubes

These may be sucked, but the number should be limited if the patient has a restricted oral intake.

Saliva Substitutes

These are useful for the treatment of a dry mouth (Health Education England 2016).

Soft Paraffin/Lip Salves

These prevent the lips becoming dry and cracked. Water-soluble gels are recommended for patients receiving oxygen therapy (NICE 2018).

Solutions for Mouth Cleaning

Any mouthwash solution can be used for mouth cleaning, as can solutions that actively stimulate the flow of saliva. The most efficient method of mouth cleaning remains, however, a mild toothpaste applied with a soft, small-headed toothbrush (Health Education England 2016).

Mouth-Care Packs

A prepared sterile pack is used when intensive mouth care is needed when a mouthwash alone or tooth-brushing is not appropriate. The pack may contain:

- a plastic tray divided into compartments to hold the mouth-cleaning solution
- gauze swabs.

If a pack is not available, a sterile mouth-care tray can be assembled using:

- a foil tray
- a gallipot
- gauze swabs.

Please refer to the local policy in relation to the use of foam sticks or cotton sticks within the clinical area.

The mouth-care pack should be covered, labelled with the patient's name and the date, cleaned and replenished after use, and replaced every 24 hours or as required. In the patient's own home, equipment can be adapted appropriately, maintaining a safe environment.

GUIDELINES AND RATIONALE FOR THIS NURSING PRACTICE

- Explain the nursing practice to the patient *to gain consent and cooperation, and to encourage participation in care,* ensuring that there is some understanding of this practice.
- Collect and prepare the equipment *to ensure an efficient use of time and resources.* Some solutions are more effective if prepared immediately before use.
- Ensure the patient's privacy *to respect their individuality and maintain self-esteem.*
- Help the patient into a comfortable sitting position, either in bed or on a chair, *to help patient cooperation and promote as much independence as possible.* It is sometimes possible for patients to sit comfortably in front of a washbasin in either their own home or an institution.
- Place some protective material over the patient's chest and under the chin *to protect the clothes.* The patient's own towel can be used.
- Observe the patient throughout this activity *to monitor any adverse effects.*
- Apply clean plastic gloves after efficient hand-washing *to prevent contamination with body fluids and to maintain a safe environment.*
- It is advisable to wear gloves for all mouth care, as it may involve direct contact with the oral mucosa and oral secretions.

- Ask or help the patient to remove their dentures and place them in a bowl of clean water (labelled if necessary) *to gain access and a clear view of the oral cavity.*
- Examine the patient's mouth and tongue using the torch and spatula, *to observe the condition of the teeth, dentures, tongue, lips, gums and mucous membrane.* Note any food debris, any ulcers or sores, and the condition of the lips (Health Education England 2016).
- If possible, discuss with the patient the most suitable and acceptable mouth care for their particular needs *to promote individualized care and aid compliance.*
- Help patients to clean their teeth or dentures with their toothbrush and toothpaste.
- Offer a suitable mouthwash, explaining that it should not be swallowed, and help to hold the equipment as necessary to rinse the mouth until all the debris and cleaning paste have been removed.
- Offer tissues for drying the mouth.
- Help to apply lubrication to the lips as required *to maintain the integrity of the skin of the lips.* This can be done by placing the lubricant on a gloved finger and applying it directly, or patients may apply it themselves, *to encourage independence.*
- Return the patient's clean dentures in a bowl of clean water and encourage the patient to wear them *to maintain the shape of the oral cavity.*
- Ensure that the patient is left feeling as comfortable as possible. A period of rest should ideally be encouraged after this nursing practice.
- Dispose of equipment safely *to maintain a safe environment.*
- Document the nursing practice appropriately and immediately report any deterioration or improvement in the condition of the mouth, as well as abnormal findings. Do this *to enable changes in practice to be implemented to maintain optimum mouth care for each patient.*
- In undertaking this practice, nurses are accountable for their actions, the quality of care delivered and record-keeping according to *The Code* (Nursing and Midwifery Council 2018).

Intensive Mouth Care for Dependent Patients

- Explain the nursing practice *to gain the patient's consent and cooperation* if possible.
- Ensure the patient's privacy *to respect individuality.*
- Help the patient into a comfortable position *to help them tolerate the practice.*
- Collect and prepare the equipment, including the mouth-cleaning pack or tray.
- Put on clean plastic gloves *to prevent contamination with body fluids.*

- Remove dentures if present *to gain access and a clear view of the oral cavity.*
- Examine the patient's mouth as before.
- Clean all round the mouth, gums and tongue with the mouth-cleaning solution, using a soft toothbrush if possible, *to help to dislodge debris and remove plaque* (Daly & Smith 2015).
- Help the patient to use a mouthwash if possible, or rinse the mouth with a gauze swab soaked in mouthwash solution, allowing the patient to suck it. For patients with a wired mandible following oral surgery, a syringe of mouthwash in conjunction with suction may be used. This will require good cooperation from the patient and an adequate swallowing reflex to prevent inhalation of the rinsing fluid.
- Help the patient to clean their dentures, or clean them for the patient, using a toothbrush and toothpaste, and under a running tap if possible, *to retain a healthy oral mucosa.*
- Proceed with the nursing practice as before.

Mouth Care for an Unconscious Patient

The dentures should have been removed, cleaned, appropriately labelled and stored with the patient's belongings on admission (*see* 'The Patient with Impaired Consciousness', Ch. 37). Mouth-care guidelines are as for a dependent patient, with the following exceptions:

- Position the patient on their side, with no pillow and the head supported, *to prevent secretions or mouth-cleaning solution flowing into the trachea and being inhaled.*
- Place waterproof material on the bed before arranging tissues under the lower side of the patient's face *to absorb solution and saliva draining from the mouth.*
- Check that suction equipment is at hand and in working order; if required, perform oral suction before commencing and during the nursing practice *to prevent any danger of fluid being inhaled.*

PATIENT/CARER EDUCATION: KEY POINTS

In partnership with the patient and/or carer, ensure that they are competent to carry out any practices required. Information should be given on an appropriate point of contact for any concerns that may arise.

Health promotion with regard to mouth care should be multidisciplinary from childhood to old age: the public health nurse, school nurse, practice nurse and district nurse, as well as the dentist and dental hygienist, may be involved. The correct use of dental floss can be

PATIENT/CARER EDUCATION:
KEY POINTS—cont'd

included when discussing dental hygiene. General oral hygiene advice should include:

* the importance of good care of the mouth, teeth and gums related to general health
* good tooth-cleaning technique and care of the dentures
* nutritional advice about the relationship of the incidence of dental caries to food and drink with a high sugar content
* the importance of removing debris from the teeth and fornices of the mouth after meals
* the influence of fluoride in the development of teeth
* the correct method of brushing and flossing the teeth.

  Patients with a suppressed immune system should be taught oral hygiene procedures to prevent mucosal infection.

Health Education England, 2016. Mouth Care Matters. A guide for hospital healthcare professionals. Available at: https://www.mouthcarematters.hee.nhs.uk/wp-content/uploads/2016/10/MCM-GUIDE-2016_100pp_OCT-16_v121.pdf.

Medicines and Healthcare Products Regulatory Agency, 2012. Medical Device Alert: Oral Swabs With a Foam Head. MHRA, London.

National Institute for Health and Care Excellence (NICE), 2018. British National Formulary. Treatment summary. Oropharyngeal fungal infections. NICE, London. Available at: https://bnf.nice.org.uk/treatment-summary/oropharyngeal-fungal-infections.html.

NHS Quality Improvement Scotland, 2004. Working With Dependent Older People to Achieve Good Oral Care. NHS/QIS, Edinburgh.

Nursing and Midwifery Council, 2018. The Code: Professional Standards of Practice and Behaviour for Nurses, Midwives and Nursing Associates. NMC, London. Available at: https://www.nmc.org.uk/globalassets/sitedocuments/nmc-publications/nmc-code.pdf.

REFERENCES

Best, C., Hitchings, H., 2015. Improving nutrition in older people in acute care. Nursing Standard 29 (47), 50–57.

Bissett, S., Preshaw, P., 2011. Guide to providing mouth care for older people. Nursing Older People 23 (10), 14–21.

Daly, B., Smith, K., 2015. Promoting good dental health in older people: role of the community nurse. British Journal of Community Nursing 20 (9), 431–436.

 SELF-ASSESSMENT

1. When may a patient require oral hygiene?
2. What is the most appropriate equipment for carrying out mouth care?
3. What other aids may be used for mouth care?

Oxygen Therapy and Humidification of Gases

Oxygen therapy should be administered by staff trained in its administration, who know how to use the most appropriate devices and flow rates to achieve the prescribed target saturation range. It is important for staff to be aware of the range of different oxygen delivery devices to ensure patient safety.

INDICATIONS AND RATIONALE FOR OXYGEN THERAPY

Oxygen therapy is the introduction of increased oxygen to the air available for respiration to treat hypoxaemia (low concentrations of oxygen in the blood) (British National Formulary 2018) and prevent hypoxia. Hypoxia is a condition in which insufficient oxygen is available for the cells of the body, especially those in the brain and vital organs. Hypoxia may occur in the following circumstances:
- Respiratory disease in which the area available for respiration is reduced by, e.g.:
  - infection
  - chronic conditions such as chronic obstructive pulmonary disease (COPD) and carcinoma
  - pulmonary infarction or embolus
  - asthma.
- Chest injuries following trauma, in which the mechanism of respiration is impaired.
- Heart disease, when the cardiac output is reduced by, e.g.:
  - congestive cardiac failure
  - myocardial infarction.
- Haemorrhage, which reduces the oxygen-carrying capacity of the blood.
- Preoperatively and postoperatively, when analgesic drugs, such as morphine (an opiate), may have an effect on respiratory function.
- In emergency situations, e.g. cardiac or respiratory arrest and hypovolaemic, septic or cardiogenic shock, as the cardiac output falls, reducing the amount of oxygenated blood available to the vital organs.
- Head or spinal injuries.

Except in emergency situations, oxygen therapy should be prescribed by a medical practitioner, who will specify the target oxygen saturation (SpO_2) (British Thoracic Society 2017) and method of administration (British National Formulary 2018). The concentration of oxygen prescribed should be specific to each individual patient and their condition, as the delivery of inappropriate concentrations of oxygen can have serious and potentially fatal consequences (British National Formulary 2018).

Some patients with chronic lung conditions, such as COPD, chronic bronchitis or emphysema, have low oxygen levels in their blood (Cranston et al. 2005). Oxygen therapy can be administered in the patient's own home under the care of the community nurse after careful and detailed evaluation in hospital by respiratory experts (British National Formulary 2018), or in an institutional setting. Regardless of the setting, however, the underlying principles of this nursing practice remain the same, wherever oxygen administration takes place.

At home, the oxygen cylinder and its associated equipment will be delivered regularly to the patient's home from a central supply. This may vary, depending on the local health board/authority policy; however, it must always be prescribed and ordered by a medical practitioner. Alternatively, oxygen may be administered via an oxygen concentrator, which is an effective and economical way to deliver therapy to a patient who requires long-term intervention (British National Formulary 2018).

Advice on the monitoring of patients outside institutional settings is provided by the National Institute for Health and Care Excellence (NICE) in its COPD guidelines (2007). The *British National Formulary* (2018) further advocates that this must include patient education relating to the risks of continuing to smoke and the potential fire hazards that this can pose. The recommendations are that smoking cessation therapy should be provided prior to the prescription of oxygen (British National Formulary 2018).

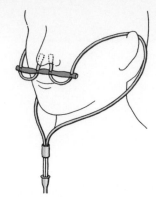

Fig. 28.1 Oxygen therapy: nasal cannulae in position.

EQUIPMENT

- Oxygen supply, e.g. piped oxygen or oxygen cylinder
- Oxygen concentrator (for use in the community)
- Reduction gauge, as required
- Flow meter
- Oxygen delivery device, e.g. mask or nasal cannulae as appropriate
- Oxygen tubing
- Humidifier, as appropriate
- 'No smoking' signs
- Receptacle for soiled disposable items

OXYGEN DELIVERY DEVICES

For a patient who is breathing spontaneously the main devices for oxygen delivery include (British Thoracic Society 2017):

- nasal cannulae
- simple face masks (medium-concentration, variable-performance)
- Venturi or fixed-performance masks
- high-concentration reservoir masks
- humidified masks
- tracheostomy masks.

Nasal Cannulae

Nasal cannulae are suitable and recommended for most patients requiring routine delivery of oxygen therapy. Nasal cannulae consist of light plastic tubes that are inserted into

each nostril and shaped to fit over the ears to maintain their position (Fig. 28.1). The advantage of nasal cannulae is that patients find them more comfortable and less claustrophobic than a conventional mask. The performance of nasal cannulae varies according to the oxygen flow rate, the patient's minute volume (volume of gas inhaled or exhaled per minute) and the patient's breathing pattern (British Thoracic Society 2017). Nasal cannulae devices can be set at a minimum of 1 L/min and a maximum of 6 L/min, which will provide an oxygen concentration range of 24–50% oxygen (British Thoracic Society 2017).

Simple Face Masks (Medium-Concentration, Variable-Performance)

Variable-performance masks are economical and – depending on the oxygen flow rate, the patient's respiratory rate and depth of respiration – will deliver a variable oxygen concentration of 35–60%. The flow of oxygen with these masks can vary between 5 and 10 L/min, but should not fall below 5 L/min to avoid accumulation of CO_2 (British Thoracic Society 2017). This type of mask is particularly useful for patients with type I respiratory failure (hypoxic respiratory failure) (Fig. 28.2).

Venturi or Fixed-Performance Masks

Fixed-performance masks provide a concentration of oxygen that does not vary with the patient's rate and depth of breathing, and are designed to deliver a constant concentration of oxygen within and in between breaths (British Thoracic Society 2017). They are normally colour-coded and the oxygen concentration range is 24–60%, with the minimum oxygen flow displayed on the mask. In cases where a patient is tachypnoeic (respiratory rate over 30 breaths/min), the oxygen flow should be increased by 50%; however, as these devices are fixed-concentration, this will not alter

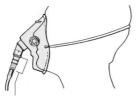

Specific adaptor for prescribed
oxygen percentage

Fig. 28.2 Oxygen therapy: mask in position.

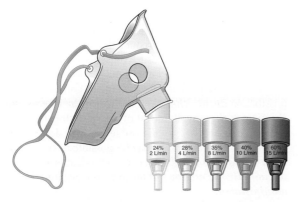

24% 2 L/min 28% 4 L/min 35% 8 L/min 40% 10 L/min 60% 15 L/min

☐ 24% Venturi - 2 L/min - Use 3 L/min if RR >30
☐ 28% Venturi - 4 L/min - Use 6 L/min if RR >30
☐ 35% Venturi - 8 L/min - Use 12 L/min if RR >30
☐ 40% Venturi - 10 L/min - Use 15 L/min if RR >30
☐ 60% Venturi - 15 L/min - Change to RM if 60%
Venturi is not sufficient

Fig. 28.3 Venturi mask. *RM*, reservoir mask; *RR*, respiratory rate. Note: the colours used in this figure do not correlate with the colours of venturi masks in practice.

the percentage of oxygen delivered (Fig. 28.3). These masks are particularly useful in patients with COPD, who require close titration of their oxygen to a specific target SpO_2 of 88–92%.

High-Concentration Reservoir Masks

Often referred to as non-rebreathing reservoir masks, these are used as a short-term measure in emergency situations (e.g. critical illness, trauma, post cardiac or respiratory arrest). With the flow meter at 15 L, these masks deliver concentrations of 60–80% (British Thoracic Society 2017).

Humidified Masks

The upper airway normally warms, moistens and filters inspired air (Waugh et al. 2014). When these functions are impaired and high flows or high concentrations of oxygen are required, humidification of gases is common practice

to prevent drying of the mucosa of the respiratory tract (British Thoracic Society 2017). Without humidification, the patient is at risk of producing secretions that are difficult to expectorate, which can lead to infection or alveolar collapse and impaired gas exchange. Various humidifiers that use hot or cold water or heat moisture exchange membranes are available. Heat moisture exchangers are used predominantly in the critical care setting for patients who are breathing with the aid of a mechanical ventilator. Hot or cold water systems involve the attachment of the oxygen delivery tubing to the humidifier. Moisture is gathered by the gas as it passes either through or over the water, and is nebulized and delivered to the patient. Single-use humidifiers are now advocated to prevent the transmission of pathogens that cause nosocomial pneumonia (La Fauci et al. 2017).

T-Pieces

Oxygen may be delivered directly into an endotracheal tube or tracheostomy tube via wide corrugated tubing and a T-piece. Adequate humidification is essential.

Emergency Situations

For emergency resuscitation procedures, when a patient is not breathing normally, oxygen should be delivered using a bag–valve–mask device (*see* 'Cardiopulmonary Resuscitation and Anaphylaxis', Ch. 8).

GUIDELINES AND RATIONALE FOR THIS NURSING PRACTICE

- Identify and check the prescription for oxygen therapy *to ensure that you are aware of the correct target range of* SpO_2.
- Explain the nursing practice *to the patient to gain consent and cooperation, and to encourage participation in care.* Oxygen masks can be a barrier to communication by making it more difficult for the patient to speak and be heard, and so there is a risk of misunderstanding. This may cause the patient to remove the mask and so the nurse needs good communication skills *to help the patient tolerate the therapy while it is necessary.* The use of closed (direct) questions, to which only a 'yes' or 'no' answer is needed, may be of help.
- Explain the dangers of smoking to the patient, family and friends, and display appropriate 'No smoking' signs, *to make sure that all understand the increased risk of fire when oxygen is administered.* Oxygen is a gas that readily supports combustion, and so in areas where it is used the risk of fire is greatly increased. **Every precaution to prevent fire should be taken.** The patient should, if possible, be aware of the problem and help in maintaining a safe environment. The dangers of smoking should be

explained to the patient, family and visitors. 'No smoking' signs can help to reinforce this precaution. Health board/authority policy on fire precautions should be familiar to all staff and carers.

- Alcohol-based solutions, oils and grease should not be used in areas where oxygen is being administered, as these volatile substances are readily flammable and the presence of oxygen increases the risk of fire. All such precautions should also be part of patient education when therapy is being administered in a community setting, involving all the family and the associated carers as well.
- At home, hang the 'No smoking' notice on the oxygen cylinder, *to act as a reminder to all the family and visitors.*
- Collect and assemble the equipment as required, *to have everything on hand.*
- Help the patient into a comfortable position *to help them tolerate the oxygen therapy without distress.* A need for oxygen therapy usually indicates that the patient has some difficulty with breathing. This dyspnoea may be relieved by helping the patient into an appropriate and comfortable position as the condition allows, e.g. sitting upright, leaning over a bed table supported on a pillow, or sitting in a chair.
- Record and document the type of oxygen delivery device, percentage of oxygen and flow rate, and aim to achieve the target SpO_2 quickly.
- Adjust the flow rate of oxygen *to ensure that the correct percentage is administered that will maintain SpO_2 within the prescribed target range.* Patients who have COPD have permanently altered respiratory physiology: the respiratory drive or stimulus to respiration responds only to a low arterial blood level of oxygen. This means that the SpO_2 target range should be 88–92%. **Higher SpO_2 levels in these patients could cause respiratory arrest.** It is important for the patient and family to understand the importance of not altering the prescribed flow rate and the danger of increasing the amount of oxygen administered.
- Sign the medication chart, according to local policy.
- Observe the patient's vital signs, including type and depth of respirations, throughout this activity *to monitor any adverse effects, as well as any improvement in respiratory function.* The patient's general condition should be observed *to identify any deterioration or improvement in the hypoxic state,* e.g. degree of drowsiness, level of orientation or level of consciousness. The colour and condition of the patient's skin should be observed for cyanosis, clamminess or sweating.
- Connect the single-use humidifier to the oxygen point and, using the correct tubing, attach an appropriate mask.

- Observe the flow of oxygen and water vapour through the mask or cannulae before administration *to check that the equipment is working efficiently.*
- Place the mask in the correct position, and adjust it to fit firmly and comfortably over the patient's nose and mouth (see Fig. 28.2), *to ensure that all the oxygen prescribed is administered and as little as possible escapes from the mask.*
- Remain with the patient as necessary and help them to keep the equipment in position.
- Change the bottle when required *to maintain humidification.*
- Check the oxygen tubing regularly for any build-up of condensation, which may reduce the flow.
- Monitor the SpO_2 levels using pulse oximetry (*see* Ch. 32) *to evaluate the effect of the oxygen administered.*
- Ensure that the patient is left feeling as comfortable as possible *to ensure that they will continue to tolerate the oxygen therapy.* Removal of the mask for drinking should be supervised by the nurse and will depend on the patient's condition. It may be possible to change to nasal cannulae at mealtimes, using a mask at other times *to maintain the accuracy of the oxygen percentage being administered.*
- Oxygen, even when adequately humidified, causes the mouth and nasal passages to become dry. Frequent oral and nasal hygiene will therefore be required *for the patient's comfort and to maintain a healthy oropharyngeal mucosa.* Oral fluids should be encouraged, *to counteract the drying effect on the mucosa.*
- The inside of the oxygen mask may become wet with condensation and so the patient's face can be washed and the inside of the mask dried as appropriate. Do this *to increase the patient's comfort and tolerance of this nursing practice greatly.*
- Wean the patient off the oxygen, as instructed by the medical staff.
- Dispose of the equipment safely *to prevent any transmission of infection.*
- Document the nursing practice appropriately, monitor the after-effects and report any abnormal findings immediately, *to ensure safe practice and enable prompt appropriate medical and nursing intervention to be initiated as soon as possible.*
- In undertaking this practice, nurses are accountable for their actions, the quality of care delivered and record-keeping in accordance with *The Code* (Nursing and Midwifery Council 2018).
- While receiving oxygen therapy, patients should be monitored *to check that the predetermined oxygen saturation is maintained and to ensure the safety of the patient;* it is vital for nurses to be able to monitor

accurately and to be aware of the limitations of this, *to ensure the quality of this practice.* Pulse oximetry is considered as the 'fifth vital sign' (O'Driscoll et al. 2017) and allows continuous non-invasive measurement of the oxygen saturation levels (Chan et al. 2013).

• In acute and critical care environments, the effectiveness of oxygen therapy may also be monitored by assessing the arterial blood gases (*see* Ch. 3).

PATIENT/CARER EDUCATION: KEY POINTS

In partnership with the patient and/or carer, ensure that they are competent to carry out any practices required. Information should be given on an appropriate point of contact for any concerns that may arise. The reason for the administration of oxygen therapy should be explained to the patient and the family and carers involved. They should understand that it is a specific part of the treatment.

At home, the patient and carers should be shown how to adjust the flow rate to the prescribed rate only, how to fill the humidifier, maintaining a safe environment, and how to connect the mask and tubing. The procedure for changing oxygen cylinders or using an oxygen concentrator, and the personnel involved, will depend on health authority/board policy; in some instances, carers may be instructed in this.

The increased risk of fire should be explained and simple instructions about fire precautions given. The danger of smoking when oxygen is used should be continually reinforced: patient and family cooperation is needed. They can choose where the 'No smoking' signs should be displayed.

For patients with COPD, everyone should understand the importance of never increasing the prescribed flow of oxygen delivered to the patient. This may need reinforcing if there is a change of carer in the community setting. The reason for this should be part of patient education.

The patient should understand the importance of immediately reporting any changes in respiratory function, such as increased dyspnoea, cough, sputum or a general feeling of distress.

REFERENCES

British National Formulary/National Institute for Health and Care Excellence, 2018. Oxygen. BNF/NICE. Available from: https://bnf.nice.org.uk/treatment-summary/oxygen.html.

British Thoracic Society, 2017. British Thoracic Society Guideline for oxygen use in healthcare and emergency settings: Key messages for nurses and PAMs (Professions Allied to Medicine). May 2017. Available from: https://www.brit-thoracic.org.uk/standards-of-care/guidelines/bts-guideline-for-emergency-oxygen-use-in-adult-patients/.

Chan, E.D., Chan, M.M., Chan, M.M., 2013. Pulse oximetry: understanding its basic principles facilitates appreciation of its limitations. Respiratory Medicine 107 (6), 789–799.

Cranston, J.M., Crockett, A.J., Moss, J.R., Alpers, J.H., 2005. Domiciliary oxygen for chronic obstructive pulmonary disease. The Cochrane Database of Systematic Reviews (4), CD001744.

La Fauci, V., Costa, G.B., Facciolà, A., et al., 2017. Humidifiers for oxygen therapy: what risk for reusable and disposable devices? Journal of Preventive Medicine and Hygiene 58 (2), E161.

National Institute for Health and Clinical Excellence, 2007. Chronic Obstructive Pulmonary Disease in Adults. NICE, London.

Nursing Midwifery Council, 2018. The Code: Professional Standards of Practice and Behaviour for Nurses, Midwives and Nursing Associates. NMC, London. Available at: https://www.nmc.org.uk/globalassets/sitedocuments/nmc-publications/nmc-code.pdf.

O'Driscoll, B.R., Howard, L.S., Earis, J., Mak, V., 2017. BTS guideline for oxygen use in adults in healthcare and emergency settings. Thorax 72 (Suppl. 1), ii1–ii90.

Waugh, A., Grant, A., 2014. Ross and Wilson Anatomy & Physiology in Health and Illness, 12th ed. Churchill Livingstone, London.

SELF-ASSESSMENT

1. What oxygen delivery devices may be used with patients who require supplementary oxygen?
2. What factors would influence your choice of oxygen delivery device?
3. What is the target oxygen saturation for a patient who has chronic obstructive pulmonary disease?
4. What safety precautions should be taken while caring for a patient receiving oxygen therapy either at home or in hospital?
5. Which vital signs would the nurse monitor during oxygen therapy?

29

Patient Admission, Transfer and Discharge

LEARNING OUTCOMES

By the end of this chapter, you should be able to:
- prepare the patient and carer for transfer to another care setting
- complete patient transfer documentation.

BACKGROUND KNOWLEDGE REQUIRED

- Children and Young People's Act (Scotland) (2014) (Scottish Parliament 2014)
- Policy guidance on discharge planning for your area
- Revision of local policy on the transfer of patients
- *The Royal Marsden Manual of Clinical Nursing Procedures* (Dougherty et al. 2015)

INDICATIONS AND RATIONALE FOR PATIENT TRANSFER

Healthcare reform and the nationwide introduction of health and social care integration have resulted in a much greater focus on the appropriate use of the services available for patient care. Thus, the patient may be transferred between institutional and community settings within the statutory health and social care agencies or in the voluntary or private/independent sectors, as is judged appropriate for their individual needs and benefit.

OUTLINE OF THE PROCEDURE

'Patient transfer' (rather than discharge) is the term used in this chapter, as it demonstrates a continuum rather than a cessation of care. The procedure may be simple or complex, depending on the needs of the patient and carer. The systematic approach to care – namely, assessment, planning, implementation and evaluation – may, however, be used as a framework for the patient transfer process.

- The assessment phase involves the collection of data pertinent to the patient and/or carer. A variety of sources may be used to build up a holistic picture of the patient and the caring environment. Some of this information will already have been collected during the patient admission assessment.
- The planning stage utilizes the assessment data to provide a plan of transfer. Liaison with other agencies to request and discuss their input will also be carried out at this stage of the process.
- The implementation phase involves putting the plan into action and completing patient transfer documentation.
- The evaluation stage of the transfer procedure is essential in order to assess the effectiveness of the process and to identify any difficulties or problems.

GUIDELINES AND RATIONALE FOR THIS NURSING PRACTICE

General principles will be given first, followed by guidelines for planning and implementing the transfer process. Some of the guidelines may not be applicable to patients transferring from community to institutional settings.

Transfer and discharge to and from hospital can be a distressing time for individuals and their families and friends (Oxtoby 2016). As health professionals, it is important that nurses develop and adapt practice and respond to the ever-changing needs of the service provided (Department of Health 2016; Scottish Government 2017). The multidisciplinary team can make a significant difference to the speed and quality of the patient journey (Department of Health 2017). A crucial factor in planning transfer and discharge is the process of communication, cooperation and collaboration between health and social care, the multidisciplinary team, patients and relatives.

Principles

- The patient and carer should be involved in all stages of the transfer process, *to enable consideration and discussion of their needs prior to the transfer plan being completed and implemented* (NICE 2015). Older people in particular often find it a major life transition, particularly when it means having to move home or establish new routines.

- Patient transfer is normally a multidisciplinary procedure that may involve social, voluntary and independent care agencies, as well as different healthcare professionals, *to ensure a holistic approach to patient transfer.*
- Good communication is an essential part of the patient transfer process, *as poor communication patterns affect continuity of care* on transfer from community to institutional settings, as well as from institutional to community care (Department of Health 2016).
- It is essential for there to be early involvement of, and liaison with, staff from the receiving care setting (which may be a hospital ward, an intermediate care facility, a nursing home or the patient's own home). Some areas have a designated liaison nurse who provides a link between institutional and community care *to promote continuity of care* (Oxtoby 2016).
- The multidisciplinary team can speed up the transfer process and manage the care pathway to an expected or predicted date of transfer (including weekends), and there are some examples of other agencies supporting discharges within the community setting (Department of Health 2017).
- Evaluation systems are in place *to monitor the effectiveness of the patient transfer process.* These differ, depending on your geographical area.

Planning Patient Transfer

- Discuss care needs with the patient and carer *to ascertain their views and requirements,* and involve them in the decision-making process.
- Information related to risk factors should be recorded and shared between care settings (e.g. the patient being at risk of falls or any sensory deficit that may put the patient at risk).
- Plan and initiate any teaching programmes for the patient and/or carer. Examples include a self-medication programme for patients being transferred from institutional to community care (Department of Health 2017) *to prepare the patient and carer for tasks that they will be required to undertake in the community.*
- Consult, liaise with and refer to the appropriate care agencies (health, social, voluntary or independent). If the patient has complex care needs, it may be necessary to invite all the relevant personnel, including the patient and/or carer, to a case conference *to ensure that support services are in position prior to transfer* (Department of Health 2016).

- Order any equipment or patient aids (e.g. moving and handling equipment or oxygen cylinder) *to ensure that the receiving care setting meets the patient's needs.*
- If the patient has complex needs and is being transferred from institutional care, it is valuable to organize a home assessment visit prior to transfer. This will involve the patient, carer and district nurse, as well as other relevant personnel such as the liaison nurse, occupational therapist, physiotherapist and social care staff, *to enable the patient's needs to be assessed within their own environment and to enable an assessment of the carer's ability to provide care.*
- Arrange for transport between care settings *to ensure that the transport is appropriate for the patient's needs.*
- Information related to any infection that may put the patient, carers or other healthcare personnel at risk should be recorded. If appropriate, the meticillin-resistant *Staphylococcus aureus* (MRSA) status of the patient should be stated (*see* Ch. 20).
- Order a small supply of continence, dressing or medicinal products *to ensure that products are available for the immediate transfer period.*
- Assess the patient's ability to administer medication. If deficits are identified, a teaching programme may have to be initiated for the patient and carer, and/or patient compliance devices can be introduced. This should be carried out in conjunction with the pharmacist *to check that the patient and carer are able to administer the medicines correctly.*
- Consult with the carers about access arrangements to the patient's home on the day of transfer *to enable access arrangements to be made in advance.*
- Give an approximate expected time of arrival to the patient, carer and any other personnel who require this information (e.g. the district nurse and home help, or the continuing care facility) *to enable the caring network to be organized.*

Implementing the Transfer Process

- Complete the patient transfer documentation (Box 29.1) and retain a copy *to provide a permanent record of the transfer process.*
- Ensure that the medical staff have completed a transfer form to give to the patient's general practitioner. This usually comprises a summary of diagnoses, treatments, medication and follow-up appointments, *to provide a permanent summary of the admission details.*
- Send the documentation to the personnel in the receiving care setting. This should be carried out according to local health authority policy but may involve an internal mailing system, the postal service, delivery by the patient/carer, faxing or a computer network. In the future,

BOX 29.1 Example of a Checklist of Contents for Transfer Documentation

Social Data
- Patient details: name, date of birth, address, telephone number, occupation, housing and any dependants
- Carer details: name, address, telephone number, occupation, any relevant health problems or disabilities, other dependants and ability/willingness to care

Health Data
- Diagnosis (including patient/carer's knowledge and understanding of the diagnosis)
- Disability/impairment
- Prognosis (if applicable)
- Medication (including any specialized instructions or medicine aids)
- Treatment (this might include details of procedures such as wound care, catheter management or continence products)
- Investigations carried out and results if known

Current Status
- Information relating to assessed needs and planned care of the patient

Patient/Carer's Needs
- These will be specific to the service user and should be decided in conjunction with the patient/carer
- A multidisciplinary assessment of the patient's current status is essential to establish their needs

Support Services
- Details of care/therapy provided by professionals from other services (such as dietitians, physiotherapists or occupational therapists) in the current care setting
- Information: name, contact number and type of input, on any support services arranged for the post-transfer period (including the date of commencement)
- Most care settings will have a directory of services in the local area; for information on national services, contact the NHS Helpline (see 'Patient/Carer Information' later)

Financial Data
- Details of welfare benefits (either in place or applied for)

Equipment Data
- Details of equipment, either in place or requested (indicating the source of the equipment)
- Equipment should be in place prior to transfer

Health Promotion/Patient Education
- Provide a summary of:
  - health promotion activities
  - information on any education programmes
- Enclose a copy of the patient education or health promotion literature given to the patient

All documentation should be signed and dated by the nurse responsible for the patient's care.

---

patient-held records (which stay with the patient as they move between care areas) may be the way in which information is communicated, *to enable the sharing of information between care settings.*

- Discuss any medication with the patient. This includes reinforcing information provided by the medical staff, such as the reason for the drug, its dosage, timing or frequency and route of administration, and any special instructions. The use of a personal medical record card may be of value to some patients *to reinforce the information given on the container label and to facilitate understanding.*
- Follow-up care can be offered by pharmacists, general practitioners or nurses, and is an important aspect of discharge planning *to ensure that patients understand the types of medication they are taking,* especially with regard to new medication (NICE 2015).
- Check that the patient has all their personal belongings *to ensure that no property is lost during transfer.*

- Arrange any follow-up outpatient appointment *to ensure that the patient and carer are aware of follow-up care.*
- Provide details of the receiving care setting (the named nurse and contact number).
- In undertaking this practice, nurses are accountable for their actions, the quality of care delivered and record-keeping according to *The Code* (Nursing and Midwifery Council 2018).

ADDITIONAL INFORMATION

Information related to any risk factors should be recorded. This might include:
- moving and handling factors
- difficulties related to the self-administration of medication
- the patient being at risk of falls
- any infection that may put the patient or carers at risk
- any sensory deficit that may put the patient at risk.

Whereas patients may function effectively within their existing environment, they may be at risk (e.g. by becoming disorientated) in a new care setting.

The patient's ability to communicate and understand information, as well as any deficits in hearing, sight or speech, for example, should be noted. Information on equipment such as hearing aids or spectacles that the patient may require to communicate effectively should be provided.

It is essential for staff to communicate with the patient/carer to ensure that they are fully informed and understand all aspects of the transfer. Any anxieties or concerns should be discussed and documented.

If transfer is taking place to a continuing care facility, the patient should, whenever possible, visit the facility prior to transfer.

Record any difficulties that the patient has with breathing, as well as treatments such as inhalers or oxygen therapy. For the patient being transferred to the community, arrangements should be made for the delivery of oxygen cylinders or a concentrator, teaching being given to the patient and carer on its use and precautions.

The nutritional status of the patient can affect the healing process and so any problems should be documented. Information should be provided on any special dietary requirements and whether there has been input from a dietitian. Information is also needed on patients' ability to feed themselves and on the equipment required to aid this activity.

Equipment and feeding regime details should be provided for patients with enteral feeding requirements. Carers or patients will usually be taught this procedure prior to leaving hospital.

Bladder and bowel function are essential activities. Like nutrition, they may be affected by a change in environment or illness. A record of the patient's current bladder and bowel pattern should therefore be given, together with a note of any difficulties related to function, including abnormal patterns such as diarrhoea, constipation or urinary incontinence. Any investigations should be documented, and a record of necessary continence aids or toilet equipment should be given.

The patient may be at risk of pressure sores. The risk factors and score (see 'Integrity of the Skin', Ch. 21) should be documented, along with the plan of care and any special equipment required. If pressure sores are present, a full description (including tracings) should be documented as baseline data for the staff in the receiving care setting.

The condition of the patient's mouth may affect their health. Thus, any problems such as ulceration, oral infection or problems with dentition, plus details of treatment, should be described.

The following should be documented:
- deficits in the patient's ability to mobilize
- information on any rehabilitation programmes
- the equipment required to aid mobility
- the level and type of assistance required from another person
- any active or passive exercises that need to be followed up in the receiving care setting.

Concerns regarding a change in body image caused by the illness should be discussed and documented. Sexual issues require sensitivity and diplomacy. The patient may discuss issues of a highly confidential nature, and it may not always be appropriate to document this information.

Patients may contemplate death during an episode of illness. Such thoughts may be transitory or may be longer-lasting when the patient has a life-threatening or terminal illness. It is important for the staff in the receiving care environment to be aware of the information and understanding that the patient has about their condition and prognosis. Counselling initiated with the patient should be outlined.

PATIENT/CARER EDUCATION: KEY POINTS

In partnership with the patient and/or carer, ensure that they are competent to carry out any practices required. Information should be given on an appropriate point of contact for any concerns that may arise.

Education for the patient and carer will depend on the needs identified in the planning phase of transfer. Patient education may take the form of:
- health promotion initiatives
- the teaching, demonstration and supervision of a practical procedure, such as the administration of insulin
- literature on a specific illness or disease such as myocardial infarction, to be used in conjunction with discussion
- verbal discussion to evaluate understanding (e.g. of an illness or medication), as verbal advice is not always assimilated by patients.

Information on support groups is available from local health, social and voluntary agencies or at a national level from the Patient Advice and Support Service (Scotland; 0800 9172127) or the number 111 (whole of the UK), or via the internet (https://www.nhs.uk).

Details of patient education programmes should be recorded in the transfer documentation.

REFERENCES

Department of Health, 2016. Discharging older people from hospital. National Audit Office, London.

Department of Health, 2017. Discharge to assess: Transforming urgent and emergency care services in England. NHS England, London.

Dougherty, L., Lister, S., 2015. The Royal Marsden Manual of Clinical Nursing Procedures, ninth ed. Professional ed. John Wiley & Sons, Chichester.

National Institute for Health and Care Excellence, 2015. Older people with social care needs and multiple long-term conditions. NICE. Available at: https://www.nice.org.uk/guidance/ng22/resources/older-people-with-social-care-needs-and-multiple-longterm-conditions-pdf-1837328537797.

Nursing and Midwifery Council, 2018. The Code: Professional Standards of Practice and Behaviour for Nurses, Midwives and Nursing Associates. London, NMC. Available at: https://www.nmc.org.uk/globalassets/sitedocuments/nmc-publications/nmc-code.pdf.

Oxtoby, K., 2016. Preventing unsafe discharge from hospital. Nursing Times 25 (112), 14–15.

Scottish Government, 2017. 2030 Nursing: a vision for nursing in Scotland. Scottish Government, Edinburgh.

Scottish Parliament, 2014. Children and Young People (Scotland) Act, Edinburgh. Available at: https://togetherscotland.org.uk/pdfs/Together_response_Part_4_5_18_guidance_v1.pdf.

SELF-ASSESSMENT

1. What are the four main areas within the framework for the patient transfer process?
2. Who would be involved in the patient transfer process?
3. List the areas that may involve patient carer education.
4. What types of information should be shared with staff in the receiving care area?

30

Preoperative Nursing Care

LEARNING OUTCOMES

By the end of this chapter, you should be able to:
- explain the standard preoperative preparation of a patient who is undergoing elective surgery
- describe the nurse's role in preparing a patient for surgery.

BACKGROUND KNOWLEDGE REQUIRED

- Revision of the cardiopulmonary system
- Review of local health authority and trust policy on the preoperative preparation of patients
- Review of local health authority and trust policy on preoperative venous thromboembolism (VTE) prophylaxis

The guidelines in this nursing practice apply to patients undergoing day surgery, those being admitted on the day of surgery and those requiring a longer hospital stay.

INDICATIONS AND RATIONALE FOR PREOPERATIVE CARE

Preoperative nursing care is required to prepare the patient physically and emotionally for surgery and therefore *reduce the risk of complications and promote optimal recovery* (Hinkle & Cheever 2014).

GUIDELINES AND RATIONALE FOR THIS NURSING PRACTICE

- Explain the pre- and postoperative routines to the patient and answer any questions appropriately; the discussion of any fears or anxieties that the patient may have should be encouraged. *High levels of anxiety have a negative impact on postoperative outcomes (Kagan & Bar-Tal 2008) and studies have demonstrated that patients' anxiety levels are reduced if they receive information and explanation (Alanazi 2014).*

- Record the temperature, pulse, respiration rate, blood pressure, oxygen saturation and urinalysis, if required, *to give baseline findings with which to compare postoperative observations and detect abnormalities.* Any abnormalities should be discussed with the nurse in charge and medical staff.

- Withhold solid food from patients for 6 hours before elective surgery but encourage the patient to drink clear fluids up to 2 hours before surgery. Clear fluids are defined as water, pulp-free juice and tea or coffee, without milk (European Society of Anaesthesiology 2011). Do this *to reduce the risk of regurgitation and aspiration of gastric contents at induction of general anaesthetic* (Murray & Clayton 2012).

- Ensure that patients participating in an Enhanced Recovery After Surgery (ERAS) pathway have access to a carbohydrate drink 2 hours before their surgery (Smith et al. 2014).

- Prepare the patient's skin according to local health authority and trust policy. This may involve the patient showering on the day of surgery *to reduce the number of microorganisms on the skin surrounding the incision and may therefore reduce the risk of surgical site infection* (National Institute for Health and Care Excellence 2013). Hair removal should not be routinely undertaken. If it is required, use electric clippers with a single-use head. Undertake hair clipping as close to the time of surgery as possible (Association for Perioperative Practice 2016).

- Assist the patient in changing into a theatre gown and ensure that all underwear has been removed, although paper pants may be worn on some occasions. Nail varnish and make-up should be removed so that the true colour of the patient's skin can be observed during the perioperative period. Evidence that the nail varnish interferes with the accuracy of pulse oximetry readings is contradictory.

- Measure the patient for anti-embolism stockings, if these have been recommended, and help the patient to them to put on. Do this *to reduce the risk of deep vein thrombosis* (Scottish Intercollegiate Guidelines Network 2010).
- Dentures are usually removed *because of the danger of inhaling them during induction of anaesthesia.* Health authority policies vary regarding the removal of spectacles, hearing aids and other prostheses, e.g. wigs and artificial eyes. Generally, they may remain in situ until the patient arrives in the operating theatre*, to maintain the patient's dignity.*
- Tape the patient's wedding ring into place. All other jewellery, including body piercings, should be removed if it is practicable to do so, *to reduce the risk of burns from electrosurgical equipment and of localized tissue trauma* (Association for Perioperative Practice 2016). Any jewellery or piercings that cannot be removed must be clearly documented in the preoperative checklist.
- Complete the preoperative checklist with the patient. This must include a check of the patient's identification both verbally and from the identification band, and confirmation that the patient has given informed consent for the procedure. Confirm with the patient that the correct site and procedure are noted on the consent form. The surgeon performing the operation should mark the site of surgery in cases involving laterality or multiple structures or levels (e.g. a finger, toe, skin lesion, vertebra) (World Health Organization 2009). This is done *to comply with legal requirements and local hospital policy, and to reduce the risk of surgery being performed on the incorrect site.*
- When the theatre personnel arrive to take the patient to the operating theatre, a comprehensive handover of care is undertaken. Confirm all of the details on the preoperative checklist with the theatre personnel and the patient. Ensure that all relevant documentation accompanies the patient, i.e. preoperative checklist, case notes, consent form, prescription chart, nursing documentation and so on. The patient may walk to theatre or travel on a hospital bed or theatre trolley, according to local health authority policy.
- The appropriate information should have been given to the relatives before the patient leaves the ward, so that they can, with the patient's permission, telephone to check progress *to help reduce the relatives' anxiety.*
- In undertaking this practice, nurses are accountable for their actions, the quality of care delivered and record-keeping in accordance with *The Code* (Nursing and Midwifery Council 2018).

PATIENT/CARER EDUCATION: KEY POINTS

In partnership with the patient and/or carer, ensure that they are competent to carry out any practices required. Information should be given on an appropriate point of contact for any concerns that may arise.

It is important for patients being admitted on the day of their surgery to receive all of the necessary preoperative information and knowledge prior to their admission. This will probably involve nurses working in the pre-assessment and outpatient clinics. Written material should be provided to reinforce the verbal information given. Patients may be required to undertake some preoperative preparations at home, such as skin preparation and preoperative fasting.

REFERENCES

Alanazi, A., 2014. Reducing anxiety in preoperative patients: a systematic review. British Journal of Nursing 23 (7), 387–393.

Association for Perioperative Practice, 2016. Standards and Recommendations for Safe Perioperative Practice, 4th ed. AfPP, Harrogate.

European Society of Anaesthesiology, 2011. Perioperative fasting in adults and children: guidelines from the European Society of Anaesthesiology. European Journal of Anaesthesiology 28, 556–569.

Hinkle, J.L., Cheever, K.H., 2014. Preoperative Nursing Management. Brunner & Suddarth's Textbook of Medical-Surgical Nursing, 13th ed. Lippincott Williams & Wilkins, Philadelphia.

Kagan, I., Bar-Tal, Y., 2008. The effect of preoperative uncertainty and anxiety on short-term recovery after elective arthroplasty. Journal of Clinical Nursing 17 (5), 576–783.

Murray, H., Clayton, T., 2012. Regurgitation and aspiration. Anaesthesia & Intensive Care Medicine 13 (12), 617–620.

National Institute for Health and Care Excellence, 2013. Surgical Site Infection – Quality Standard [QS49]. Available at: https://www.nice.org.uk/guidance/qs49.

Nursing and Midwifery Council, 2018. The Code: Professional Standards of Practice and Behaviour for Nurses, Midwives and Nursing Associates. NMC, London. Available at: https://www.nmc.org.uk/globalassets/sitedocuments/nmc-publications/nmc-code.pdf.

Scottish Intercollegiate Guidelines Network, 2010. Prevention and management of venous thromboembolism: Guideline No 122. SIGN, Edinburgh.

Smith, M.D., McCall, J., Plank, L., et al., 2014. Preoperative carbohydrate treatment for enhancing recovery after elective surgery. The Cochrane Database of Systematic Reviews (8), CD009161.

World Health Organization, 2009. WHO guidelines for safe
surgery 2009: safe surgery saves lives. WHO, Geneva.

WEBSITES

https://www.afpp.org.uk *Association for Perioperative Practice*
https://www.rcn.org.uk *Royal College of Nursing*
https://www.sign.ac.uk *Scottish Intercollegiate Guidelines Network*
https://www.who.int/patientsafety/safesurgery/en/ *World Health
   Organization: Safe Surgery*

SELF-ASSESSMENT

1. Why is it important to ensure that patient's anxiety is reduced preoperatively?
2. What is the preoperative fasting requirement for healthy patients?
3. Describe the current guidelines for prophylaxis of venous thromboembolism.

Postoperative Nursing Care

By the end of this chapter, you should be able to:
- explain the general postoperative care of a patient
- describe the nurse's role in carrying out general postoperative care.

BACKGROUND KNOWLEDGE REQUIRED

- Revision of airway management strategies
- Revision of the signs of difficulty in breathing, including changes in respiratory rate, colour, hypoxia, stridor and the use of accessory muscles
- Revision of the signs and symptoms of haemorrhage
- Revision of the strengths and weaknesses of pulse oximetry
- Revision of the effects of postoperative hypothermia
- Revision of the types and clinical features of shock
- Revision of the physiology of wound healing
- Review of local health authority and trust policy on postoperative care

INDICATIONS AND RATIONALE FOR POSTOPERATIVE CARE

Postoperative nursing care is required to monitor the patient's condition *in order to prevent and identify any problems that may occur after a surgical procedure.*

GUIDELINES AND RATIONALE FOR THIS NURSING PRACTICE

Receiving the Patient back into the Ward

- Handover of the patient's care to the ward nurse should take place at the patient's bedside *so that their condition can be adequately observed and assessed.* The patient will have already met the recovery room discharge criteria, so should be conscious and comfortable on their return to the ward. No patient should be returned to the ward until control of postoperative nausea and vomiting, and of pain is satisfactory (Association of Anaesthetists of Great Britain and Ireland 2013).
- Undertake an assessment of the patient's condition:
  - Airway – Ensure the airway is clear and patent, and that there are no signs of airway obstruction.
  - Breathing – Measure the patient's respiratory rate and rhythm, and look, listen and feel for signs of respiratory distress. Monitor the oxygen saturation, and note the colour of the skin, lips and nailbeds, *to observe for signs of cyanosis.*
  - Circulation – Record the pulse (rate, rhythm and strength), blood pressure, temperature and urinary output. Compare the results with the patient's preoperative and intraoperative recordings.
  - Disability – Speak to the patient *to assess their level of consciousness.*
  - Exposure – Observe the wound site *to note any staining or bleeding on to the dressing.* Observe any surgical drains that may be present, *to monitor their patency and to note the amount and nature of any drainage.* This will ensure prompt recognition of problems such as haemorrhage or blockage.

Initial Postoperative Nursing

- Read the patient's theatre notes to confirm that the surgical procedure that has been carried out and to ascertain any instructions from the surgeon or anaesthetist, e.g. the positioning of the patient or any oxygen therapy required.
- On the patient's initial return to the ward, 15-minute observations should be performed; this may vary from patient to patient. Observation of respiratory rate, oxygen saturations, temperature, blood pressure, pulse rate and level of consciousness should be recorded using the National Early Warning System (NEWS), which has been shown *to improve the detection and response to clinical deterioration in adult patients* (NHS England 2017).

- Changes in the patient's NEWS score will trigger changes in the frequency of observations and/or the escalation of care to medical staff. Patients with a NEWS score of 7 or more need continuous monitoring of vital signs, and emergency assessment by a team with critical care competencies; they may require transfer to a level 2 or 3 critical care facility (Royal College of Physicians 2017).
- Monitor the patient's pain score (resting and moving) and administer analgesics as required by the patient and as prescribed by the medical staff, *to relieve pain and anxiety.* Check the intraoperative and recovery record for type and last dose of analgesia *to ensure that overdosage of analgesia is avoided.* Regularly reassess the patient's pain score following administration of analgesia. Refer the patient to the acute pain team if the pain cannot be adequately controlled.
- Assess if the patient has signs of nausea or vomiting. Opioid drugs are a potent cause of nausea and vomiting (Hatfield 2014). If the patient is nauseated, it is safer to nurse them in the recovery position (*see* Ch. 18), if possible. Administer prescribed anti-emetics and monitor their effect.
- If an intravenous infusion is present, check that it is functioning according to medical staff instructions. The insertion site should be inspected at each shift change *to minimize peripheral vascular catheter-related complications* (Loveday et al. 2014).

Continuing Postoperative Nursing

- Assist the patient to wash and change into their own clothing and offer a mouthwash, *to aid comfort and the recovery of a sense of individuality.* If the patient has been wearing anti-embolic stockings, the continued benefit of these is to be emphasized.
- Encourage the patient to sit up in bed well supported by pillows (unless contraindicated) and move around as much as possible, helping them out of bed when the blood pressure recordings are satisfactory. These measures help *to minimize the risk of complications, such as skin breakdown, deep venous thrombosis and postoperative chest infection.*
- Unless contraindicated, allow the patient to drink, gradually increasing the amounts of clear fluids; then gradually introduce solid food if there is no vomiting and if bowel sounds are present, *in order to rehydrate the patient and to help restore the blood glucose level to within the normal range.*
- Ensure that patients who are participating in an Enhanced Recovery After Surgery (ERAS) programme comply with all the programme's postoperative requirements, e.g. early and progressive mobilization, early feeding, and discontinuation of intravenous fluids (Carmichael et al. 2017).

- Record the amount and time when the patient passes urine and has a first bowel movement, *as constipation is a common postoperative problem because of immobility, dehydration and the use of opioid analgesics.*
- Regularly assess the patient's pain using a validated scale, such as a numerical, verbal or visual rating scale (Ingadóttir & Zoëga 2017). Effective pain management can *enhance the patient's postoperative recovery.*
- Ensure that the patient has adequate periods of rest, *as this will aid recovery.*
- Give encouragement and support to the patient and provide any explanation or information that may be requested. It is important to remind the patient of the measures they may take to reduce the risk of complications, such as chest, urinary and wound infections or venous thromboembolism formation (Liddle 2013).
- In undertaking this practice, nurses are accountable for their actions and the quality of care delivered; they must keep clear and accurate records in accordance with *The Code* (Nursing and Midwifery Council 2018).

PATIENT/CARER EDUCATION: KEY POINTS

Depending on the surgical procedure performed, the patient may require a planned education programme delivered by an appropriately experienced nurse. All patients should be informed of ways of reducing the risk of occurrence of the common postoperative complications.

Day surgery patients and their carers assume a large degree of responsibility for postoperative care, and staff must ensure that they are able to cope with this before allowing the patient to be discharged. Close liaison should be maintained with the community healthcare team (*see* 'Patient Admission, Transfer and Discharge', Ch. 29). The patient needs to be provided with high-quality information and communication, *as this is vital for a smooth and uneventful recovery at home* (Mitchell 2015). As a minimum, the patient and/or carer should receive information about normal postoperative convalescence, what complications might occur and who to contact if they have any concerns. This is particularly important for patients who are following an ERAS pathway, as their length of hospital stay is likely to have been reduced (Jones et al. 2017).

Discharge medications, including analgesia, should be clearly explained, especially if they are new to the patient. Involvement of the family and carers can help to ensure compliance.

REFERENCES

Association of Anaesthetists of Great Britain and Ireland, 2013. AAGBI Safety Guideline – Immediate Postanaesthesia Recovery 2013. AABGI, London.

Carmichael, J., Keller, D., Baldini, G., et al., 2017. Clinical Practice Guidelines for Enhanced Recovery After Colon and Rectal Surgery from the American Society of Colon and Rectal Surgeons and Society of American Gastrointestinal and Endoscopic Surgeons. Society of American Gastrointestinal and Endoscopic Surgeons.

Hatfield, A., 2014. The Complete Recovery Room Book, fifth ed. Oxford University Press, Oxford.

Ingadóttir, B., Zoëga, S., 2017. Role of patient education in postoperative pain management. Nursing Standard 32 (2), 50–63.

Jones, D., Musselman, R., Pearsall, E., et al., 2017. Ready to go home? Patients' experiences of the discharge process in an Enhanced Recovery After Surgery (ERAS) program for colorectal surgery. Journal of Gastrointestinal Surgery: Official Journal of the Society for Surgery of the Alimentary Tract 21 (11), 1865–1878.

Liddle, C., 2013. How to reduce the risk of deterioration after surgery. Nursing Times 106 (23), 16–17.

Loveday, H.P., Wilson, J.A., Pratt, R.J., et al., 2014. Epic3: national evidence-based guidelines for preventing healthcare-associated infections in NHS hospitals in England. The Journal of Hospital Infection 86 (Suppl. 1), S1–S70. (V).

Mitchell, M., 2015. Home recovery following day surgery: a patient perspective. Journal of Clinical Nursing 24 (3–4), 415–427.

NHS England, 2017. National Early Warning Score (NEWS). Available at: https://www.england.nhs.uk/nationalearlywarningscore/.

Nursing and Midwifery Council, 2018. The Code: Professional Standards of Practice and Behaviour for Nurses, Midwives and Nursing Associates. NMC, London. Available at: https://www.nmc.org.uk/globalassets/sitedocuments/nmc-publications/nmc-code.pdf.

Royal College of Physicians, 2017. National Early Warning Score (NEWS) 2: Standardising the assessment of acute-illness severity in the NHS. RCP, London.

❓ SELF-ASSESSMENT

1. What are the signs and symptoms of respiratory distress?
2. What observations are undertaken as part of the NEWS scoring system?
3. What are the signs and symptoms of hypovolaemia?
4. How might the patient's level of consciousness be assessed?

32

Pulse Oximetry

LEARNING OUTCOMES

By the end of this chapter, you should be able to:
- list the indications for using pulse oximetry
- describe how to monitor patients requiring pulse oximetry
- describe how to interpret pulse oximetry readings in clinical practice
- demonstrate an awareness of the limitations of this monitoring modality
- state the complications of pulse oximetry.

BACKGROUND KNOWLEDGE REQUIRED

- Revision of the physiology of oxygen transport in the blood
- Revision of the principles of oxygen administration (*see* Ch. 28)

INDICATIONS AND RATIONALE FOR PULSE OXIMETRY MONITORING

Pulse oximetry is a simple and reliable monitoring modality that continuously measures how much haemoglobin is carrying oxygen; it is used in both primary and secondary care. Safe interpretation of readings is effective only if the care provider understands how it works and knows its limitations (World Health Organization 2011). Pulse oximetry is now regarded as vital in the safe administration of oxygen therapy and is sometimes termed the fifth vital sign (Tierney et al. 1997; Woodrow 1999; British Thoracic Society 2017).

The indications for pulse oximetry include its use:
- *as a baseline indicator of a patient's oxygenation status,* e.g. in the assessment of possible hypoxaemia in clinical situations such as new-onset confusion in the elderly

- *as an evaluation of a patient's response to therapy,* e.g. in the management and safe use of oxygen therapy in both adults and neonates
- *in continuous monitoring during anaesthesia and procedures requiring sedation*
- *in the diagnosis of obstructive sleep apnoea,* where it is of diagnostic value.

Advantages of Pulse Oximetry

- It is less painful than invasive arterial puncture.
- It provides a continuous non-invasive method of monitoring.
- It is inexpensive.
- It provides a real-time/point-of-care testing method with immediate results.

What Does a Pulse Oximeter Measure?

A pulse oximeter is a simple, inexpensive and non-invasive technique for monitoring oxygenation.

The two numerical values obtained from a pulse oximeter are:
- the oxygen saturation of haemoglobin in arterial blood, described as SpO_2
- the pulse rate in beats per minute.

Some oximeters also display a pulse waveform or a signal indicator that provides information on the strength of the pulse being detected. This display signifies how well the tissues are perfused (Figs 32.1 and 32.2).

What is Oxygen Saturation?

Haemoglobin, within red blood cells, carries oxygen; one molecule of haemoglobin can carry up to four molecules of oxygen on its binding sites. If all the binding sites on the haemoglobin molecule are carrying oxygen, then it is considered to be 100% saturated. Oxygen saturation is a measure of how much oxygen the blood is carrying as a percentage of the maximum it could carry. For example, 100 haemoglobin molecules could together carry a maximum of 400 oxygen molecules (100×4); if these 100 haemoglobin molecules were carrying 380 oxygen molecules, they would

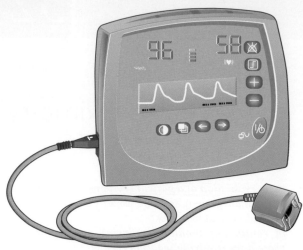

Fig. 32.1 Pulse oximeter with pulse waveform.

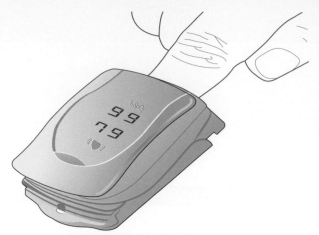

Fig. 32.3 Self-contained pulse oximeter.

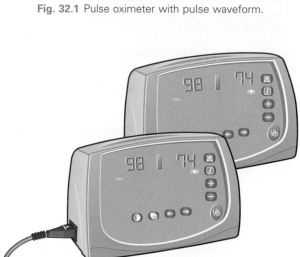

Fig. 32.2 Pulse oximeter showing bar signal strength.

be carrying $(380 \div 400) \times 100 = 95\%$ of the maximum number of oxygen molecules that they could carry, and so together would be 95% saturated.

PULSE OXIMETER

Numerous models of pulse oximeters are available. Some are built into multi-parameter monitors, which are used in critical care areas, while others are stand-alone monitors consisting of a monitor and a probe (see Figs 32.1 and 32.2) or self-contained units (Fig. 32.3).

The monitor contains the microprocessor and display, which shows the oxygen saturation, the pulse rate and the waveform. It is connected to the patient via a probe that senses the patient's pulse.

Probe

This consists of two parts:
- light emitting diodes (LEDs)
- a light detector (photo-detector)

The probe is the most fragile component of the pulse oximeter and is easily damaged; its link to the main unit is via a connector with a series of very fine pins that can be easily damaged. It is essential to ensure that the pins are aligned correctly before attempting to insert it into the monitor. Do not remove the probe from the machine by pulling on the cable; always grasp the connector firmly.

There are a variety of oximetry probes, such as ear, finger or toe probes, which can be reusable or disposable. Fig. 32.4 shows reusable probes (used in adults) and Fig. 32.5 shows disposable probes (used in children).

How Does the Pulse Oximeter Work?

Although pulse oximeters are relatively easy to use, the physics behind this monitoring modality are complex and so this is a simple overview of the principles behind calculation of pulse oximetry reading.

Oximeters work on:
- the laws of spectrophotometry (light absorption) using two types of light: red and infrared
- the Beer–Lambert law, which states that deoxygenated blood absorbs red light while oxygenated blood absorbs infrared light.

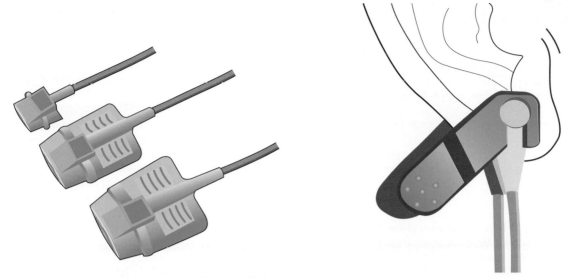

Fig. 32.4 Finger, toe and ear probes.

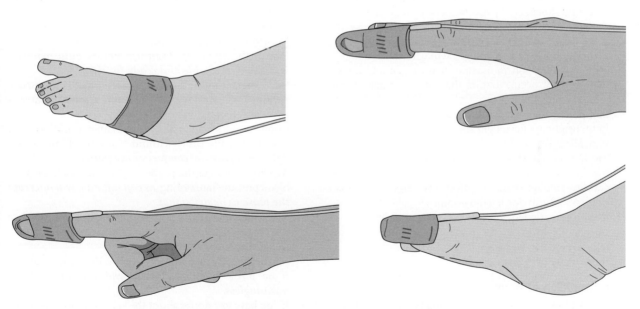

Fig. 32.5 Disposable probes for use on babies and children.

Two LEDs in the probe emit red and infrared light and the oximeter measures the absorption of these two specific wavelengths of light. The probe is positioned either on the fingertip or on the earlobe, and its LEDs transmit red and infrared through pulsing arterial blood to the photodetector. As already stated, oxygenated blood absorbs the infrared light, whereas deoxygenated blood absorbs red light. During systole, in the pulse cycle, there is an influx of oxygenated blood to the tissues, causing more infrared light to be absorbed and reducing the amount of light reaching the photodetector. The oxygen saturation of blood is determined by the degree of light absorption; the results are processed by the microprocessor within the oximeter and a result is displayed.

Plethysmography Trace

Many pulse oximeters display pulsatile changes in light absorbance on a graph that is termed a 'plethysmographic trace' or, more commonly, the 'pleth'. The pleth shows the quality of the pulsatile signal but is affected by many factors such as:

- peripheral blood flow, e.g. low blood pressure will reduce accuracy
- peripheral temperature, e.g. a low temperature will also reduce accuracy.

A poor pleth tracing can easily mislead the computer into calculating the oxygen saturation incorrectly (Moyle 2002).

Limitations

Pulse oximetry only measures haemoglobin oxygen saturation and gives no information about respiratory rate or ventilation: therefore it is not a complete measure of respiratory sufficiency. In order to assess ventilation, arterial blood gases must be measured (*see* Ch. 3). Factors that can affect the accuracy of pulse oximetry include:

- poor perfusion: this may be due to hypotension, hypovolaemic shock, cold peripheries or cardiac failure
- darker skin: deeply pigmented skin may decrease the pulse oximeter's accuracy, although the effect is minor
- carbon monoxide poisoning: haemoglobin has a higher affinity for carbon monoxide than oxygen and a high reading may occur, despite the patient actually being hypoxaemic
- nail polish, dirt and artificial nails
- light: bright artificial light shining directly on the probe may affect the reading
- motion, such as shivering: seizures may make it difficult for the probe to pick up a signal
- certain anti-retroviral medications: these can affect oxygen's affinity for haemoglobin
- dyes: e.g. methylene blue lowers saturation levels
- cardiac arrhythmias: these may cause very inaccurate measurements, especially if there are significant apex/radial deficits (Moore 2009).

Interpretation of Results

For most adult patients the SpO_2 should be 94–98% (British Thoracic Society 2017).

For patients at risk of hypercapnic respiratory failure, such as those with chronic obstructive pulmonary disease (COPD), the SpO_2 should be 88–92% (British Thoracic Society 2017).

Complications

Continuous use of finger probes can cause blisters on the finger pad, as well as pressure damage to the skin or nailbed.

Burns have also been reported from continuous use of the probe and it is recommended that the probe should be repositioned every 2–4 hours (Medical Devices Agency 2001). It is also recommended that the probe is not placed on a paralysed limb, as the patient may not be able to inform staff of any discomfort experienced (Woodrow 1999).

Important Practice Points

Accurate pulse oximetry readings depend on the fact that staff using this equipment are able to do so correctly and that they understand how to document and interpret the results in relation to the patient's clinical status. Assess and treat the **patient** and not the oximeter:

- Use oximetry as an adjunct to patient assessment and treatment evaluation.
- **Never** withhold oxygen if the patient has signs or symptoms of hypoxaemia, regardless of oximetry readings.

GUIDELINES AND RATIONALE FOR THIS NURSING PRACTICE

- Explain the nursing practice to the patient *to gain consent and cooperation.*
- Wash your hands *to reduce the risk of cross-infection* (World Health Organization 2018).
- Prepare the equipment *to ensure that the pulse oximeter is checked, available and ready for use.*
- Select the appropriate probe *to obtain the best possible readings.* If used on a finger or toe, ensure the area is clean and remove any nail varnish.
- Connect the probe to the pulse oximeter and position it so that it fits easily without being too loose or too tight, *to ensure the comfort of the patient.*
- Avoid positioning the probe on the arm being used for blood pressure monitoring, *as cuff inflation will interrupt the pulse oximeter signal.*
- Allow the pulse oximeter to detect the pulse and calculate the oxygen saturation (this may take several seconds), *to obtain an accurate reading.*
- Ensure that the display indicator has detected a pulse as *if no pulse is detected, any readings obtained are meaningless.*
- If you have any doubt about the accuracy of the reading, check your patient, escalating any concerns you have to a more experienced member of the healthcare team *to ensure patient safety.*
- If the oximeter is equipped with alarms, ensure that these are on *to detect any reduction in saturation and possible deterioration in the patient's condition.*
- If no signal is obtained:
  - The function of the oximeter probe can be checked by placing it on your own finger.

- Try another location, e.g. the ear lobe.
- Check the temperature of the patient: if the patient is cold, gentle rubbing of the digit or ear lobe may restore a signal.
- Document the saturation in the patient's observation chart and report any abnormal findings immediately *to provide a written record and assist in the implementation of any actions taken in response to the abnormal finding.*
- In undertaking this practice, nurses are accountable for their actions, the quality of care delivered and record-keeping in accordance with *The Code* (Nursing and Midwifery Council 2018).

PATIENT/CARER EDUCATION: KEY POINTS

It is important for patients to know the reason for this practice and, if continuous monitoring is required, why the probe must stay on for accurate readings. Patients should be given information on the practice to ensure cooperation and they should be asked to let the nursing team know if the probe is causing discomfort so that the site may be changed.

REFERENCES

British Thoracic Society, 2017. BTS guideline for oxygen use in adults in healthcare and emergency settings. Thorax 72 (Suppl. 1, June 2017), i1–i90.

Medical Devices Agency, 2001. MDA SN2001(08): Tissue Necrosis Caused by Pulse Oximeter Probes. MDA, London.

Moore, T., 2009. Pulse oximetry. In: Moore, T., Woodrow, P. (Eds.), High Dependency Nursing Care: Observation, Intervention and Support for Level 2 Patients, second ed. Routledge, London, pp. 147–153.

Moyle, J., 2002. Pulse Oximetry, second ed. BMJ Books, London.

Nursing and Midwifery Council, 2018. The Code: Professional Standards of Practice and Behaviour for Nurses, Midwives and Nursing Associates. NMC, London. Available from: https://www.nmc.org.uk/globalassets/sitedocuments/nmc-publications/nmc-code.pdf.

Tierney, L.M., Jr., Whooley, M.A., Saint, S., 1997. Oxygen saturation: a fifth vital sign? Western Journal of Medicine 166, 285–286.

Woodrow, P., 1999. Pulse oximetry. Nursing Standard 13 (42), 42–46.

World Health Organization, 2011. Pulse Oximetry Training Manual. Patient Safety. A World Alliance for Safer Healthcare. WHO, Geneva.

World Health Organization, 2018. 5 moments for hand hygiene. WHO, Geneva. Available from: https://www.who.int/gpsc/5may/background/5moments/en/.

SELF-ASSESSMENT

1. What are the indications for pulse oximetry monitoring?
2. Which sites may be used for the pulse oximetry probe?
3. What are the normal ranges of SpO_2 for a patient with chronic obstructive pulmonary disease?
4. What are the potential complications of continuous pulse oximetry monitoring?

33

Recognizing and Responding to Signs of Abuse

LEARNING OUTCOMES

By the end of this chapter, you should be able to:
* identify a vulnerable adult at risk of abuse
* identify different types of adult abuse
* recognize and respond to signs of harm or abuse.

BACKGROUND KNOWLEDGE REQUIRED

* Revision of policy and legislation relating to the protection or safeguarding of vulnerable adults (Department of Health 2011; Royal College of Nursing 2018)
* Revision of the local safeguarding policy: this will provide specific details for your area of practice, including useful contacts
* Nurses, midwives, students and healthcare support workers: understand *The Code* (Nursing and Midwifery Council 2018), as it is the foundation of good nursing and midwifery practice, and a key tool in protecting the health and well-being of the public

INDICATIONS AND RATIONALE FOR RECOGNIZING AND RESPONDING TO SIGNS OF ABUSE

Safeguarding means protecting everyone's right to be safe while receiving care (Royal College of Nursing 2018). It is part of everyday healthcare practice in any setting.

Nurses and other healthcare professionals must be able to identify vulnerable patient groups who may be at risk of abuse from family members, carers or practitioners. They must be able to recognize the different types of abuse that patients may experience, including institutional abuse and the associated signs to watch out for, and to identify factors that may contribute to a person's vulnerability.

This chapter will enhance your skills to recognize confidently and manage effectively those situations where you suspect a person in your care is at risk of harm, abuse or neglect.

OUTLINE OF THE PROCEDURE

A vulnerable adult is someone who is over 18 and cannot look after or protect themselves. The definition could include people who:
* have a physical or sensory disability
* have a learning disability
* have a mental health problem
* are older
* live in a care home (Department of Health 2013).

IDENTIFYING DIFFERENT TYPES AND SIGNS OF ABUSE

Seven core categories of abuse may be identified (Department of Health & Home Office 2000; Social Care Institute for Excellence 2018). The list of signs is not exhaustive.

Physical

This category may include: rough handling; hitting; punching; pushing; inappropriate or unlawful use of restraint; making someone purposefully uncomfortable (e.g. opening a window and removing blankets); misuse of medication (e.g. over-sedation); forcible feeding or withholding food.

Sexual

This category may include: inappropriate looking; sexual teasing or innuendo or sexual harassment; indecent exposure; inappropriate touch anywhere; any sexual activity that the person lacks the capacity to consent to.

Psychological/Emotional

This category may include: enforced isolation – preventing someone accessing services or educational and social opportunities; removing mobility or communication aids or intentionally leaving someone unattended when they need assistance; preventing the expression of choice and opinion;

failure to respect privacy; preventing someone from meeting their religious and cultural needs.

Neglect and/or Acts of Omission

This category may include: failure to provide or allow access to food, shelter, clothing, heating, or personal or medical care; providing care in a way that the person dislikes; ignoring or isolating the person; not taking account of an individual's cultural, religious or ethnic needs.

Discriminatory

This category may include: unequal treatment based on age, disability, gender reassignment, marriage and civil partnership, pregnancy and maternity, race, religion and belief, sex or sexual orientation (known as 'protected characteristics' under the Equality Act (GOV.UK 2010); verbal abuse, derogatory remarks or inappropriate use of language related to a protected characteristic; denying access to communication aids, or not allowing access to an interpreter, signer or lip reader; deliberate exclusion on the grounds of a protected characteristic.

Financial and/or Material

This category may include: theft of money or possessions; fraud, scamming, preventing a person from accessing their own money, benefits or assets; employees taking a loan from a person using the service; misuse of personal allowance in a care home; false representation, using another person's bank account, cards or documents.

Organizational or Institutional

This category may include: not offering choice or promoting independence; lack of respect for dignity and privacy; poor-quality care; lack of leadership and supervision; rigid regimes; discouraging visits or involvement of relatives or friends.

RECOGNIZING AND RESPONDING TO SIGNS OF HARM OR ABUSE

Nurses have a duty to recognize the signs and symptoms of abuse and to act on any concerns they may have. They are required to make patient care their primary concern and to ensure that protecting vulnerable adults is an integral part of everyday nursing practice (Royal College of Nursing 2018).

Nurses have a key role in the protection of vulnerable adults. Abuse can occur in a range of environments, including the NHS, voluntary organizations, private care homes and patients' personal residences. Nurses can help recognize abuse and respond accordingly, if they are knowledgeable and aware of adults in their care who could be vulnerable to, and at risk of, abuse. To safeguard the vulnerable adult, nurses also need to understand the different types of adult abuse and the associated signs and symptoms, ensuring that any abuse is reported appropriately (Straughair 2011)

Reporting of any concerns will be explicit in local health board policies. It is a worthwhile exercise to locate and become familiar with the policy for protecting and/or safeguarding vulnerable adults in your area of practice. Familiarize yourself with the reporting process and identify the key personnel with designated responsibility for adult safeguarding. Access adult safeguarding resources to develop your professional knowledge and understanding (*see* Royal College of Nursing 2018).

PREVENTING ABUSE

Preventing abuse and neglect should be done in the context of person-centred support and personalization, empowering individuals to make choices and supporting them to manage risks. This should lead to the services that people might wish to use, with the potential to prevent abuse and neglect within healthcare settings (Social Care Institute for Excellence 2018).

One way in which governments are being proactive is to implement policy regarding adult support and abuse prevention that highlights the need for inter-agency working. For example, the Adult Support and Protection (Scotland) Act 2007 ('The Act') seeks to protect and benefit adults at risk of being harmed. The Act requires councils and a range of public bodies to work together to support and protect adults who are unable to safeguard themselves, their property and their rights. The Act provides a range of measures that agencies can use to identify those at risk. The public bodies are collectively required to take steps to decide whether a person is at risk of harm while balancing the need to intervene with an adult's right to live as independently as possible (The Scottish Government 2017). Similar policy is in place in other countries within the United Kingdom.

REFERENCES

Adult Support and Protection (Scotland) Act 2007. Available from: https://www.legislation.gov.uk/asp/2007/10/contents.

Department of Health, 2011. Safeguarding adults: the role of health service practitioners. The Stationery Office, London.

Department of Health & Home Office, 2000. No Secrets; Guidance On Developing And Implementing Multi-Agency Policies and Procedures to Protect Vulnerable Adults From Abuse. The Stationary Office, London.

GOV.UK, 2010. Equality Act. Available from: https://www.gov.uk/guidance/equality-act-2010-guidance.

Nursing and Midwifery Council, 2018. The Code: professional standards of practice and behaviour for nurses, midwives and nursing associates. NMC, London. Available from: https://www.nmc.org.uk/globalassets/sitedocuments/nmc-publications/nmc-code.pdf.

Royal College of Nursing, 2018. Adult safeguarding: roles and competencies for health care staff. Available from: https://www.rcn.org.uk/professional-development/publications/pub-007069.

Social Care Institute for Excellence, 2018. Safeguarding adults. Available from: https://www.scie.org.uk/safeguarding/adults/introduction.

Straughair, C., 2011. Safeguarding vulnerable adults: the role of the registered nurse. Nursing Standard 25 (45), 49–56.

The Scottish Government, 2017. Adult support and protection. Available from: https://www2.gov.scot/Topics/Health/Support-Social-Care/Adult-Support-Protection.

WEBSITE

https://www.gov.uk/government/publications/report-of-the-mid-staffordshire-nhs-foundation-trust-public-inquiry *Report of the Mid Staffordshire NHS Foundation Trust Public Inquiry 2013*

SELF-ASSESSMENT

1. What is expected of nurses and other healthcare professionals in terms of protecting the health and well-being of the public?
2. How would you identify a vulnerable adult at risk of abuse?
3. What are the main types of adult abuse?

34

Rectal Examination and Removal of Faeces (Digital)

There are two parts to this chapter:
1. Digital rectal examination
2. Digital removal of faeces.

LEARNING OUTCOMES

By the end of this chapter, you should be able to:
- prepare the patient for this procedure
- collect and prepare the equipment
- assist the practitioner performing this procedure as requested.

BACKGROUND KNOWLEDGE REQUIRED

- Revision of the anatomy and physiology of the sigmoid colon, rectum and anus
- A basic understanding of the potential complications for spinal injury patients in relation to bowel care

1. DIGITAL RECTAL EXAMINATION

INDICATIONS AND RATIONALE FOR RECTAL EXAMINATION

Rectal examination is used as a diagnostic aid to:
- assess anal/rectal sensation
- assess if faecal matter is present and its amount and consistency (Fig. 34.1)
- assess the need for, and outcome of, digital stimulation to trigger defaecation by stimulating the recto-anal reflex
- assess the need for manual removal of faeces
- evaluate bowel emptiness post procedure
- assess rectal bleeding
- assess severe constipation
- assess severe diarrhoea
- assess pain in the anal or rectal area
- assess a suspected enlarged prostate gland
- assess a suspected rectocele.

An experienced nurse who has undergone appropriate training may perform a digital rectal examination (DRE) as part of the assessment process for severe constipation (Royal College of Nursing 2012). This procedure assists the nurse practitioner in the decision-making process when choosing an appropriate laxative or enema. The nurse practitioner may also use this procedure to remove faeces present in the lower rectum if appropriate.

OUTLINE OF THE PROCEDURE

DRE must be performed with caution on patients with a spinal injury at T6 or above. DRE can stimulate the vagus nerve, causing the heartbeat to slow and blood pressure to fall. The patient may demonstrate a flush over the upper body and experience a sense of impending doom. This is known as 'autonomic dysreflexia' and requires prompt medical attention.

Prior to the procedure, it is recommended that physical observations are conducted, whether this is a first-time or an ongoing intervention; signs of autonomic dysreflexia in patients with spinal cord injury should be sought. **If, at any time, the heart rate drops or signs of autonomic dysreflexia are seen, the procedure should be stopped** (Multidisciplinary Association of Spinal Cord Injury Professionals 2012; Royal College of Nursing 2012).

Verbal consent should be obtained from the patient prior to the procedure and this should be documented in the patient's notes. Chaperoning is also essential.

The medical or nursing practitioner will put a disposable glove on the dominant hand and apply some lubricant to the fingertips. They will then insert an index finger into the patient's rectum and perform the examination. On completing the examination, the practitioner will remove the glove by turning it inside out as they take it off. A lubricated rectal speculum may be inserted by a **medical practitioner** (Fig. 34.2) and, with the aid of the light source, a visual examination is carried out. An anal or rectal swab may also be taken for laboratory examination.

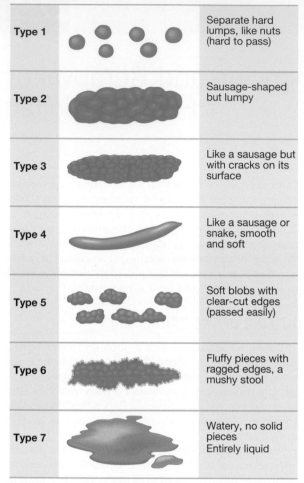

Type 1		Separate hard lumps, like nuts (hard to pass)
Type 2		Sausage-shaped but lumpy
Type 3		Like a sausage but with cracks on its surface
Type 4		Like a sausage or snake, smooth and soft
Type 5		Soft blobs with clear-cut edges (passed easily)
Type 6		Fluffy pieces with ragged edges, a mushy stool
Type 7		Watery, no solid pieces Entirely liquid

Fig. 34.1 Bristol Stool Chart. Reproduced with permission from Ralston SH, Penman ID, Strachan MWJ, Hobson RP: Davidson's Principles and Practice of Medicine, 23rd edn, Edinburgh, 2018, Elsevier Ltd, and adapted from Lewis SJ, Heaton KW: Stool form scale as a useful guide to intestinal transit time, Scandinavian Journal of Gastroenterology 32:920–924, 1997.

It is important to note that this is an invasive and embarrassing procedure for the patient. Care and consideration should be exercised by the practitioner at all stages of this procedure, remaining alert to potential issues that could arise, such as previous radiotherapy to this area, detection of a previously undiagnosed rectal carcinoma or a past history of sexual abuse. The examiner also needs to be sensitive to any cultural or religious needs that the patient may have. DRE should not be confused with digital stimulation or digital removal of faeces (manual evacuation), which can be performed on a regular basis in patients with neurogenic bowel dysfunction as part of a bowel management programme. DRE is often used to ensure that the rectum is empty following defaecation or to note the effect of suppositories and enemas.

◎ EQUIPMENT

- Tray/flat surface
- Disposable gloves
- Apron
- Sterile rectal speculum (*see* Fig. 34.2) (if required)
- Water-soluble lubricant
- Protective covering for the bed
- Receptacle for soiled disposable items
- Swabs
- Sterile laboratory swab in a container (if required)
- Light source

GUIDELINES AND RATIONALE FOR THIS NURSING PRACTICE

- Help to explain the procedure to the patient *to gain consent and cooperation.*
- **The consent for the procedure should be documented, particularly if this is a first-time intervention for the patient** (Steggal 2008; Steggal & Cox 2009; Kyle 2011).
- Collect and prepare the equipment *to maintain efficiency of practice.*
- Obtain a baseline pulse *to allow for quick identification of any complications related to stimulating the vagus nerve during the procedure.*
- Assist the patient into the required position, adopting the left lateral position with both knees bent (Fig. 34.3), *to allow good visualization of the anus and facilitate easier insertion of the index finger* (Royal College of Nursing 2012).
- Apply a disposable apron; wash and dry your hands before applying disposable gloves.
- Explain to the patient that the external and internal areas will be examined, *to observe and note the following:*

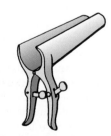

Fig. 34.2 Rectal speculum.

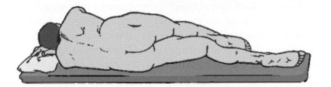

Fig. 34.3 Lateral position.

- rectal prolapse: document size, colour and any ulceration
- haemorrhoids: note size, position and grade; haemorrhoids can appear on the external side of the anus
- anal fissures: appear as breaks or cuts at the anal opening
- gaping anus: suggests that internal and external anal sphincter tone has been reduced or lost
- anal skin tags: note number, position and condition
- other conditions, such as threadworm or excoriation: document and treat accordingly
- foreign bodies: include objects that the person has inserted.
- Having completed an observational examination, the nurse should palpate the perianal area, feeling for any irregularities, *to identify any tenderness or the presence of abscesses.* With a gloved finger, start at the 12 o'clock position and move clockwise to 6 o'clock. Return to 12 o'clock and in an anticlockwise direction move to 6 o'clock (Royal College of Nursing 2012).
- Lubricate a gloved index finger with lubricant gel and inform the patient that you are about to commence the examination.
- Prior to finger insertion, encourage the patient to breathe out and talk; place the gloved finger on the anus for a few seconds *to prevent the anal sphincter from going into spasm on insertion.* Gently placing a finger on the anus initiates the anal reflex, causing the anus to contract and then relax (Royal College of Nursing 2012).
- Insert one finger only. The index finger assesses anal sphincter control. Resistance on insertion indicates good internal sphincter tone; only during defaecation does the sphincter relax (Royal College of Nursing 2012).
- With the finger inserted in the anus, sweep in a clockwise motion and then anticlockwise, noting any irregularities. Palpate around the anus for 360 degrees *to establish whether there is any tenderness or swelling in the rectum* (Steggal 2008; Steggal & Cox 2009).
- Assess for faecal matter in the rectum. Note consistency, amount and type, using the Bristol Stool Chart (*see* Fig. 34.1), *to allow for assessment of faecal loading/ constipation and the need for further interventions.*

- Observe the patient throughout the procedure *to detect any signs of discomfort, distress or autonomic dysreflexia; stop if the anal area is bleeding, or if the patients asks you to stop or is demonstrating signs of autonomic dysreflexia.*
- Once the procedure is completed, clean any residual lubricating gel from the perianal area *to provide comfort and dignity, and to prevent excoriation to the patient's skin.*
- Remove gloves and apron (Loveday et al. 2014) and dispose of them according to local policy. Wash hands according to local policy.
- Ensure that the patient is left feeling as comfortable as possible.
- If any bleeding is likely as a result of the examination, ensure that the patient's underwear is protected.
- Offer the patient the toilet/commode, as the procedure may have stimulated the anorectal reflex and the urge to defaecate.
- Dispose of the equipment safely in accordance with local policy and infection control procedures *to protect others.*
- Document the procedure in the patient's records, including patient consent for the examination, the reason for DRE, the outcome and the review date, *to assess the need for a repeat DRE, to provide a written record and to assist in the implementation of any action, should an abnormality or adverse reaction to the practice be noted.*

2. DIGITAL REMOVAL OF FAECES

INDICATIONS AND RATIONALE FOR DIGITAL REMOVAL OF FAECES

Digital removal of faeces (DRF) is considered an invasive procedure and, according to the Royal College of Nursing (2012), should only be performed if necessary. Culture and religious beliefs must be taken into consideration before undertaking the procedure (Royal College of Nursing 2012).

According to Solomons & Woodward (2013), nurses in acute hospital settings should familiarize themselves with the Royal College of Nursing (2012) guidelines on DRF, along with the Multidisciplinary Association of Spinal Cord Injury Professionals' (2012) *Guidelines for the Management of Neurogenic Bowel Dysfunction in Individuals with Central Neurological Conditions*. Some patients, e.g. those with a spinal cord injury or multiple sclerosis, may require DRF as a regular part of their care package. The National Patient Safety Agency (2004; 2018) has highlighted the fact that some people with an established spinal cord lesion are dependent on DRF as part of their routine bowel care; however, when admitted to the acute setting, there may be a failure to perform the procedure for such individuals. This can place them at risk of developing autonomic dysreflexia. They further assert that, no matter what the clinical setting is, nurses have a duty of care to any patient with a spinal cord injury to provide DRF or to ensure that there is a colleague who is competent in this procedure. This is particularly important if DRF is part of the patient's routine bowel care or if it is otherwise indicated (National Patient Safety Agency 2004; Nursing and Midwifery Council 2015; Nursing and Midwifery Council 2018b; National Patient Safety Agency 2018).

DRF is indicated:

- when other methods of bowel management have failed
- to assess stool consistency
- to assess faecal impaction or loading
- when there is an incomplete ability or an inability to defaecate
- in neurogenic bowel dysfunction
- in spinal cord injury.

◎ EQUIPMENT

- Disposable gloves (several pairs)
- Incontinence pad/bed protection
- Plastic apron
- Tissues or toilet paper
- Cleaning wipes
- Lubricating gel/local anaesthetic gel (as indicated and as per local health guidelines)
- Disposable bag
- Bedpan/commode

GUIDELINES AND RATIONALE FOR THIS NURSING PRACTICE

This is a two-person procedure *to ensure accurate and timely monitoring of observations and of the patient's condition during the procedure.* The use of automated sphygmomanometers may be helpful in monitoring vital signs in this instance. Manual pulse and blood pressure should also be recorded to note rate, rhythm and amplitude.

- Explain the procedure and obtain verbal consent, documenting the consent in the patient's records, *to reduce anxiety and gain consent.*
- Ensure that the procedure is carried out in privacy, selecting an area that can be screened, *to maintain the patient's privacy and dignity.*
- Take the patient's pulse rate at rest prior to the procedure *to record a baseline pulse and monitor for changes.*
- Take the patient's blood pressure, particularly if it is a spinal patient, *to record baseline blood pressure and monitor for changes.*
- Wash your hands and apply apron and gloves. Local health policy may indicate the use of double gloves *to prevent possible contact with body fluids and to minimize the risk of cross-infection.*
- Position the patient in the left lateral position (*see* Fig. 34.3), with their back to the edge of the bed and their knees flexed. Place an absorbent pad underneath the buttocks and cover the rest of the patient. Use this positioning *to allow easy of entry into the rectum, following the natural curve of the colon.*
- Examine the perianal area for any abnormalities before starting the procedure, *to ensure that it is safe to proceed* (see 'Digital Rectal Examination' earlier).
- For patients who receive this procedure on a regular basis, use lubricating gel on the gloved index finger *to minimize discomfort and avoid anal mucosal trauma.*
- If this is a first-time or an acute procedure, a local anaesthetic gel (Instillagel) may be topically applied to the anal area.
- Wait 5 minutes to allow the gel to take effect *to ensure that the patient is as pain-free and comfortable as possible, and to allow the anaesthetic gel to have the required effect.* Do not apply the gel if the anal mucosa is damaged and check for contraindications.
- Reassure the patient throughout the procedure *to avoid unnecessary stress or embarrassment and to ensure consent.*
- Insert a lubricated and gloved index finger into the rectum for 4–5 cm *to minimize patient discomfort and avoid anal mucosal trauma.*
- Assess for the presence of faecal matter using the Bristol Stool Chart (*see* Fig. 34.1) *to check for the presence of faecal matter and to establish the consistency of the stool.*
- Bristol Stool Chart type 1: remove a lump at a time until the rectum is empty *to minimize discomfort and facilitate easier removal of stool.*
- Bristol Stool Chart type 2: push a finger into the middle of the faecal mass and split it. Remove small sections of faeces at a time and place in a receptacle *to minimize discomfort and facilitate easier removal of faeces.*

- Do not overstretch the sphincter by using a hooked finger to remove large pieces of stool, *to avoid trauma to the rectal mucosa and sphincter.*
- If the rectum is full of soft stool, continuous gentle circling of the finger may be used to remove it; this is still considered as DRF (Royal College of Nursing 2012).
- If the top glove becomes very soiled, remove it and replace with a new top glove *to avoid soiling of the patient's skin and to maintain cleanliness.*
- Lubricate a gloved finger with each change of glove, using extra lubrication as required, *to facilitate easier insertion and minimize friction and discomfort.*
- **If the faecal mass is too hard or larger than 4 cm across, or you are unable to break it up, stop and inform the medical team** *to minimize the risk of autonomic dysreflexia.*
- If the patient becomes distressed, check the pulse again, against the baseline reading; **stop if the pulse rate has dropped, or if there is pain or bleeding in the anal area.** Check blood pressure for patients with spinal injury *to monitor the condition of the patient and to establish whether it is necessary to stop.*
- When the rectum is empty, remove the top glove, and clean and dry the patient's perianal area *to maintain cleanliness and to leave the patient comfortable.*
- Observe the skin on completion of the procedure *to monitor skin condition.*
- Dispose of the gloves, apron and other equipment in the correct clinical waste bag and wash your hands *to prevent cross-infection.*
- Offer the patient the toilet/commode, as the procedure may have stimulated the anorectal reflex and the urge to defaecate.
- Ensure that the patient is comfortable and check the pulse (and blood pressure in spinal patients) *to observe for any adverse reactions.*
- Record the bowel results in the patient's record and communicate the results to the patient and medical team, if appropriate. Consistency of stool, volume, date and time should all be noted *to establish the effectiveness of the procedure and to ensure continuity of care.*
- *The Code* (Nursing and Midwifery Council 2018a), under the heading of 'Preserve Safety', states that nurses must make sure that patients' and public safety are protected. Nurses must work within the limits of their competence, exercising a professional 'duty of candour' and raising concerns immediately whenever situations are encountered that could potentially put patients or public safety at risk. **It is essential to recognize and understand this, and to work within the limits of your competence.** Information and advice provided should be evidence-based, and knowledge and skills must be updated *to ensure safe and effective practice at all times.*

 PATIENT/CARER EDUCATION: KEY POINTS

In partnership with the patient and/or carer, ensure that they are competent to carry out any practices required. Information should be given on an appropriate point of contact for any concerns that may arise. A careful explanation should help to gain the patient's cooperation and aid relaxation, which will in turn reduce the discomfort of the examination.

The patient should be informed of whom to contact if severe pain, discharge or bleeding is experienced after the examination. Contact numbers for appropriate counselling services should be available in the event of distress caused by issues that relate to any history of sexual abuse experienced by the patient.

The nurse may also advise the patient post examination about fluids, fibre and dietary requirements.

Other factors that might be explained to the patient include the prevention of constipation, performance of pelvic floor exercises, achievement of an effective positioning technique to enable less straining at stool and self-administration of rectal medications.

REFERENCES

Kyle, G., 2011. Digital rectal examination. Nursing Times 107 (12), 50–51.

Loveday, H.P., Wilson, J.A., Pratt, R.J., et al., 2014. Epic3: National evidence-based guidelines for preventing healthcare-associated infections in NHS hospitals in England. Journal of Hospital Infection 86, S1–S36.

Multidisciplinary Association of Spinal Cord Injury Professionals, 2012. Guidelines for Management of Neurogenic Bowel Dysfunction in Individuals with Central Neurological Conditions. MASCIP, Middlesex.

National Patient Safety Agency, 2004. Patient Briefing: Ensuring the Appropriate Provision of Manual Bowel Evacuation for Patients with an Established Spinal Cord Lesion. NPSA, London.

National Patient Safety Agency, 2018. Patient Briefing: Resources to support safer bowel care for patients at risk of autonomic dysreflexia. NPSA, London.

Nursing and Midwifery Council, 2015. Guidelines for Records and Record Keeping. NMC, London.

Nursing and Midwifery Council, 2018a. The Code: Professional Standards of Practice and Behaviour for Nurses, Midwives and Nursing Associates. NMC, London. Available at: https://www.nmc.org.uk/globalassets/sitedocuments/nmc-publications/nmc-code.pdf.

Nursing and Midwifery Council, 2018b. Future Nurse: Standards of Proficiency for Registered Nurses. NMC, London. Available at: https://www.nmc.org.uk/globalassets/sitedocuments/education-standards/future-nurse-proficiencies.pdf.

Royal College of Nursing, 2012. Management of Lower bowel Dysfunction including DRE and DRF - guidance for nurses. RCN, London.

Solomons, J., Woodward, S., 2013. Digital Removal of faeces in the bowel management of patients with spinal cord injury: a review. British Journal of Neuroscience Nursing 9 (5), 216–221.

Steggal, M., 2008. Digital rectal examination. Nursing Standard 22 (47), 46–48.

Steggal, M., Cox, C., 2009. A step by step guide to performing complete digital rectal examination. Gastrointestinal Nursing 7 (2), 28–32.

WEBSITES

https://www.bladderandbowel.org/ *Bladder and Bowel Support Community*

https://improvement.nhs.uk/documents/3074/Patient_Safety_Alert_-_safer_care_for_patients_at_risk_of_AD.pdf *NHS Improvement: Resources to support safer bowel care for patients at risk of autonomic dysreflexia*

https://www.rcn.org.uk/professional-development/publications/pub-003226 *Royal College of Nursing: Management of lower bowel dysfunction, including DRE and DRF*

https://rcni.com/hosted-content/rcn/continence/home *Royal College of Nursing: Continence*

https://www.rnoh.nhs.uk/sites/default/files/sia-mascip-bowelguidenew2012.pdf *Guidelines for management of neurogenic bowel dysfunction in individuals with central neurological conditions*

https://www.spinal.co.uk/wp-content/uploads/2017/05/Autonomic-Dysreflexia.pdf *Spinal Injuries Association: Living with Spinal Cord Injury factsheet: autonomic dysreflexia*

SELF-ASSESSMENT

1. Describe the complications associated with performing a digital rectal examination on a patient with a spinal injury.
2. Describe and justify the correct positioning of the patient prior to a rectal examination.
3. Explain why a patient may be apprehensive prior to undergoing a rectal examination.
4. Discuss the reasons why this procedure may not be carried out.

35

Respiration, Including Nebulizers and Inhalers

There are two parts to this chapter:
1. Respirations
2. Inhalers, nebulizers (inhaled therapies) and peak flow measurement.

1. RESPIRATIONS

LEARNING OUTCOMES

By the end of this chapter, you should be able to:
• prepare the patient for this nursing practice
• assess, measure and record respiration
• recognize any abnormalities in the patient's condition.

BACKGROUND KNOWLEDGE REQUIRED

• Revision of the functions of the main respiratory organs (upper and lower respiratory tract)
• Revision of the position of the respiratory system, in relation to the circulatory system
• Revision of the neurological control of respiration

INDICATIONS AND RATIONALE FOR ASSESSING RESPIRATION

The basic function of the respiratory system is to supply sufficient oxygen for the body's metabolic needs and to remove carbon dioxide (Waugh & Grant 2014). This is achieved through inspiration and expiration. The importance of accurately recording the respiratory rate should never be underestimated, as the respiratory rate will often increase and be the first vital sign to alter when a patient's physical condition is deteriorating (Philip et al. 2013; Mølgaard et al. 2016).

Assessment of respiration may be made for the following reasons:

• to obtain a baseline measurement *to gather information regarding the patient's presenting condition and to allow any alteration in the patient's breathing pattern to be promptly noticed*
• to monitor a patient who has breathing problems *to help with diagnosis*
• to compare against baseline measurements *to help evaluate the effect of treatment on patients who have pulmonary disease and to establish any alteration in the patient's condition.*

OUTLINE OF THE PROCEDURE

Be discreet and avoid informing the patient when respirations are being taken. Count the respiratory rate for 60 seconds, and throughout the procedure, observe for signs of respiratory compromise (e.g. skin colour, signs of increased respiratory effort, additional sounds).

Accurately and correctly record respirations on the appropriate chart. Report any abnormal reading or observation to a mentor or the nurse in charge.

When you have finished with the equipment, clean it and return it to storage. Cleanse your hands.

EQUIPMENT

• Appropriate hand-cleansing equipment
• Watch with a second hand
• Correct vital sign documentation charts

GUIDELINES AND RATIONALE FOR THIS NURSING PRACTICE

• On approach, observe the patient to establish how much effort is required for them to breathe (work of breathing) and for signs of respiratory distress. You may notice flaring of the nostrils, pursed lips or use of the accessory muscles of breathing. These include the sternocleidomastoid muscle or scalene muscles in the neck, the intercostal muscles (in between the ribs) and the diaphragm at the top of the abdomen.

- Recording the respiratory rate is best carried out without the patient's knowledge; *if the patient becomes aware that the respiratory rate is being assessed, they may inadvertently try to control their breathing, giving a false reading.*
- Ensure that you can see the chest clearly and that the patient is in a comfortable position and as relaxed as possible, *to help ensure an accurate assessment.*
- Observe the patient throughout for any signs of discomfort or distress, *to monitor any adverse effects and establish the presence of any underlying physical conditions.*
- Respiratory assessment is usually carried out immediately after assessment of the patient's pulse, while the nurse still has a finger in position to palpate the radial pulse, *to reduce the risk of the patient becoming aware that the respiration rate is being assessed.*
- Count the respirations for 60 seconds by observing the rise and fall of the patient's chest. One respiration consists of one breath in (inspiration) and one breath out (expiration). The normal respiratory rate for an adult is 12–20 respirations per minute (Royal College of Physicians 2017).
- Observe the rhythm, depth and noise of respiration. Normally, respiration should be effortless and quiet, with a regular rhythm and adequate depth.
- Observe for unusual noises. A high-pitched sound on inspiration (stridor) usually indicates an upper respiratory tract obstruction and a whistling sound on expiration (wheeze) usually indicates a lower respiratory tract obstruction. Other sounds may include gurgling (caused by secretions), grunting or snoring (caused by the soft tissues of the airway losing muscle tone).
- Observe the patient's skin colour for signs of low oxygen levels in the tissues (hypoxia). The patient may be pale (pallor) or there may be a blue tinge to the skin (cyanosis).
- Carry out the assessment for 60 seconds, *as this is required for an accurate assessment* (Mølgaard et al. 2016).
- Document the findings accurately on the correct chart, comparing them against past recordings. Report any abnormal findings immediately, according to local policy, and be aware of any possible complications *to allow immediate intervention if it is required* (Nursing and Midwifery Council 2010).
- In undertaking this practice, nurses are accountable for their actions, the quality of care delivered and record-keeping, in accordance with *The Code* (Nursing and Midwifery Council 2018).

👪 PATIENT/CARER EDUCATION: KEY POINTS

Information should be given on an appropriate point of contact for any concerns that may arise.

Explain techniques that may help to ease breathing difficulties to patients who have respiratory problems. Such advice may include the avoidance of restrictive clothing, resting positions and breathing techniques.

The effects of exercise on breathing rates and patterns should also be explained.

2. INHALERS, NEBULIZERS (INHALED THERAPIES) AND PEAK FLOW MEASUREMENT

LEARNING OUTCOMES

By the end of this chapter, you should be able to:
- prepare the patient for this nursing practice
- collect and prepare the equipment
- administer drugs via a pressurized metered-dose inhaler (pMDI) or nebulizer
- maintain equipment safely before and after administration
- document administration of medicines (NMC 2010).

BACKGROUND KNOWLEDGE REQUIRED

- Revision of the anatomy and physiology of the respiratory system
- Revision of 'Oxygen Therapy' (*see* Ch. 28)
- Revision of 'Administration of Medicines' (*see* Ch. 2)
- Revision of local policy on inhaled therapies

INDICATIONS AND RATIONALE FOR USING INHALED THERAPIES

Patients with underlying respiratory conditions, such as asthma and chronic obstructive pulmonary disease (COPD), may be prescribed medication that needs to be taken by inhalation. Inhaled therapies come in a variety of forms, including pressurised Metered Dose Inhaler (pMDI), breath-actuated inhalers, dry powder inhalers (DPI) and nebulizers (British National Formulary/National Institute for Health and Care Excellence 2018). While some may contain similar medication, the dose and way in which they are delivered vary according to each device.

INHALER THERAPY

The patient's inhaler technique should always be checked when the opportunity presents itself (British Thoracic Society/Scottish Intercollegiate Guidelines Network 2016; White et al. 2018), as even those who have been using inhalers for a long period of time may not be using the correct technique. Indeed, it is believed that a number of acute asthma attacks could be avoided with correct inhaler technique (White et al. 2018).

OUTLINE OF THE PROCEDURE

The procedure will depend on which type of inhaler is being administered. The three main types of inhaler are:
- pMDI, which requires a 'press and breathe' technique
- breath-actuated MDI, which requires a 'breathe in normally' technique
- DPI, which requires a 'breathe in hard' technique (Asthma (UK) 2018).

Regardless of the type of inhaler, the principles of safe administration of medication apply to all (Nursing Midwifery Council 2018).

◉ EQUIPMENT

- Prescribed inhaler device
- Prescription chart
- Pen

GUIDELINES AND RATIONALE FOR THIS NURSING PRACTICE

- Introduce yourself to the patient *to value the person and help establish a therapeutic relationship* (O'Dowd 2016).
- Explain the procedure to the patient *to obtain consent and cooperation. Patients should be encouraged to be active partners in their care.*
- Cleanse your hands, according to national policy, *to prevent cross-infection between patients* (World Health Organization 2018).
- Check the prescription chart and identity of the patient *to minimize medication errors and optimize patient safety* (Nursing Midwifery Council 2018).
- Ensure the patient is standing or sitting as upright as possible *to optimize lung expansion.*

For a pMDI

- Remove the mouthpiece cover *to allow access to the mouthpiece.*

- Shake the inhaler *to mix together the asthma medication and propellant, and to ensure that the correct dose of medication is released.*
- Ask the patient to breathe out gently *to allow more space in the airways and to optimize inhalation of the medication to reach the small airways.*
- The patient should then hold the inhaler upright and put the mouthpiece into their mouth, with their lips and mouth closed around the inhaler *to prevent escape of medication.*
- Observe as the patient breathes in deeply and slowly and presses the canister, while continuing to breathe in slowly and deeply, *to optimize the delivery of medication to the lungs.*
- Observe as the patient removes the inhaler from their mouth, closes their mouth and holds their breath for 10 seconds (or as long as they comfortably can) *to allow the medication more time to reach the small airways deep in the lungs.*
- Breathe out gently and, if a second dose is required, repeat these steps after approximately 30–60 seconds (Asthma (UK) 2018) *to give adequate rest between doses, and to optimize the effect of the medication, which will provide maximum control of symptoms with the minimum required dose* (Joels 2012).
- Replace the mouthpiece cover after use *to prevent foreign bodies entering the mouthpiece,* which would then be at risk of being inhaled by the patient.
- Observe the patient throughout this activity for any signs of discomfort or distress *to allow immediate intervention in the event of an adverse reaction.*
- Document administration of the medication according to local policy.
- If this is a preventer inhaler, provide facilities for oral hygiene *to reduce the risk of compromising the patient's oral health* (Godara et al. 2011).
- Cleanse your hands according to national policy *to prevent cross-infection between patients* (World Health Organization 2018).

For a pMDI with a Spacer Device

Occasionally, patients may need to use a spacer device for the administration of inhaled therapies. While this may be due to a patient's lack of the dexterity and coordination required to self-administer an inhaler (British National Formulary/National Institute for Health and Care Excellence 2018), Godara et al. (2011) suggest that this also reduces the medication deposits in the oral cavity that can cause oral health problems (e.g. thrush infections). The time delay in delivery using a spacer device allows more of the particles to evaporate, which then increases the amount inhaled into the lung (Godara et al. 2011).

- Take off the cap and shake the inhaler *to mix the medicine inside the inhaler with the propellant.*
- Position the inhaler in the end of the spacer.
- Ask the patient to breathe out gently for as long as feels comfortable, *to allow more space in the airways and to optimize inhalation of the medication to reach the small airways.*
- Put the spacer mouthpiece between the patient's teeth and lips, making a seal *to prevent the escape of medication.*
- Press the canister *to put one puff of the medicine into the spacer.*
- Ask the patient to breathe in slowly and steadily (not hard and fast) through the mouthpiece *to optimize the delivery of medication deep into the lungs.*
- Remove the spacer from the patient's mouth and ask them to hold their breath for 10 seconds (or for as long as is comfortable), and then breathe out slowly through their nose *to allow the medication more time to reach the small airways deep in the lungs.*
- N.B. In situations where a patient is unable to hold their breath, they can keep the spacer in their mouth, sealing their lips around the end of this, while they breathe in and out of the mouthpiece five times. This is as effective as holding the breath for 10 seconds (Lavorini & Fontana 2009).
- If the patient requires a second dose, wait 30 seconds, remove the inhaler, shake it and repeat the steps above *to give adequate rest between doses, and to optimize the effect of the medication, which will provide maximum control of symptoms with the minimum required dose* (Joels 2012).

It is worth noting that using spacers to administer inhalers is at least as effective as a nebulizer in the treatment of acute, severe asthma with hypoxia (Cates et al. 2006). In addition to their being more cost-effective and convenient, the advantages of this approach include lower pulse rate increase in comparison to nebulizers, a more rapid administration and improved efficiency of delivery of medication (Lavorini & Fontana 2009). However, it is important to note the difference between asthma attacks and lung attacks of COPD. Van Geffen et al. (2016) conducted a Cochrane review that concluded that there was no clear evidence to favour one method over the other. Their findings established that while there was no difference in lung function or undesirable side-effects after 1 hour, the secondary outcome in terms of lung function did favour nebulizer over inhaler in COPD.

NEBULIZER THERAPY

Nebulizers allow drugs to be administered directly into the lower respiratory tract. Drugs are usually available in solution, in single-use containers called nebules. When a nebulizer is attached to a flow of air or oxygen, it converts the solution of a drug into an aerosol for therapeutic inhalation (British National Formulary/National Institute for Health and Care Excellence 2018). The nebulizer will convert the drug into respirable particles that are small enough (2–5 microns in diameter) to reach the bronchioles, and is used to deliver a higher dose of medication than can be achieved with standard inhalers. However, lung deposition of the drug will be dependent on the particle and droplet size, the type of nebulizer chamber, the volume of fluid, and the flow rate of gas driving the nebulizer, as well as the patient's respiratory pattern.

Treatment with nebulizers aims to deliver a therapeutic dose of a drug within a reasonably short period of time, i.e. between 5 and 10 minutes (British National Formulary/National Institute for Health and Care Excellence 2018). Nebulizers can be useful when a large dose of a drug is required, or if a patient is unable to use any other device to inhale a drug, often in an acute situation. Nebulized drugs can be used without the need for the patient to coordinate breathing with inhalation, unlike using inhalers. Occasionally, drugs for inhalation are unavailable in other forms of inhaler.

Nebulized drugs are used for patients with primary respiratory diseases, such as asthma (British National Formulary/National Institute for Health and Care Excellence 2018), and also for patients with other diseases that have respiratory symptoms, such as cancer or heart failure. Thus, the nebulizer can be used in acute, emergency situations such as acute asthma or COPD, in primary healthcare or institutional settings. Equally, routine use for chronic disease management or palliative care can also occur in different care settings.

Common reasons for using nebulizers include:
- *to administer bronchodilators*, e.g. in asthma or COPD
- *to administer nebulized sodium chloride 0.9%* to aid expectoration, e.g. in palliative care
- *to administer an antibiotic*, e.g. in cystic fibrosis or *Pneumocystis carinii* pneumonia.

The drug and driving gas for the nebulizer are prescribed by a medical practitioner and often administered by a nurse. Sometimes, treatment will be coordinated with chest physiotherapy. Compressed air is the most common driving gas used, although high-flow oxygen may be chosen during an acute asthmatic event. A flow rate of 6–8 L/min is required for either air or oxygen, to ensure that the drug particle size is small enough to allow lung deposition and drug effectiveness (British National Formulary/National Institute for Health and Care Excellence 2018). For patients who have acute severe asthma, it is recommended that the driving gas is oxygen, to prevent a reduction in blood oxygen levels (desaturation) during nebulization. For patients who have COPD, it is recommended that the driving gas is air, to prevent diminution of the hypoxic drive, leading to an abnormally high level of carbon dioxide in the blood (hypercapnia).

If long-term domiciliary nebulizer treatment is needed, the patient may become efficient in their own self-care using nebulizer treatment at home, with access to a local nebulizer service for ongoing support and education, as well as maintenance of equipment.

There are currently three main types of nebulizer available, although research is ongoing to create ones that have improved efficiency of drug delivery (British National Formulary/National Institute for Health and Care Excellence 2018):

- jet is the most commonly used
- ultrasonic is a more expensive system
- adaptive aerosol delivery provides more precise drug delivery.

The decision to use a mask or mouthpiece depends on the individual patient and the drug being administered. Some patients may be unable to hold a mouthpiece and so a mask is more suitable. Some drugs have side-effects and it is recommended that they be used in conjunction with either a mask or a mouthpiece. For example, an uncommon side-effect of anti-cholinergic drugs (e.g. ipratropium bromide) is angle-closure glaucoma (an eye problem) (Kalra and Bone 1988) and so this medication is better suited to a mouthpiece (British Thoracic Society 2004). It is important to follow the manufacturer's instructions to ensure that the most appropriate delivery devices and equipment are used, to maximize drug delivery and minimize side-effects for the patient.

For some patients needing nebulization, it is important to measure peak expiratory flow rate (PEFR) before and after nebulization to check the effectiveness of drug administration (see 'Guidelines and Rationale' later). This is commonly required in patients with asthma (Rees & Kanabar 2006).

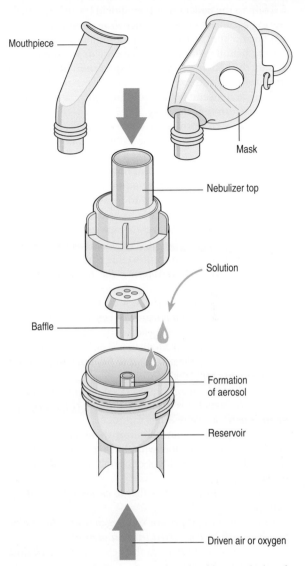

Fig. 35.1 Jet nebulizer. Reproduced with permission from Brooker C, Nicol M: Nursing Adults: The Practice of Caring. Edinburgh, 2003, Mosby.

⊚ EQUIPMENT

- Prescribed air supply: most commonly, an electric or battery-operated air compressor
- Prescribed oxygen supply, either piped or in cylinders
- Oxygen tubing
- Nebulizer (Fig. 35.1)
- Mouthpiece or appropriate oxygen mask (*see* Fig. 35.1)
- Prescribed drugs
- Sputum carton, as required
- 'No smoking' signs, as appropriate (*see* Ch. 28)
- Receptacle for soiled disposable items

For Peak Flow Measurement
- Single-patient use peak flow meter *or, if unavailable,*
- Peak flow meter with disposable mouthpiece
- Specific chart for documenting results

GUIDELINES AND RATIONALE FOR THIS NURSING PRACTICE

- Explain the nursing practice to the patient *to gain consent and cooperation, to encourage participation in care and to reduce anxiety.*

- Explain to the patient that they should breathe normally during nebulization *to enhance drug deposition.*
- Explain to the patient that they should avoid talking during nebulization *to enhance drug deposition.*
- Ensure the patient's privacy *to respect individuality and maintain self-esteem.*
- Prepare and assemble the equipment *to ensure efficient administration of the drug.*
- If oxygen is the driving gas for nebulization, explain the dangers of smoking to the patient and family/carers, positioning the 'No smoking' signs as appropriate, *to make sure that they understand that there is an increased risk of fire when oxygen is being administered.*
- If indicated, help the patient to measure their PEFR by recording the best of three results on the peak flow meter before commencing nebulizer therapy, *to help to evaluate the effects of the treatment* (Fig. 35.2).
- Help the patient into a comfortable position, upright if possible, *to help them tolerate the therapy without distress.*
- Prepare the patient for the noise of the nebulizer *to minimize anxiety and encourage concordance.*
- Identify and check the drug administration prescription (see 'Administration of Medicines', Ch. 2) *to ensure safe administration of the drug and to fulfil the professional requirements for drug administration.*
- If more than one drug is prescribed, follow the manufacturer's instructions *to ensure that the correct equipment is used,* as some drugs cannot be mixed and some drugs require particular nebulizer chambers.
- Fill the nebulizer chamber with the prepared medication, keeping the nebulizer chamber upright *to avoid spillage of the drug* (Fig. 35.3).
- Connect the equipment together *to ensure efficient drug delivery.*
- Turn on the air compressor or oxygen source *to ensure the drug will be converted into an aerosol.*
- Observe the fine spray from the nebulizer *to check that the equipment is working.*
- Encourage the patient to breathe the nebulized aerosol through the mouthpiece or mask *to achieve the maximum effect.*
- Observe the patient closely during nebulization *to monitor the effects and observe for side-effects such as tremor or tachycardia.*
- Time the nebulization, which should take no more than 10 minutes. There may still be solution in the nebulizer chamber after this time; however, when the noise of the nebulizer changes from a hissing to a spluttering of the solution, turn off the nebulizer.
- Encourage the patient to expectorate if the medication has been prescribed *to loosen the bronchial secretions.*

1. Fit disposable mouthpiece to peak flow meter

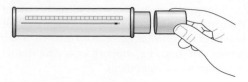

2. Ensure patient stands up or sits upright and holds peak flow meter horizontally without restricting movement of the marker. Ensure the marker is at the bottom of the scale

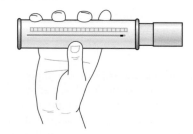

3. Ask patient to breathe in deeply, seal lips around mouthpiece and breathe out as quickly as possible

4. Repeat steps 2 and 3 twice more. Choose and record the highest of the three readings

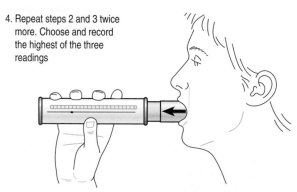

Fig. 35.2 Measuring peak expiratory flow rate. Note that in some countries, and in acute care, peak flow meters are single patient use. The technique outlined in this figure is only used in primary care or instances where they do not have single patient use peak flow meters. Reproduced with permission from Brooker C, Nicol M: Nursing Adults: The Practice of Caring. Edinburgh, 2003, Mosby.

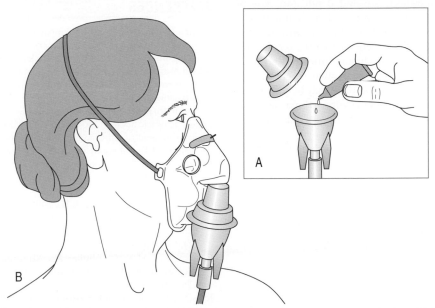

Fig. 35.3 Adding the nebulizer solution. (A) Fill the nebulizer with the prepared medication. (B) Encourage the patient to breathe the nebulized aerosol through the mouthpiece or mask. Reproduced with permission from Nicol M, Bavin C, Bedford-Turner S et al.: Essential Nursing Skills, 2nd edn. London, 2003, Mosby.

- Offer the patient oral hygiene, as some drugs can cause huskiness and oral candidiasis.
- Ensure that the patient is left feeling as comfortable as possible.
- Measure and record the patient's PEFR, if indicated, *to monitor the effect of treatment.*
- Wash and dry the nebulizer, tubing and mask or mouthpiece, according to manufacturer's instructions and local policy, *to minimize the risk of infection and ensure that equipment remains functional.*
- Follow the manufacturer's instructions and local policy for safe storage of the equipment *to comply with health and safety needs regarding infection control.*
- Monitor the patient's respiratory rate and pulse, according to instructions, *to provide ongoing information about their clinical status.*
- Document the nursing practice appropriately, monitor after-effects and report any abnormal findings immediately *to ensure safe practice and to enable prompt, appropriate medical and nursing intervention to be initiated.*

- In undertaking this practice, nurses are accountable for their actions, the quality of care delivered and record-keeping in accordance with *The Code* (Nursing Midwifery Council 2018).

ADDITIONAL INFORMATION

If oxygen is used, all precautions to prevent the risk of fire should be maintained, as with oxygen therapy.

This is not a sterile procedure but adequate standards of cleanliness should be maintained. The nurse should wash their hands before commencing and on completing this nursing practice. The equipment for each patient should be kept clean and dry when not in use. It should be changed according to manufacturer's instructions to prevent infection.

Regular maintenance checks of all equipment should be carried out as per local policy.

During the nursing practice itself, the patient is not encouraged to speak.

The solution is normally administered over a period of up to 10 minutes, which can be explained to the patient.

Monitor the respiration rate and depth and type of respiration, taking readings as frequently as required. The patient should take deep regular breaths through the mouthpiece of the nebulizer to ensure that the medication reaches the mucosa of the bronchi and bronchioles, rather than just the oropharynx. Patients will often experience less dyspnoea after this procedure, and there may be a dramatic relief of bronchospasm for patients with asthma. This can be monitored by taking peak flow recordings over a period of time.

Observe and record the amount, colour and type of any sputum.

A healthy mouth and oropharyngeal mucosa is essential for maximum absorption of the medication. Frequent oral hygiene should therefore be performed as appropriate. A mouthwash after expectorating may be appreciated and should be available if desired.

👥 PATIENT/CARER EDUCATION: KEY POINTS

In partnership with the patient and/or carer, ensure that they understand the goals of treatment. The reason for the inhaler or nebulizer therapy should be carefully explained to the patient and family, so that concordance is continued and patients feel empowered.

If oxygen is used for nebulization, information about fire risks and the precautions needed should be provided (see Ch. 28).

If the patient is self-caring, instructions about preparing the medication and using the equipment should be given, and the nurse should ensure that these continue to be followed correctly.

At home, the nurse should ensure that the patient and carers keep the equipment clean and separate from other household equipment, in order to maintain a safe environment. In the home, patient and family should have written instructions regarding the care and maintenance of the equipment. Contact with the provider of the nebulizer should be made available to encourage regular servicing of equipment to ensure its effectiveness. A telephone contact for an appropriate member of the healthcare team should be provided. The patient should understand the importance of immediately reporting any changes in respiratory function, such as increased dyspnoea, cough or sputum, or any general feeling of distress (NICE 2010).

REFERENCES

Asthma (UK), 2018. Using your inhalers. Available from: https://www.asthma.org.uk/advice/inhalers-medicines-treatments/using-inhalers/#Typesofasthmainhalersandhowtousethem.

British National Formulary/National Institute for Health and Care Excellence, 2018. Respiratory system, drug delivery. Available from: https://bnf.nice.org.uk/treatment-summary/respiratory-system-drug-delivery.html.

British Thoracic Society, 2004. British Guideline on the Management of Chronic Obstructive Airways Disease: A National Clinical Guideline. BTS, London.

British Thoracic Society/Scottish Intercollegiate Guidelines Network, 2016. British guideline on the management of asthma. Thorax 63, iv1.

Cates, C.J., Crilly, J.A., Rowe, B.H., 2006. Holding chambers (spacers) versus nebulisers for beta-agonist treatment of acute asthma. The Cochrane Database of Systematic Reviews (2), CD000052.

Godara, N., Godara, R., Khullar, M., 2011. Impact of inhalation therapy on oral health. Lung India: Official Organ of Indian Chest Society 28 (4), 272.

Joels, C., 2012. Protocol for assessing inhaler technique in patients with asthma. Nursing Standard (through 2013) 26 (19), 43.

Kalra, L., Bone, M.F., 1988. The effect of nebulized bronchodilator therapy on intraocular pressures in patients with glaucoma. Chest 93 (4), 739–741.

Lavorini, F., Fontana, G.A., 2009. Targeting drugs to the airways: the role of spacer devices. Expert Opinion on Drug Delivery 6 (1), 91–102.

Mølgaard, R.R., Larsen, P., Håkonsen, S.J., 2016. Effectiveness of respiratory rates in determining clinical deterioration: a systematic review protocol. JBI Database of Systematic Reviews and Implementation Reports 14 (7), 19–27.

National Institute for Health and Care Excellence, 2010. Chronic obstructive pulmonary disease in over 16s: diagnosis and management. NICE, London. Available from: https://www.nice.org.uk/guidance/CG101/chapter/1-Guidance#managing-stable-copd.

Nursing and Midwifery Council, 2010. Standards for Pre-Registration Nursing Education. NMC, London.

Nursing and Midwifery Council, 2018. The Code: Professional Standards of Practice and Behaviour for Nurses, Midwives and Nursing Associates. NMC, London. Available at: https://www.nmc.org.uk/globalassets/sitedocuments/nmc-publications/nmc-code.pdf.

O'Dowd, A., 2016. Kate granger. BMJ : British Medical Journal / British Medical Association 354.

Philip, K., Richardson, R., Cohen, M., 2013. Staff perceptions of respiratory rate measurement in a general hospital. The British Journal of Nursing 22 (10), 570–574.

Rees, J., Kanabar, D., 2006. The ABC of Asthma, fifth ed. Blackwell, Oxford.

Royal College of Physicians, 2017. National Early Warning Score (NEWS) 2: Standardising the Assessment of Acute-Illness Severity in the NHS. Royal College of Physicians, London.

van Geffen, W.H., Douma, W.R., Slebos, D.J., Kerstjens, H.A.M., 2016. Bronchodilators delivered by nebuliser versus pMDI with spacer or DPI for exacerbations of COPD. The Cochrane Database of Systematic Reviews (8), Art. No.: CD011826.

Waugh, A., Grant, A., 2014. Ross and Wilson Anatomy & Physiology in Health and Illness, twelveth ed. Churchill Livingstone, Edinburgh.

White, J., Paton, J.Y., Niven, R., Pinnock, H., 2018. Guidelines for the diagnosis and management of asthma: a look at the key differences between BTS/SIGN and NICE. Thorax 73 (3), 295.

World Health Organization, 2018. Five moments for hand hygiene. Available from: http://www.who.int/gpsc/5may/background/5moments/en/.

SELF-ASSESSMENT

1. You are asked to measure and record your patient's respirations. What other indicators of respiratory function can be assessed at the same as counting the respiratory rate?
2. What is the normal respiratory rate and why is it necessary to count respirations with the patient unaware that you are doing so?
3. What are the advantages and disadvantages of administering drugs via an inhaler?
4. What are the advantages and disadvantages of administering drugs via a nebulizer?
5. What factors would influence your choice of device?
6. How would you assist the patient to self-administer an inhaler?

Stoma Care

INDICATIONS AND RATIONALE FOR STOMA CARE

A stoma is an artificial opening from the small or large intestine on to the surface of the abdomen, through which the bowel contents or urine are/is diverted for excretion (Fig. 36.1). The stoma is formed after surgical intervention for the treatment of intestinal or bladder disease. Different names are used, according to the site of the stoma.

Stoma care involves cleansing the stoma and surrounding skin, and providing a suitable appliance for the safe collection and disposal of excreta. Nurses either perform this on the patient's behalf, or educate and support patients until they are able to look after the stoma competently or a carer (i.e. healthcare support worker, social services carer or family member) is able to do this for them.

A stoma may be temporary or permanent. A temporary stoma is often created to divert faeces away from an operation site (anastomosis) to allow healing to occur. The stoma is then reversed by the surgeon with minimal or no loss of intestinal function. A permanent stoma implies that the bowel cannot be reconnected.

Colostomy

A colostomy is an opening from the colon, usually the transverse or descending colon. It is commonly positioned in the left iliac fossa and may be required for patients who:
- have malignant disease of the rectum or colon
- have diverticular disease of the colon
- have inflammatory disease of the intestine, e.g. Crohn's disease or ulcerative colitis
- have suffered trauma to the abdomen or rectum
- suffer faecal incontinence.

Ileostomy

An ileostomy is an opening from the ileum. It is commonly positioned in the right iliac fossa and may be formed for the same reasons as a colostomy, although it is more often seen in patients who have inflammatory disease of the intestine, e.g. Crohn's disease or ulcerative colitis. In some cases, a temporary stoma may be created so that, once the disease has resolved, the stoma may be closed and the intestine anastomosed to function as before.

Jejunostomy

A jejunostomy is an opening from the jejunum.

Urostomy

A urostomy is an opening from the bladder or ureter into a segment of the ileum. It is commonly positioned in the right iliac fossa, this being used as a channel for the urine to be diverted through an abdominal stoma. This is also known as an ileal conduit, and may be required for the treatment of malignant disease of the bladder or in the management of the neuropathic bladder or urinary incontinence.

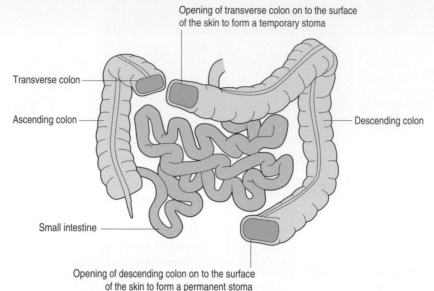

Opening of transverse colon on to the surface of the skin to form a temporary stoma

Transverse colon

Ascending colon

Descending colon

Small intestine

Opening of descending colon on to the surface of the skin to form a permanent stoma

Fig. 36.1 Sites that may be chosen for colostomy.

⊚ EQUIPMENT

- Trolley or tray
- Bowl of warm water (or warm water in a sink if the patient is mobile enough to reach the toilet)
- Soft wipes
- Adhesive removal spray
- Suitable appliance (stoma pouch)
- Scissors
- Measuring guide
- Measuring jug or bowl (if appropriate)
- Gloves (non-sterile) and apron
- Disposal bag

STOMA APPLIANCES

There is a wide range of appliances available and, with the guidance of a stoma care nurse, the patient will choose the one most suitable for their needs. Stoma pouches may have pre-cut apertures or may have to be cut to fit individually. They may be closed pouches or open-ended to allow emptying (Fig. 36.2).

The pouches may be one-piece or two-piece appliances. A one-piece appliance is one in which the adhesive flange and pouch are sealed together. The backing paper is removed from the adhesive ring prior to application and the whole pouch is removed and discarded when appropriate. A two-piece appliance consists of a baseplate that is placed around the stoma and is secured on to the abdomen. The pouch is

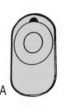

A

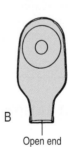

B

Open end

Fig. 36.2 Examples of disposable stoma bags. (A) Closed pouch. (B) Open lower end to permit emptying of the contents.

then clipped or secured (stuck) on to the baseplate. The pouch can be renewed without changing the baseplate.

Postoperatively, the surgeon will place a transparent appliance over the stoma. This allows observation of the stoma and its function by nursing staff and aids patient teaching. The appliance will be changed for the first time on the first or second postoperative day to commence teaching and facilitate enhanced recovery after surgery (ERAS).

GUIDELINES AND RATIONALE FOR THIS NURSING PRACTICE

- Explain the nursing practice to the patient *to gain consent and cooperation.* Patients should be encouraged to be active partners in their care.
- Ensure the patient's privacy *to maintain self-esteem and prevent embarrassment.*
- Wash your hands *to reduce the risk of cross-infection* (World Health Organization 2018).
- Collect and prepare the equipment *to have everything ready to hand.*
- Help the patient into a comfortable position *to reduce any distress and to help them see the area of the stoma.*
- Help the patient to adjust their clothing *to expose the abdomen in the area of the stoma for easy access and so that the patient can observe the practice.*
- Put on gloves and apron *to prevent any contamination from body fluids.*
- Place soft wipes appropriately *to protect the surrounding area from spills or leakage.*
- Observe the patient throughout this activity for any signs of discomfort or distress. Do this *to allow the nurse to intervene immediately in the event of an adverse reaction.*
- Empty the appliance and, if required, measure its contents *to permit evaluation of the elimination fluid balance.*
- Using an adhesive remover spray *to prevent skin damage and discomfort,* gently remove the appliance *to expose the stoma area.*
- Wash the skin around the stoma with soft wipes and warm water only: *soap may cause skin irritation.*
- Encourage the patient to look at the stoma and explain what you are doing *to help them gradually accept the change of body image and to encourage early independence.*
- Observe the colour and condition of the stoma and the surrounding skin *to evaluate the wound healing process.*
- Dry the skin around the stoma thoroughly *to maintain healthy, intact skin, ensure adhesion of the flange and prevent excoriation.*
- Prepare the appliance as required by measuring the size and shape of the stoma, cutting the aperture of the pouch *to tailor it to fit the individual stoma.*
- Place the new appliance in position *to make sure that it fits comfortably and does not permit any leakage round the stoma* (Fig. 36.3).
- Seal an open-ended bag with an appropriate closure, such as a Velcro closure for ileostomy pouches, *to prevent leakage.*
- Ensure that the patient is left feeling as comfortable as possible *to limit distress and promote the healing process.*
- Dispose of any waste products and soiled appliances, according to health authority policy, *to prevent the transmission of infection.*
- Wash your hands *to reduce the risk of cross-infection* (World Health Organization 2018).
- Document the nursing practice in the patient's care plan, monitor the after-effects and report any abnormal findings immediately, *to ensure safe practice and enable prompt, appropriate medical and nursing intervention to be initiated.*
- In undertaking this practice, nurses are accountable for their actions, the quality of care delivered and record-keeping in accordance with *The Code* (Nursing and Midwifery Council 2018).

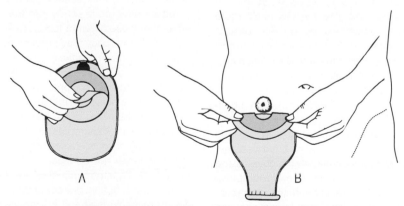

Fig. 36.3 Positioning an appliance over a stoma. (A) Removing the protective covering from the adhesive ring before placing the appliance over the stoma. (B) Applying a stoma pouch. The open-ended pouch is sealed with a clip ready for use. When the clip is removed, the stoma pouch can be emptied without removing the appliance from the skin.

PATIENT/CARER EDUCATION: KEY POINTS

Patient support and education begin prior to surgery. As the presence of a stoma completely changes the way in which bodily waste is eliminated from the body, patients need education and support to adjust to this change. Ideally, the stoma nurse should meet with the patient and a relative before surgery to discuss the forthcoming procedure, the likelihood of a stoma, the implications this will have for lifestyle and some potential postoperative complications. The patient should be shown an appropriate appliance and be given written literature relative to the surgery. By being offered preoperative support and education, patients are less likely to develop psychological problems following surgery.

Stoma siting is also a vital preoperative role of the stoma nurse, as the site where the stoma is placed on the abdomen can have an effect on the recovery process. Attention must also be paid to the patient's employment status, leisure activities, and religious and cultural influences, and these must be taken into consideration when siting (Humphrys 2017).

Before, during and after admission, stoma support and education are shared with stoma nurses and with nurses from both the acute and the community settings. The main aim of stoma education is to provide patients with the right skills and support to enable them to be independent in the care of their own stoma. Where this is unlikely, a relative or carer may be taught the skills to carry this out on the patient's behalf.

The presence of a stoma has a major impact on the patient's sexuality and body image. Body image has been described as the way in which we see ourselves in the world (Humphrys 2017), and the presence of a stoma can place challenges on an individual's physical, emotional and psychological well-being. Sexuality involves much more than the physical act of sexual expression. For some, it is a measure of self-worth, acceptance, security, comfort and human contact, as well as cohesion in a relationship. Nurses involved in the care of a patient with a stoma should demonstrate knowledge of actual and potential problems with sexuality and body image. Nurses should create an environment that encourages patients to talk about the stoma and any worries or concerns they may have regarding the threat to their body image and sexuality. Effective listening skills can be used to ensure that both the physical and the psychological needs of the patient are met (Humphrys 2017). The patient may wish to discuss with the stoma care nurse any concerns they may have about emotional and psychological adjustment to life with a stoma.

The practical aspect of stoma education encourages patients to be fully prepared prior to starting to change the pouch. They will need to gather all the necessary equipment and to carry out the step-by-step process of removing the old pouch, washing and drying the peristomal skin area, and then reapplying and securing the new pouch. Pouches should be emptied or changed as often as necessary to prevent overfilling and leakage on to the surrounding skin area. This is usually when they are one-third to one-half full, to prevent them becoming heavy. In hospital the contents of the pouch should be emptied into the toilet or Clinimatic. The soiled pouch should be treated as clinical waste. The faecal output from the stoma should initially be measured and observed for any abnormality.

Following discharge home, the patient will be instructed to place the soiled pouch in a disposal bag and place it in the dustbin outside their house. Stoma care should be regarded as a form of toileting, and appropriate hand-washing should be performed to reduce the incidence of cross-infection (Health Protection Scotland 2016).

All stoma patients should have contact details for their nearest stoma care nurse, who can review them in the hospital or at home if necessary, should they experience any problems.

Patients should also be encouraged to contact local and national support groups by attending meetings or using the internet.

Nutritional Advice

During the first few days after surgery, the patient will have nothing orally and will receive nutrition via intravenous infusion. Oral fluids will be gradually introduced and increased to light diet when the stoma becomes active. Once the patient is allowed a normal diet, the stoma will discharge faecal material more frequently. By a process of observation, the patient should be encouraged to introduce new foods slowly into their diet and notice the effect that these different foods have on faecal elimination (output). Some foods may produce more undesired flatus while others may make the effluent looser or bulkier (thick). This may help the patient to manage their own output from their stoma. This process may take a few weeks and the stoma nurse can provide some written information and advice regarding diet following surgery.

Patients with ileostomies should be aware that foods like mushrooms, nuts, sweetcorn, coconut and some tough fruit skins may not be digested properly and may block the stoma. Ileostomy patients are also advised to drink about 1–1.5 L of fluid per day and to add extra salt to their diet to maintain fluid and electrolyte balance. Urostomy patients are advised to drink 1.5–2 L of fluid per day to keep the urine as dilute as possible and to prevent urinary tract infections. Cranberry juice or capsules may also be taken to prevent the growth of bacteria in the urinary tract.

Potential Postoperative Complications

Patients and carers should be aware that there are some potential complications that may occur following stoma formation.

Oedema

All stomas are swollen immediately after surgery due to handling of the bowel, but this oedema should reduce gradually over the following weeks and the stoma size should be established at 6 weeks. During this time the stoma should be observed. The size of the stoma has to be measured regularly so that the aperture of the flange is cut correctly. If it is cut too big, any leakage of effluent on to the peristomal skin area may cause irritation or leakage; if cut too small, ischaemia may occur. Leakage may also be caused by the flange resting on stoma mucosa.

Necrosis

This is most common in the first 48 hours following surgery and is caused by inadequate blood supply to part of the bowel that is used to form the stoma. Initially the stoma will become a dusky-purple colour due to the impaired blood supply. Ischaemia may develop into necrosis, which results in a black, odorous bowel. The necrosis may be superficial, which will result in sloughing off of the tissue, or it may be deep, which will require surgical excision.

Mucocutaneous Separation

This occurs when there is a breakdown of the suture line securing the stoma to the abdominal surface, leaving a wound cavity. Management is by use of stoma pastes and an adhesive washer.

Dermatitis

This is defined as inflammation or excoriation of the peristomal skin. Contact dermatitis is seen when there is a sensitivity or allergy to the appliance and can occur at any time. It is easily identified, as the outline of the pouch remains visible on the skin after the pouch has been removed. Effluent dermatitis occurs when the patient has suffered from leakages from the pouch or when the pouch has been cut too big. Barrier wipes or sprays or hydrocolloid dressings can be used to protect the area after assessment by the stoma nurse. Topical steroids may be prescribed in extreme circumstances.

Retraction

This is when the stoma lies on or recedes below the surface of the abdominal wall and is caused by the bowel being under tension. Retraction can cause leakages of effluent and contact dermatitis. Management may be through convexity appliances, which should be used only after assessment by the stoma nurse specialist. A convexity appliance is one where the outward curving of the adhesive on the flange begins at the stoma. This helps to secure a seal around the stoma, providing security and promoting physical and psychological well-being (Cheetham & Catte 2013). Washers and pastes may also be used to fill in any dips or creases on the abdominal wall.

Prolapse

Prolapse occurs when a length of the bowel protrudes from the abdomen. This can be very alarming for the patient, can cause leakages of effluent and odour from the appliance, and can lead to body image problems. Some patients may require a larger pouch and the aperture has to be resized. The prolapsed stoma can sometimes be reduced manually when the patient is supine, but always prolapses again when the patient mobilizes (Liao & Qin 2014). A support belt or garment can then be worn to prevent future prolapse in the short term. However, the stoma may have to be surgically refashioned for long-term management if the prolapse proves to be a major problem for the patient.

Stenosis

Stenosis occurs when the opening of the stoma narrows. It can be caused by non-elastic scar tissue forming around the stoma following retraction, mucocutaneous separation and necrosis. It is characterized by abdominal pain and difficulty of the stoma expelling the stool. Management of stenosis is to educate patients to maintain soft stools through diet and stool-softening agents (such as lactulose), and also by introducing a dilator into the lumen of the stoma to keep it patent. The long-term management may involve surgical refashioning of the stoma.

Hernia

When a stoma is formed, a potential site of weakness in the abdominal muscle is created. A hernia occurs when the peritoneum bulges through the weakened muscle wall. A parastomal hernia occurs when a hernia develops around the stoma. Patients can present with anything from a slight swelling around the stoma to a large, uncomfortable mass that is causing pain and discomfort. Patients with parastomal hernias have problems with body image, as the swelling may be obvious and some may have to wear a hernia support. Patients should be informed that the presence of a hernia may cause bowel obstruction. Signs and symptoms may include non-function of the stoma and abdominal pain and discomfort. This should therefore be explained to the patient, who should be provided with information on who to contact, should they experience these signs and symptoms. Some patients with larger hernias may have them surgically repaired (Cronin 2014).

REFERENCES

Cheetham, M., Catte, C., 2013. The Problem - A Retracted Stoma. The Association of Coloproctology of Great Britain. Available from: https://www.acpgbi.org.uk.

Cronin, E., 2014. Stoma siting: why and how to mark the abdomen in preparation for surgery. Gastrointestinal Nursing 12 (3), 12–19.

Health Protection Scotland, 2016. Standard Infection Control Precautions Literature Review: Hand Hygiene: Hand washing version 2. National Health Services Scotland. Available at: https://www.nipcm.hps.scot.nhs.uk/documents/sicp-hand-hygiene-hand-washing-in-the-hospital-setting/.

Humphrys, N., 2017. Sexual health and sexuality in people with a stoma: a literature review. Gastrointestinal Nursing 15 (10), 18–26.

Liao, C., Qin, Y., 2014. Factors associated with stoma quality of life among stoma patients. International Journal of Nursing Sciences 1 (2), 196–201.

Nursing and Midwifery Council, 2018. Nursing and Midwifery Council 2018b Future Nurse: Standards of Proficiency for Registered Nurses. NMC, London. Available at: https://www.nmc.org.uk/globalassets/sitedocuments/education-standards/future-nurse-proficiencies.pdf.

World Health Organization, 2018. Five moments for hand hygiene. Available at: http://www.who.int/gpsc/tools/Five_moments/en/.

WEBSITES

https://www.colostomyuk.org *Colostomy UK*
http://www.iasupport.org *Ileostomy and Internal Pouch Association*
https://www.urostomyassociation.org.uk *Urostomy Association*

SELF-ASSESSMENT

1. List the different types of stoma that can be created and name two predisposing factors for each one.
2. What equipment is necessary to renew a stoma pouch?
3. What dietary advice would you give an ileostomy patient?
4. What advice would you give a patient with a parastomal hernia?
5. What can happen if the aperture of the flange is cut wrongly after surgery?

37

The Patient With Impaired Consciousness

There are three parts to this chapter:
1. Airway maintenance
2. Glasgow Coma Scale assessment
3. Protective care of the patient with impaired consciousness.

LEARNING OUTCOMES

By the end of this chapter, you should be able to:
- maintain an adequate airway for the patient with impaired consciousness
- assess and record the level of consciousness using the Glasgow Coma Scale
- care for the patient with impaired consciousness.

BACKGROUND KNOWLEDGE REQUIRED

- Revision of the anatomy and physiology of the nervous system, with special reference to the brain and consciousness
- Review of local policy and national guidelines relating to the care of the patient with impaired consciousness

INDICATIONS AND RATIONALE FOR CARE DURING A STATE OF IMPAIRED CONSCIOUSNESS

Consciousness is a state of awareness of self and the environment, and depends on arousal and awareness (Patel & Hirsch 2014). Nursing intervention is required when a patient's level of consciousness is such that, unaided, they can no longer maintain a clear airway, the normal protective reflexes are so reduced that the patient can no longer maintain safety of their environment, and the patient is unable to perform activities of living (Hickey 2013). In this context, clinical observation of the patient is needed and the nurse has a primary responsibility to detect and report any alteration in the patient's condition (Nursing and Midwifery Council 2018). Patients with impaired consciousness are *'extremely vulnerable … [and] should be protected in every possible way'* (Wijdicks 2017: p. 117).

There are four main causes of impaired consciousness (Box 37.1):
- neurological
- metabolic
- diffuse physiological brain dysfunction, e.g. drugs or alcohol
- psychiatric or functional, considered when organic causes have been excluded (Cooksley et al. 2018).

EQUIPMENT

Equipment for Assessing Level of Consciousness
- Level of consciousness assessment chart: e.g. the Glasgow Coma Scale
- Pen torch: to assess eye pupil size and reaction to light
- Sphygmomanometer and stethoscope: to measure blood pressure
- Thermometer: to measure temperature
- Pulse oximeter: to measure peripheral oxygen saturation (SpO_2)

Additional Equipment
- Bed with a detachable head
- Padded cot sides (see local clinical environment policy for bed rails risk assessment protocol)
- Disposable airway: either Guedel oropharyngeal or nasopharyngeal
- Self-inflating bag-valve mask resuscitator
- Equipment for endotracheal intubation if required
- Equipment for oral, pharyngeal or tracheal suction
- Equipment for oxygen therapy administration (*see* Ch. 28)
- Equipment for nasogastric, percutaneous endoscopic gastrostomy or total parenteral nutrition feeding (*see* Ch. 26)
- Equipment for mouth care (*see* Ch. 27)
- Equipment for eye care (*see* Ch. 17)
- Equipment for catheter care (*see* Ch. 11)

BOX 37.1 Some Common Causes of Impaired Consciousness

Neurological
- Trauma
- Vascular events, e.g. ischaemic stroke, haemorrhagic stroke and subdural haematoma
- Brain tumour
- Central nervous system infection
- Hydrocephalus

Metabolic
- Hypoglycaemia and hyperglycaemia
- Hyponatraemia and hypernatraemia
- Uraemia

Diffuse Physiological Brain Dysfunction
- Seizures
- Alcohol intoxication
- Opioid toxicity
- Drug overdose
- Poisoning
- Hypothermia

Psychiatric/Functional
- Considered when organic causes have been excluded

1. AIRWAY MAINTENANCE

GUIDELINES AND RATIONALE FOR THIS NURSING PRACTICE

The most important aspect of nursing in impaired consciousness is the maintenance of a clear airway and oxygenation while the reason for the patient's impaired consciousness is being diagnosed and treated. This will help *to ensure that the patient's respiratory function is as efficient as possible in the circumstances.*

- Explain the necessity for airway intervention to the patient *to offer reassurance.*
- Remove any dentures that may be present *to avoid obstruction of the airway.*
- Turn the patient into a lateral recumbent position with the head of the bed elevated to 10–30 degrees *to maintain the airway and prevent restricted lung ventilation.*
- Observe the patient throughout this activity *to monitor any adverse effects.*
- Perform oral and pharyngeal suction, through the oral airway if necessary – endotracheal suction being carried out only by an appropriately skilled practitioner – *to prevent the aspiration of bronchial or oral secretions* (*see* 'Tracheostomy Care', Ch. 38).
- Insert an airway if required, *to help to maintain an adequate airway.*
- Measure peripheral oxygen saturation *to detect hypoxia.*
- Administer oxygen therapy as prescribed, *to prevent hypoxia* (*see* 'Oxygen Therapy', Ch. 28).
- Assess and record a Glasgow Coma Scale score *to establish the patient's baseline level of consciousness.*
- Monitor and record the Glasgow Coma Scale score *to monitor and evaluate the patient's level of consciousness,* until it is equal to 15 or the clinical judgement of the multidisciplinary team determines that this is no longer necessary.

2. GLASGOW COMA SCALE ASSESSMENT

The Glasgow Coma Scale (GCS) was developed in 1974 to provide a tool for the assessment of impaired consciousness (Teasdale & Jennett 1974). It is a long-established and universally accepted consciousness assessment method (Braine & Cook 2016). In 2014, the fortieth anniversary of implementation of the GCS, the tool was updated with a view to minimizing ambiguity and enhancing consistency of assessment (Teasdale et al. 2014). The revised GCS clearly displays assessment criteria and associated scoring (Fig. 37.1).

The principle of assessing the patient's level of consciousness *'is about determining the degree of (increasing) stimulation that is required to elicit a response from them based on three modes of behaviour: eye opening, verbal response and motor response'* (Teasdale et al. 2014: p. 13).

As shown in Fig. 37.1, there are a number of eye-opening ranges:
- spontaneous opening, i.e. in the absence of stimulation
- opening in response to sound
- opening in response to stimulation
- eyes do not open.

Verbal response also has a range of possible responses, including:
- orientated to time, place and person
- confused responses
- words
- sounds
- no verbal response.

Motor response ranges include:
- obeys commands
- localizing
- normal flexion
- abnormal flexion

GLASGOW COMA SCALE : Do it this way

Institute of Neurological Sciences NHS Greater Glasgow and Clyde

CHECK	OBSERVE	STIMULATE	RATE
For factors Interfering with communication, ability to respond and other injuries	Eye opening, content of speech and movements of right and left sides	**Sound** : spoken or shouted request **Physical** : Pressure on finger tip, trapezius or supraorbital notch	Assign according to highest response observed

Eye opening

Criterion	Observed	Rating	Score
Open before stimulus	✔	Spontaneous	4
After spoken or shouted request	✔	To sound	3
After finger tip stimulus	✔	To pressure	2
No opening at any time, no interfering factor	✔	None	1
Closed by local factor	✔	Non testable	NT

Verbal response

Criterion	Observed	Rating	Score
Correctly gives name, place and date	✔	Orientated	5
Not orientated but communication coherently	✔	Confused	4
Intelligible single words	✔	Words	3
Only moans / groans	✔	Sounds	2
No audible response, no interfering factor	✔	None	1
Factor interfering with communication	✔	Non testable	NT

Best motor response

Criterion	Observed	Rating	Score
Obey 2-part request	✔	Obeys commands	6
Brings hand above clavicle to stimulus on head neck	✔	Localising	5
Bends arm at elbow rapidly but features not predominantly abnormal	✔	Normal flexion	4
Bends arm at elbow, features clearly predominantly abnormal	✔	Abnormal flexion	3
Extends arm at elbow	✔	Extension	2
No movement in arms / legs, no interfering factor	✔	None	1
Paralysed or other limiting factor	✔	Non testable	NT

Sites For Physical Stimulation

Finger tip pressure   Trapezius Pinch   Supraorbital notch

Features of Flexion Responses

Modified with permission from Van Der Naalt 2004
Ned Tijdschr Geneeskd

Abnormal Flexion
Slow Sterotyped
Arm across chest
Forearm rotates
Thumb clenched
Leg extends

Normal flexion
Rapid
Variable
Arm away from body

For further information and video demonstration visit www.glasgowcomascale.org

Graphic design by Margaret Frej based on layout and illustrations from Medical Illustration M I • 268093
(c) Sir Graham Teasdale 2015

Fig. 37.1 Glasgow Coma Scale: chart for documenting the assessment of a patient's level of consciousness. © Sir Graham Teasdale 2015.

- extension
- no motor response.

The revised GCS should be used with a four-stage standard structured assessment, namely:

- check
- observe
- stimulate
- rate.

A preliminary check should be performed to identify any factors that might interfere with assessment, including language and cultural differences, intellectual neurological deficits, sensory impediments such as hearing loss, effects of treatment such as intubation, tracheostomy or sedation, and effects of other lesions such as orbital/cranial fractures, dysphasia, hemiplegia or spinal cord injury (Teasdale et al. 2014).

The nurse should then observe for evidence of spontaneous behaviours in each of the three modes of the GCS, e.g. trying to remove an oxygen mask or nasogastric tube (Waterhouse 2017).

Stimulation is applied with increasing intensity until a response from the patient is obtained or a lack of response is evident. An auditory stimulus, such as a spoken request, should be used first and, if no response is achieved, a physical stimulus should then be applied. Recommendations for the application of physical stimulation include pressure on the fingertip (applying pressure to the distal part of the nail and varying the finger used); trapezius pinch; or pressure to the supraorbital notch (which should not be used if there is a fracture in this region). Pressure should be applied for 10–15 seconds (Teasdale & Jennett 1974). See Fig. 37.1 for pictorial guidance on the potential sites for application of physical stimulation. Best motor response is assessed by comparing the movements of each arm. Where there is variation within the assessment, the highest level of response should be noted.

Rating is performed against defined criteria. The first decision is whether patient findings meet the criterion for the top step in eye opening, verbal response and motor response (de Sousa & Woodward 2016). If this is met, the appropriate rating is allocated. If not, subsequent steps are considered in descending order until a point of no response is reached. If the initial check has identified a factor that renders a response not testable, e.g. orbital oedema preventing eye opening, this is recorded as 'NT'. Patient responses can be allocated a numerical rating or score. A decreasing numerical score equates with increasing neurological deterioration (Teasdale et al. 2014). Communicating GCS using a score can be speedy; however, caution should be exercised where a response is not testable, and best practice is evident where the scores for eye opening, verbal response and motor response are reported and documented

separately, e.g. GCS 15/15: E4, V5, M6 (Waterhouse 2017).

For patients admitted for head injury observation, GCS should be supplemented by assessment of pupil size and reaction to light, limb movements, respiratory rate, heart rate, blood pressure, temperature and blood oxygen saturation. Pupil inequality, asymmetry of limb movement and Cushing's triad of hypertension, bradycardia and abnormal respiratory patterns are indicative of neurological deterioration (Waterhouse 2017). These observations should be performed and recorded every 30 minutes until GCS is equal to 15. After assessment in the emergency department, the frequency of observations for patients with a GCS equal to 15 should be:

- half-hourly for 2 hours
- then 1-hourly for 4 hours
- then 2-hourly thereafter.

If GCS deteriorates, observations should revert to half-hourly and follow the above frequency schedule again (National Institute for Health and Care Excellence 2014).

3. PROTECTIVE CARE OF THE PATIENT WITH IMPAIRED CONSCIOUSNESS

In addition to maintenance of a clear airway, neurological assessment, and monitoring and management associated with the underlying cause of impaired consciousness, the nurse should implement protective care measures *to prevent further complications* (Geraghty 2005).

- Position the patient's limbs *to maintain their position comfortably and to allow an adequate flow of circulation to the extremities.*
- Nurse the patient on a high-dependency, pressure-relieving mattress system, and alternate the side on which the patient lies every 2 hours *to maintain healthy tissue at the pressure areas and to aid the expansion of each lung* (see 'Integrity of the Skin', Ch. 21).
- Provide all nursing care as frequently as required, explaining the care to the patient, irrespective of consciousness state and ensuring privacy before commencing care. The patient will be completely dependent for all of their needs, and the nurse must respect the patient's individuality and maintain their dignity at all times.
- Document all nursing practices appropriately, reporting abnormal findings immediately *to ensure safe practice and enable prompt, appropriate medical and nursing intervention to be initiated.*
- In undertaking these practices, nurses are accountable for their actions, the quality of care delivered and record-keeping, according to *The Code* (Nursing and Midwifery Council 2018).

PATIENT/CARER EDUCATION: KEY POINTS

According to Sisson (1990), hearing is the last sense lost when a person becomes unconscious. It is therefore imperative for the nurse to communicate with the patient, providing information and support. Information received by patients with impaired consciousness may assist in reducing stress (Othman & El-Hady 2015). In partnership with the patient and/or carer, ensure that they are competent to carry out any practices required. Information should be given on an appropriate point of contact for any concerns that may arise.

Education primarily involves the family. Explanations of the rationale for nursing interventions and the expected outcome should therefore be shared with them.

The family should be encouraged to talk to the patient about their interests and hobbies, reinforcing this with tapes and music if appropriate. The family should also be encouraged to touch the patient and hold their hand. They may provide aspects of essential care for the patient, if willing and able, as family-centred stimulation can improve patient outcomes (Salmani et al. 2017).

Healthcare professional education is also vital, as observations should be performed by staff trained to undertake these procedures and who understand their clinical relevance (Scottish Intercollegiate Guidelines Network 2014). With specific reference to the GCS, accuracy is dependent on the professional using and interpreting it correctly (Braine & Cook 2016).

REFERENCES

Braine, M.E., Cook, N., 2016. The Glasgow Coma Scale and evidence-informed practice: a critical review of where we are now and where we need to be. Journal of Clinical Nursing 26, 280–293.

Cooksley, T., Rose, S., Holland, M., 2018. A systematic approach to the unconscious patient. Clinical Medicine 18 (1), 88–92.

De Sousa, I., Woodward, S., 2016. The Glasgow Coma Scale in adults: doing it right. Emergency Nurse 24 (8), 33–38.

Geraghty, M., 2005. Nursing the unconscious patient. Nursing Standard 20 (1), 54–64.

Hickey, J.V., 2013. Management of patients with a depressed level of consciousness. In: Hickey, J.V. (Ed.), Clinical Practice of Neurological and Neurosurgical Nursing, seventh ed. Lippincott Williams and Wilkins, London.

National Institute for Health and Care Excellence, 2014. Head injury: assessment and early management (CG176). NICE, London.

Nursing and Midwifery Council, 2018. The Code: Professional Standards of Practice and Behaviour for Nurses, Midwives and Nursing Associates. NMC, London. Available at: https://www.nmc.org.uk/globalassets/sitedocuments/nmc-publications/nmc-code.pdf.

Othman, S.Y., El-Hady, M.M., 2015. Effect of implementing structured communication messages on the clinical outcomes of unconscious patients. Journal of Nursing Education and Practice 5 (9), 117–131.

Patel, S., Hirsch, N., 2014. Coma. Continuing Education in Anaesthesia Critical Care & Pain 14 (5), 213–219.

Salmani, F., Mohammadi, E., Rezvani, M., Kazemnezhad, A., 2017. The effects of family-centered affective stimulation on brain-injured comatose patients' level of consciousness: a randomized controlled trial. International Journal of Nursing Studies 74, 44–52.

Scottish Intercollegiate Guidelines Network, 2014. Care of Deteriorating Patients Consensus Recommendations. SIGN, Edinburgh.

Sisson, R., 1990. Effects of auditory stimuli on comatose patients with head injury. Heart and Lung: The Journal of Critical Care 19 (4), 373–378.

Teasdale, G., Allan, D., Brennan, P., et al., 2014. Forty years on: updating the Glasgow Coma Scale. Nursing Times 110 (42), 12–16.

Teasdale, G., Jennett, B., 1974. Assessment of coma and impaired consciousness: a practical scale. Lancet 2 (7872), 81–84.

Waterhouse, C., 2017. Practical aspects of performing Glasgow Coma Scale observations. Nursing Standard 31 (35), 40–46.

Wijdicks, E.F.M., 2017. Management of the comatose patient. In: Wijdicks, E.F.M., Kramer, A.H. (Eds.), Critical Care Neurology Part 1 Handbook of Clinical Neurology, 3rd Series, vol. 140. Elsevier, Amsterdam.

WEBSITES

www.glasgowcomascale.org *The Glasgow Structured Approach to Assessment of the Glasgow Coma Scale*

SELF-ASSESSMENT

1. List the main causes of impaired consciousness.
2. Describe the care required to manage the patient's airway safely and maintain adequate oxygenation.
3. Explain the procedure for Glasgow Coma Scale assessment.
4. Complete the self-test available at https://www.glasgowcomascale.org.
5. Describe protective care for the patient with impaired consciousness.
6. Identify the priorities for patient and family education.

38

Tracheostomy Care

There are three parts to this chapter:
1. Principles of tracheostomy care
2. Removal of respiratory tract secretions via a tracheostomy tube
3. Changing a tracheostomy tube.

LEARNING OUTCOMES

By the end of this chapter, you should be able to:
- understand the rationale for tracheostomy
- identify the equipment used in this nursing practice
- discuss the care of a patient with a tracheostomy in situ
- identify the potential problems a patient with a tracheostomy may experience.

BACKGROUND KNOWLEDGE REQUIRED

- Revision of the anatomy and physiology of the upper respiratory tract, and the anatomy of the upper gastrointestinal tract
- Review of local policy or guidelines on the care of a patient with a tracheostomy
- Revision of your knowledge in relation to wound care (*see* Ch. 40)

INDICATIONS AND RATIONALE FOR THE CREATION OF A TRACHEOSTOMY

A tracheostomy is an artificial opening that is surgically created by an incision made into the anterior wall of the trachea (Dhillon & East 2013). The incision is usually made at a level between the second and fourth cartilaginous rings of the trachea.

The indications for tracheostomy can be listed (McGrath 2014) as:
- *to secure and maintain a patent airway in upper airway obstruction (actual or potential)*

- *to secure and maintain a safe airway in patients with injuries to the face, head or neck and following certain types of surgery to the head and neck*
- *to facilitate the removal of bronchial secretions* where there is poor cough effort with sputum retention
- *to make an attempt to protect the airway of patients who are at high risk of aspiration,* i.e. those with incompetent laryngeal and tongue movement on swallowing, as in neuromuscular disorders, unconsciousness, head injuries and stroke
- *to enable long-term mechanical ventilation of patients*, either in an acute intensive care setting or sometimes chronically in hospitals or in the community
- *to facilitate weaning from artificial ventilation.*

A tracheostomy can be temporary, i.e. left in situ for a number of days, weeks or months before removal, or permanent, i.e. retained for the remainder of the patient's life. Most tracheostomies are temporary (McGrath 2014).

Temporary Tracheostomy

A temporary tracheostomy involves the opening of a surgical incision and insertion of a tracheostomy tube. The tube is then held in place by straps secured around the patient's neck (Fig. 38.1).

Permanent Tracheostomy (or Tracheostoma)

A permanent tracheostomy (or tracheostoma) involves the incision of the circumference of the trachea so that it forms a permanent stoma or opening on the surface of the skin, i.e. the trachea is incised and sutured to the skin surface. In these cases a tracheostomy tube may remain in situ until the stoma has healed or if there are any complications with healing or stoma formation.

What Is a Laryngectomy?

Laryngectomy is complete surgical removal of the larynx, which disconnects the upper airway (nose and mouth) from the lungs (McGrath 2014). This is a permanent and irreversible procedure (although partial laryngectomies are

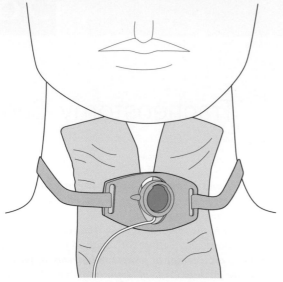

Fig. 38.1 Tracheostomy dressing and securing device in situ.

possible). The patient may or may not have a tracheostomy tube in situ.

1. PRINCIPLES OF TRACHEOSTOMY CARE

Tracheostomy is becoming more common in both acute and community settings (Paul 2010). As a nurse, you therefore need to understand the rationale for this surgical procedure and utilize evidence-based knowledge in caring for the patient who has a tracheostomy in place. In doing this, you will promote clinical effectiveness and prevent potential complications, as well as reassuring your patient and their family.

TRACHEOSTOMY TUBES

Plastic disposable tracheostomy tubes are usually used in the management of both temporary and long-term tracheostomies. Tubes are all double-lumen, consisting of two parts: an outer and an inner cannula. Each healthcare provider will have guidelines on the type of tube they prefer to use. A two-part tube can be left for up to 28 days. The inner cannula can be removed for cleaning purposes without disturbing the outer cannula, thus preserving the integrity of the stoma. The inner cannula also provides essential protection against potentially life-threatening problems, such as tube obstruction, as it can be removed quickly and safely, thus providing prompt relief for the patient (Council of the Intensive Care Society Standards 2014).

A patient may occasionally have a silver tube in situ that also incorporates an inner cannula. Silver tubes are used for patients who require long-term airway support. Other longer-length tubes are also available for patients with thicker or longer necks.

A cuffed tube (Fig. 38.2) may be used in the immediate postoperative phase of care, as it assists in airway maintenance and prevents the potential aspiration of secretions from the recently formed wound around the tube. The patient may feel the cuff pressing against their throat, so you should provide a meaningful explanation at this point. Once any secretions from the wound have ceased, an uncuffed tube may be considered.

Finally, tubes can be either fenestrated or unfenestrated. In addition to the tracheal opening, fenestrated tubes have holes on the outer cannula that allow air to pass through the patient's oral/nasal pharynx. They are used to wean a patient off the tube or to enable phonation.

Therefore, tubes (Fig. 38.3) can be:
- double-cannula
- cuffed/uncuffed
- fenestrated/unfenestrated.

Tracheostomy tubes come in a variety of sizes for adult use: 7.0 mm, 7.5 mm, 8.0 mm, 8.5 mm and 9 mm. The diameter and length of the tube selected will be dependent on your patient's needs and will always be slightly smaller than the diameter of the trachea (Everitt 2016).

EMERGENCY MANAGEMENT

Emergency tracheostomy management is illustrated in Fig. 38.4.

⦿ EQUIPMENT

The essential equipment to be at the bedside of **all** patients with a tracheostomy should include the following (McGrath 2014):
- Spare tracheostomy tubes: same size and type, as well as a tube the next size down
- Tracheal dilators
- Stitch cutter (if the tracheostomy tube is stitched to the skin)
- Suction equipment: suction catheters (no larger in diameter than half the diameter of the tracheostomy tube), connection tubing, suction container, gloves and apron
- Yankauer suction catheter (having a rigid wide-bore cannula; used for oral suction or as a preventive measure if bleeding occurs on changing the tracheostomy tube)
- Sterile water and normal saline

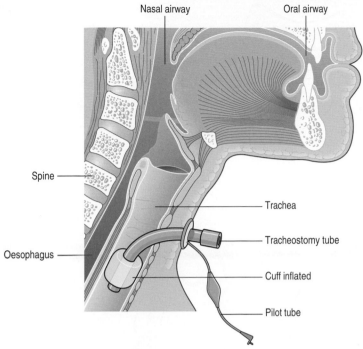

Nasal airway   Oral airway

Spine

Oesophagus

Trachea

Tracheostomy tube

Cuff inflated

Pilot tube

Fig. 38.2 Anatomy of the trachea with a tracheostomy tube in place. Reproduced with permission from the RCN Publishing Company, Woodrow P: Managing patients with a tracheostomy in acute care, *Nursing Standard*, 16 (44):39–48, 2002.

EQUIPMENT—cont'd

- Humidification equipment and tracheal masks
- Tracheostomy dressings
- Scissors
- Cuff manometer if cuffed tube in situ
- 10 mL syringe
- Tracheostomy tapes
- Catheter mount (to enable attachment to a ventilatory bag and valve, should your patient require resuscitation)
- Cuffed tube (if your patient has an uncuffed tube in situ)
- Equipment for oral hygiene
- Sticker for the patient's notes to aid in their management

GUIDELINES AND RATIONALE FOR THIS NURSING PRACTICE

The Code (Nursing and Midwifery Council 2018) states that all nurses must practise in line with the best available evidence. It is therefore imperative that you ensure that you not only are familiar with your local policies regarding tracheostomy care but also are able to identify and use all equipment related to this practice safely.

Successful tracheostomy care is dependent on a multidisciplinary approach to care, as well as collaborative care involving healthcare professionals, patients and their families. Where possible, patients should be educated regarding their treatment and care in the preoperative phase and introduced to all members of the multidisciplinary team, who will include:

- nurses
- consultant surgeon and medical team
- specialist nurse
- speech and language therapist
- physiotherapist
- dietitian
- pharmacist.

Collaborative care not only will improve communication but will assist in ensuring patient satisfaction, reduce anxiety, promote self-care, improve the patient's self-esteem and enable your patient to be an active part of the decisions made regarding their care.

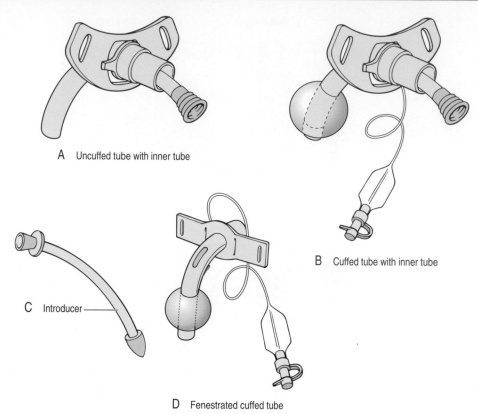

A Uncuffed tube with inner tube

B Cuffed tube with inner tube

C Introducer

D Fenestrated cuffed tube

Fig. 38.3 Tracheostomy tubes in common use.

Communication

Because a tracheostomy tube is inserted below the level of the vocal cords in the larynx, patients with a tracheostomy may encounter difficulties in communicating, which can have a psychological impact on both the patient and their family (Hashmi et al. 2010). An individualized assessment of the patient's needs must be made, along with referral to a speech and language specialist where appropriate. The initial assessment should include the patient's ability to communicate using hearing, sight and writing. An individualized care plan should be devised and implemented. Your patient, for example, may be able to use a pen and paper to communicate effectively while the tube remains in situ or until a speaking valve can be fitted.

Your patient may have a fenestrated tube (Fig. 38.5) in situ, which enables speech. Some patients may find that, with uncuffed tubes, placing a finger over the tube and forcing expired air over the vocal cords restores the voice. This latter practice should be discouraged, as it promotes the risk of respiratory infection; the use of a speaking valve should be favoured to reduce this risk (Council of the Intensive Care Society Standards 2014).

Regular evaluation of the effectiveness of a plan of care must be made, as needs may change in line with the patient's altered health status (National Confidential Enquiry into Patient Outcome and Death 2014). A call bell should be left in reach of the patient at all times. Nurses should also reflect continually on their own communication skills and be able to adapt to utilize alternative means of communication effectively.

Nutrition

The presence of a tracheostomy tube can lead to an impaired nutritional status (Eibling & Roberson 2012). It is important to remember that adequate nutritional intake will promote health and, in particular, provide the patient with energy, help prevent infection and promote healing. Everitt (2016) suggests that a minimum fluid intake of 3000 mL (unless contraindicated) is achieved to help respiratory secretions remain liquefied.

The presence of a cuffed tube can cause anxiety on the part of the patient with regard to swallowing. Hashmi et al. (2010) suggest that this problem can often be due to over-inflation of the cuff and therefore cuff pressure must be

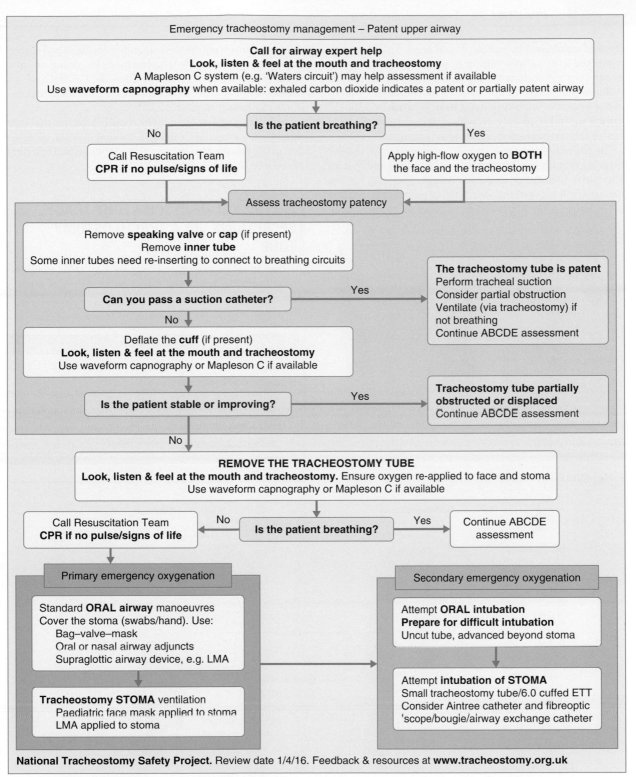

Emergency tracheostomy management – Patent upper airway

Call for airway expert help
Look, listen & feel at the mouth and tracheostomy
A Mapleson C system (e.g. 'Waters circuit') may help assessment if available
Use **waveform capnography** when available: exhaled carbon dioxide indicates a patent or partially patent airway

Is the patient breathing?

No → Call Resuscitation Team
CPR if no pulse/signs of life

Yes → Apply high-flow oxygen to **BOTH** the face and the tracheostomy

Assess tracheostomy patency

Remove **speaking valve** or **cap** (if present)
Remove **inner tube**
Some inner tubes need re-inserting to connect to breathing circuits

Can you pass a suction catheter?

Yes → **The tracheostomy tube is patent**
Perform tracheal suction
Consider partial obstruction
Ventilate (via tracheostomy) if not breathing
Continue ABCDE assessment

No → Deflate the **cuff** (if present)
Look, listen & feel at the mouth and tracheostomy
Use waveform capnography or Mapleson C if available

Is the patient stable or improving?

Yes → **Tracheostomy tube partially obstructed or displaced**
Continue ABCDE assessment

No ↓

REMOVE THE TRACHEOSTOMY TUBE
Look, listen & feel at the mouth and tracheostomy. Ensure oxygen re-applied to face and stoma
Use waveform capnography or Mapleson C if available

No ← **Is the patient breathing?** → Yes

Call Resuscitation Team
CPR if no pulse/signs of life

Continue ABCDE assessment

Primary emergency oxygenation

Standard **ORAL airway** manoeuvres
Cover the stoma (swabs/hand). Use:
    Bag–valve–mask
    Oral or nasal airway adjuncts
    Supraglottic airway device, e.g. LMA

Tracheostomy STOMA ventilation
Paediatric face mask applied to stoma
LMA applied to stoma

Secondary emergency oxygenation

Attempt **ORAL intubation**
Prepare for difficult intubation
Uncut tube, advanced beyond stoma

Attempt **intubation of STOMA**
Small tracheostomy tube/6.0 cuffed ETT
Consider Aintree catheter and fibreoptic 'scope/bougie/airway exchange catheter

National Tracheostomy Safety Project. Review date 1/4/16. Feedback & resources at **www.tracheostomy.org.uk**

Fig. 38.4 Emergency tracheostomy management algorithm. *CPR,* cardiopulmonary resuscitation; *ETT,* endotracheal tube; *LMA,* laryngeal mask airway. Reproduced with permission from the National Tracheostomy Safety Project, 2016. *Emergency Tracheostomy Management Algorithm,* 2016. Available at: https://www. tracheostomy.org.

checked regularly. The patient should remain nil by mouth when the cuff is inflated, as it places pressure on the oesophagus and anchors the larynx, thus disabling the normal swallow (Fig. 38.6). In any case, an individual assessment of the patient's swallowing status **must** be made and should involve multidisciplinary decision-making. Again, the local health care provider policy should be consulted.

In patients who are at risk of aspiration, it is recommended that the patient remains nil by mouth and that an alternative method of feeding is sought. This may involve nasogastric feeding in the short term or gastrostomy feeding in the longer term. It is therefore essential that a swallowing

assessment involving the dietitian, nurse specialist and speech and language therapist is performed. By doing so, any swallowing difficulties can be identified early and an individualized plan of care to support the patient's nutritional needs can be put in place.

In patients who remain nil by mouth, effective oral care should involve regular cleaning of the oral mucosa, observation of the condition of the mouth and tongue, and brushing of teeth or dentures (Paul 2010).

2. REMOVAL OF RESPIRATORY TRACT SECRETIONS VIA A TRACHEOSTOMY TUBE

Suction must be performed only by a suitably qualified practitioner or under the direct supervision of such a person.

◎ EQUIPMENT

- Tray
- Sterile disposable gloves
- Sterile suction catheters with a thumb control
- Sterile container and water for flushing the catheter and tubing
- Receptacle for soiled disposable items
- Suction apparatus, e.g. a portable machine or centralized suction

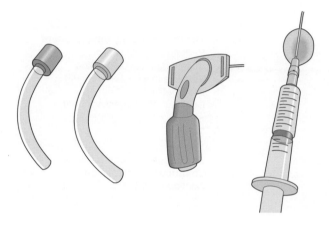

Fig. 38.5 Double-lumen, fenestrated tracheostomy tube.

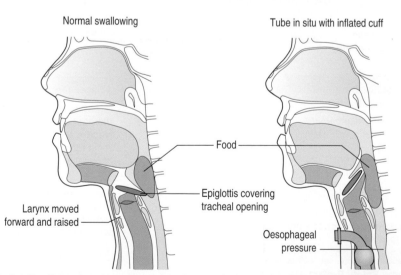

Normal swallowing

Tube in situ with inflated cuff

Food

Epiglottis covering tracheal opening

Larynx moved forward and raised

Oesophageal pressure

Fig. 38.6 Swallowing. Reproduced with permission from the British Journal of Nursing, Russell C: Providing the nurse with a guide to tracheostomy care and management, *British Journal of Nursing*, 14 (8):428–433, 2005.

GUIDELINES AND RATIONALE FOR THIS NURSING PRACTICE

- Tracheal suction should be carried out only when secretions are audible in the tracheostomy tube and the patient is unable to cough up secretions or feels that the tube is blocked, *to reduce the risk of trauma to the mucosa.*
- If possible, explain the nursing practice to the patient *to gain consent and cooperation.* Patients should be encouraged to participate actively in their care.
- Ensure the patient's privacy *to maintain dignity and a sense of self.*
- Wash your hands and collect the equipment *to maintain efficiency of practice.*
- Assist the patient into a suitable position, such as the Fowler's position, *to ensure ease of access to the tracheostomy tube.*
- If the patient has a fenestrated tube in situ, an inner tube without a hole must be inserted prior to the procedure *to prevent damage to the mucosal lining of the trachea.*
- It may be advisable to administer 100% oxygen therapy (care must be taken in patients with chronic obstructive pulmonary disease) prior to and following the procedure, *to prevent hypoxia.*
- Observe the patient throughout this activity *to note any signs of discomfort or distress.*
- Fill the sterile container with sterile water *to flush the suction catheter.*
- Open the end of the pack containing the connecting end of the suction catheter and connect it to the tubing of the suction machine. The diameter of the catheter should not exceed half the diameter of the tracheostomy tube *to ensure that hypoxia does not occur.*
- Put a disposable glove on your dominant hand.
- Slide the cover off the catheter and rinse it through with sterile water *to lubricate it.*
- Insert the catheter into the tracheostomy with the gloved hand but without any suction for the length of the tracheostomy tube.
- Withdraw the catheter, applying suction by covering the thumb control hole and rotating the catheter while this is being done. If the secretions are tenacious and difficult to remove, nebulized saline or mechanical humidification may be administered *to loosen the secretions for easier removal.* Intermittent humidification helps the patient *to expectorate spontaneously.*
- The period of suction should not exceed 10 seconds (McGrath 2014) *to minimize the risk of hypoxia.*
- Allow the patient to rest and reoxygenate before repeating insertion of the catheter *to prevent hypoxia and reduce the risk of a vasovagal response.*
- A maximum of two suctioning attempts is recommended, *as repeated attempts (more than two) place the patient at risk of cardiovascular complications.*
- Dispose of the catheter at the end of the practice after rinsing both the catheter and the tubing with sterile water.
- Ensure that the patient is left feeling as comfortable as possible.
- Dispose of the equipment safely and wash your hands *to protect others.*
- Document the nursing practice appropriately, monitor the after-effects and report any abnormal findings immediately, *to provide a written record and enable prompt intervention, should an adverse reaction to the procedure be noted.*
- Closed suction techniques are often preferred if the patient is connected to a breathing circuit on a ventilator, as repeated disconnection of the circuit is not required (McGrath 2014).
- In undertaking this practice, nurses must maintain the knowledge and skills needed for safe and effective practice, and are accountable for their actions, the quality of care delivered and record-keeping in accordance with *The Code* (Nursing and Midwifery Council 2018).

3. CHANGING A TRACHEOSTOMY TUBE/ TUBE MANAGEMENT

Effective nursing management of the stoma will aid the prevention of peristomal infection and irritation. All patients should be individually assessed and have stoma care delivered using a clean technique (McGrath 2014).

Initially, depending on the patient's condition, two nurses or carers are required for changing the tracheostomy tube holder. Following a risk assessment, this may be reduced to one person. Tube holders should be changed if visibly contaminated, or every 7 days if not visibly soiled. Holders should be tight enough to keep the tracheostomy tube securely in place, but loose enough to allow one finger to fit between the holder and the neck to reduce the possible risk of reduction in cerebral blood flow by carotid pressure.

Changing the tracheostomy tube should be a multidisciplinary decision. Tube changes should be performed by two suitably trained staff, following local guidelines.

All tracheostomy tubes are supplied with two inner cannulas, an introducer and one set of straps.

◎ EQUIPMENT

- Tray or trolley
- Sterile dressings pack
- Two tracheostomy tubes of appropriate type and make (one same size and one smaller)
- Normal saline solution (to clean around the tracheostomy site)
- Sterile water-soluble lubricating jelly
- Sterile water
- 10 mL syringe (to inflate the cuff)
- Cuff pressure manometer (if the tube has a cuff)
- Suction equipment and suction catheters
- Sterile gloves and protective eyewear
- Pen torch
- Sterile tracheal dilators (if the tube was inserted less than 6 months ago)
- Sterile scissors (to cut tapes to size)
- Tracheostomy dressing
- Disposable gloves
- Tracheostomy tube cleaning brush (silver tubes only)
- Stitch cutter (for the first tube change or as per post-insertion instructions)
- Receptacle for soiled disposable items
- Oxygen supply and appropriate masks
- Oxygen saturation monitoring
- Stethoscope

GUIDELINES AND RATIONALE FOR THIS NURSING PRACTICE

Pre-oxygenation is essential before a tube change in patients with oxygen or ventilator dependency, or those in whom the difficulty of the change is unknown (McGrath 2014).

Owing to the risk of vomiting and aspiration associated with tube changes and airway manoeuvres, patients should ideally be 'nil by mouth' for 6 hours for solids and 2 hours for clear liquids before an elective tube change.

- Explain the nursing practice to the patient *to gain consent and cooperation.* Patients should be encouraged to be active participants in their care.
- Ensure the patient's privacy *to maintain dignity and a sense of self.*
- Collect and prepare the equipment and wash your hands *to maintain efficiency of practice.*
- Assist the patient to a suitable position, such as Fowler's position, *to allow this practice to be carried out.*

- Observe the patient throughout this activity *to note any signs of discomfort or distress.*
- Open the dressings pack and the tracheostomy tube pack.
- Check that the obturator/introducer fits. Check in particular that it can be easily removed, as it blocks the airway once the tube is in situ.
- Lubricate the end of the tube and obturator with sterile water-soluble lubricating jelly *to ensure ease of insertion.*
- Wrap the tracheostomy dressing around the tube with the slit uppermost *to facilitate positioning and removal.*
- Put on the disposable gloves *to protect yourself and the patient.*
- If applicable, deflate the cuff on a cuffed tube and administer suction prior to changing the tube *to prevent trauma and remove any secretions.*
- Remove the soiled tube with a smooth outward and downward motion, discarding it in the receptacle for disposable items if it is plastic. The tube should be soaked in sterile water and/or a recognized tracheostomy tube cleaning solution and left to air-dry.
- Remove the gloves *to allow more dextrous hand movements.*
- Hold the new tube by the tapes and insert it smoothly from below in an upward, inward and then downward movement into the trachea. This follows the line of the stoma.
- Immediately remove the obturator while holding the tube in place *to free the airway and inflate the cuff,* if applicable.
- Secure the straps at the side of the patient's neck *to prevent tube dislodgement and maintain comfort.*
- If a cuffed tracheostomy tube is being changed, the cuff pressure post inflation should be checked using the cuff pressure manometer.
- *To check the tracheostomy tube is in the correct position,* confirm lung air entry using a stethoscope.
- Ensure that the patient is left feeling as comfortable as possible.
- Dispose of the equipment safely and wash your hands *to protect others.*
- Record this nursing practice appropriately, monitor the after-effects and report any abnormal findings immediately, *to provide a written record and enable prompt intervention, should an adverse reaction to the practice be noted.*
- In undertaking this practice, nurses are accountable for their actions, the quality of care delivered and record-keeping, according to *The Code* (Nursing and Midwifery Council 2018).

STRAP CHANGING

◎ EQUIPMENT

- Trolley
- Non-sterile medical examination gloves and apron
- Face mask
- Dressing pack
- Normal saline (hospital) or tap water (community) and non-woven swabs: woven gauze swabs and cotton wool must not be used for tracheostomy care, as fibres may break off and enter the respiratory tract
- Sterile tracheal dilators (should be available for the first 6 months post insertion)
- Sterile scissors
- Container of sterile water to clean the soiled inner tube
- Tracheostomy cleaning device
- Clean and dry covered container for spare inner cannula
- Appropriate tracheostomy dressing: not required if the stoma is healthy
- Velcro tube holder
- Spare clean inner cannula
- Barrier cream if required

GUIDELINES AND RATIONALE FOR THIS NURSING PRACTICE

- Explain the procedure to the patient
- Prepare a sterile dressing trolley with the items listed under 'Equipment'.
- Position the patient with the neck slightly extended.
- Apply an apron, perform hygienic hand hygiene and then put on non-sterile medical examination gloves.
- Perform suction, if required, prior to the procedure.
- Clean the stoma using non-woven swabs and normal saline, checking the area for irritation and integrity of stoma. Gently pat dry.
- Change the inner tube with a clean cannula.
- Change the straps. Practitioner 1 holds the tracheostomy tube while practitioner 2 removes the tapes and dressing.
- Discard the old straps and apply a new tracheostomy dressing.
- Resecure the tube using an appropriate tie. Allow one finger distance between the tie and neck skin (McGrath 2014).

ADDITIONAL INFORMATION

Humidification

The presence of a tracheostomy tube means that the normal route of airflow via the nose and nasal passages is bypassed. It is therefore important to ensure that air entering the tracheostomy tube is humidified and in some cases warmed. Dry humidification can be achieved by attaching a heat moisture exchange system to the end of the tube, which will conserve heat and moisture on expiration via the tube and filter air entry. By providing humidification in this way, the risk of tube blockage, crusting and damage to the lungs is reduced.

Cleaning an Inner Tube

The cleaning of the inner tube should take place every 4 hours or as required by your patient. Using a clean technique, the inner tube can be turned anti-clockwise, removed and cleansed using bottled sterile water (McGrath 2014). The tube is then dried using sterile gauze swabs and reinserted. Prior to cleansing the tube a spare inner tube should be inserted. The use of brushes is no longer advocated in the cleansing of tracheostomy tubes, as damage can be sustained to the side of the plastic tube. Current practice is to clean inner tubes using disposable tracheostomy tube-cleaning swabs, which are single-use items.

While cleaning the inner tube, take the opportunity to inspect the skin around the stoma site to determine whether it requires cleansing and a new dressing. This will avoid the need to do so later and will reduce the amount of manipulation around the tracheostomy.

PATIENT/CARER EDUCATION: KEY POINTS

Patient/carer education depends on the nurse having the necessary knowledge, skills and competence to provide meaningful explanations and support. In partnership with the patient and/or carer, ensure that they are competent to carry out any practices required. Information should be given on an appropriate point of contact for any concerns that may arise. The use of daily tracheostomy care checklists is advocated as good practice (McGrath 2014).

Patients require planned education to help them cope with the anxiety that most people experience when they first have a tracheostomy. If the tracheostomy tube does not have a speaking cap, they will need help and advice about alternative ways of communicating.

Patients who have permanent tracheostomies will require a structured teaching programme of self-care.

REFERENCES

Council of the Intensive Care Society Standards, 2014. Standards for the care of adult patients with a temporary Tracheostomy; STANDARDS AND GUIDELINES. Available from: https://www.theawsomecourse.co.uk/ICS/ICS%20Tracheostomy%20standards%20(2014).pdf.

Dhillon, R.S., East, C.A., 2013. Ear, Nose and Throat and Head and Neck Surgery, 4th ed. Churchill Livingstone Elsevier, Edinburgh.

Eibling, D., Roberson, D., 2012. Managing tracheotomy risk: time to look beyond hospital discharge. The Laryngoscope 122 (1), 23–24.

Everitt, E., 2016. Tracheostomy 3: care of patients with permanent tracheostomy. Nursing Times 112 (21/22/23), 17–19.

Hashmi, N., Ransom, E., Nardone, H., et al., 2010. Quality of Life and Self-image in Patients Undergoing Tracheostomy. The Laryngoscope 120 (S4), S196. Available from: https://doi.org/10.1002/lary.21663.

McGrath, B.A., 2014. Comprehensive Tracheostomy Care: The National Tracheostomy Safety Project Manual. Wiley-Blackwell, Sussex.

National Confidential Enquiry into Patient Outcome and Death (2014). On the Right Trach? A review of the care received by patients who underwent a tracheostomy. Available from: https://www.ncepod.org.uk/2014tc.html.

National Tracheostomy Safety Project, 2016. Emergency Tracheostomy Management Algorithm. Available at: https://www.tracheostomy.org.

Nursing and Midwifery Council (NMC), 2018. The Code: Professional Standards of Practice and Behaviour for Nurses, Midwives and Nursing Associates. NMC, London. Available at: https://www.nmc.org.uk/globalassets/sitedocuments/nmc-publications/nmc-code.pdf.

Paul, F., 2010. Tracheostomy care and management in general wards and community settings: literature review. Nursing in Critical Care 15 (2), 76–85.

? SELF-ASSESSMENT

1. List three indications as to why your patient may have a tracheostomy.
2. While nursing a patient who has a temporary double-lumen tracheostomy tube in place, the tube blocks. What do you do?
3. Identify the means by which you, the nurse, could ensure effective communication with a patient who has a tracheostomy tube in situ.
4. What kind of dressing should be applied around a tracheostomy tube?
5. Write brief notes on the key practices that will ensure that the risk of potential complications is reduced.

Venepuncture

INDICATIONS AND RATIONALE FOR VENEPUNCTURE

Venepuncture (also known as phlebotomy) is the action of extracting a sample of blood from a vein for diagnostic purposes (Hobson 2008).

Venepuncture may be performed:

- *To obtain a specimen of blood for clinical analysis.* This may include measuring electrolyte, haemoglobin or antibody levels, or checking for the presence (and type) of microbes to aid in the monitoring and diagnosis of disease.
- *To obtain a specimen of blood to monitor the therapeutic response to treatments.* This could include monitoring the levels of a drug in the body to ensure that this is an effective dose or to assess toxicity.
- *To obtain a specimen of blood as part of the process of cross-matching for blood transfusion.* This is done to ensure that the correct blood type is safely administered.

OUTLINE OF THE PROCEDURE

Venepuncture is the action of entering a vein with a needle and remains the most commonly performed invasive healthcare procedure in the United Kingdom (Dougherty 2008). In order to perform the procedure safely and effectively, the nurse must act in accordance with evidence-based guidelines and have a good level of knowledge and understanding in relation to relevant anatomy and physiology (Ahlin et al. 2017; Hobson 2008). Furthermore, the procedure requires a range of skills, including patient assessment, manual dexterity and effective communication.

The Nursing and Midwifery Council (2018a) now includes venepuncture and cannulation among the recognized nursing procedures in which the newly registered nurse must be able to demonstrate proficiency.

PSYCHOLOGICAL ISSUES AND VASOVAGAL REACTIONS

Although venepuncture and cannulation are considered to be largely routine procedures, they can still be frightening to patients, particularly if they are unfamiliar with the procedure (Weinstein 2007). Taking a confident approach and explaining the procedure can help to reduce patient anxiety (Dougherty 2012).

It is acknowledged that humans have a natural tendency to feel squeamish at the sight of blood or when experiencing pain, and that can give rise to feelings of faintness and nausea (Dougherty 2012). Furthermore, with activation of the sympathetic nervous system (through the 'fight or flight' response), heart rate and blood pressure are increased temporarily before a rapid fall in both of these occurs, which in susceptible patients can cause fainting – known as a vasovagal reaction (Ritz et al. 2010). For this reason, the nurse should ensure that the patient is in a comfortable and supported position; a reclining chair is ideal. Privacy and dignity must be maintained throughout the procedure.

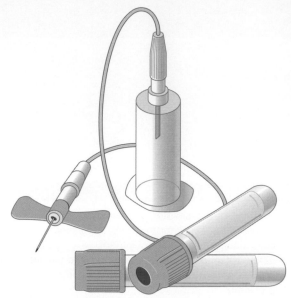

Fig. 39.1 Sterile needle device: winged infusion device – 'butterfly' needle – with safety feature.

GUIDELINES AND RATIONALE FOR THIS NURSING PRACTICE

- Prepare the equipment, ensuring that the correct blood bottles are available, as stipulated on the blood test request form, along with appropriately sized needles that are suitable to the patient's veins (you may want to have a selection of sizes available), *to ensure that you are well prepared and have all necessary equipment close to hand.*

- Check the identity of the patient, discuss the procedure and obtain informed consent *to ensure that the blood test is taken from the intended patient* (if blood is taken from the incorrect patient, this could have severe adverse consequences through misdiagnosis or the giving of the wrong blood type to a patient). An identity check should include the patient's full name and date of birth, and this should be confirmed verbally with the patient (where possible), against their identification band and against the blood sample request form – follow local policy. Encourage the patient to identify any issues that may have occurred when previously undergoing venepuncture (e.g. fainting, difficulty finding a vein, needle-phobia) *to ensure that you are well prepared for any event.*

- Position the patient appropriately so that that they are comfortable and not at risk of falling if they faint. Both arms should be exposed, and a pillow placed under the chosen arm for venepuncture will help to support the arm and facilitate easier access. Ensure good lighting to help visualize the vein. Privacy must be maintained. Follow these practices *to facilitate easier extraction of blood, to reduce risk of patient injury and to lessen anxiety and/or embarrassment.*

- Wash your hands with suitable liquid soap and warm water, and dry thoroughly; alternatively, decontaminate with alcohol gel *to reduce the risk of cross-infection*

(World Health Organization 2018). Apply a plastic disposable apron.

- Visually inspect both arms to check for any areas of bruising, infection, oedema, injury, phlebitis or the presence of any vascular access devices; these should be avoided where possible (Dougherty 2016). Apply a single-use disposable tourniquet approximately 7–8 cm above the chosen venepuncture site. The tourniquet should be tight enough to constrict the vein and promote venous distension but must not be too tight, as this can obstruct arterial blood flow; take care not to pinch the skin with the tourniquet, as this will cause pain and injury (Dougherty 2008). Work in this way *to ensure that veins are fully distended and easy to locate, and to facilitate effective venepuncture with minimal discomfort.*

- Repeated venepuncture can be traumatic for the patient and can damage blood vessels (Dougherty 2008). It is therefore important to choose an appropriate site that will give the best chance of successfully performing venepuncture with the minimum number of attempts.

- The superficial veins of the lower part of the arms are the most commonly used, as they are located close to the surface of the skin and tend to be easily accessible (Dougherty 2008). The antecubital veins (median cubital, median cephalic, and median basilica) are generally the most suitable for venepuncture, as they are large, well anchored and close to the surface (Dougherty 2008) (Fig. 39.2).

- With the tourniquet in place, palpation is used to feel the vein, assessing its quality and suitability for venepuncture; the index finger and third forefinger should normally be used. Stroking the vein downwards and watching the venous refill can help to assess the quality of the vein: a good venous refill suggests that the vein will be amenable to venepuncture. Importantly, this process also helps the practitioner to distinguish between veins and arteries (arteries must be avoided), and to feel for any valves within the veins (Dougherty 2008). On palpation the vein should ideally have soft and bouncy characteristics, refill quickly after being compressed, and be visible, straight and securely anchored to underlying supporting tissues (Dougherty 2008). Once a suitable site and vein have been selected, the tourniquet should be released, remembering that this must not be left in situ for longer than 1 minute, as this can lead to inaccuracies in the blood results and cause patient discomfort (Dougherty 2016). The nurse must have knowledge of anatomy of the lower arm and avoid nerves and arteries (*see* Fig. 39.2). Follow these practices *to ensure that the most clinically appropriate venepuncture site and vein are selected, and that arteries and nerves are avoided.*

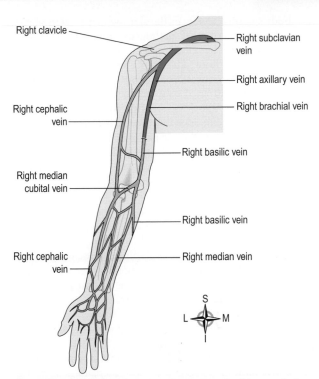

Fig. 39.2 The antecubital veins. Reproduced with permission from Waugh A, Grant A: Ross and Wilson Anatomy & Physiology in Health and Illness, ed 12, Edinburgh, 2014, Churchill Livingstone Elsevier, Fig. 5.37, p. 108.

- With an appropriate site located and the vein fully assessed, select the most appropriately sized needle for the blood extraction. A 21G needle tends to be standard, while smaller needles such as a 23G may be used for smaller, more fragile veins, e.g. in frail elderly patients. Follow these practices *to ensure that the most appropriate equipment is used to facilitate the venepuncture.*

- The hands must now be washed again (as above) *to reduce the risk of cross-infection*, and gloves applied *to reduce the risk of transmission of blood-borne infections, protecting the nurse and the patient* (World Health Organization 2018).

- Reapply the tourniquet (as detailed above) *to make the chosen vein become prominent again, facilitating easier access.*

- The patient's skin must now be cleansed using an appropriate cleansing solution. Dougherty (2008) highlights the fact that asepsis is essential when performing venepuncture, as the procedure involves breaching the body's natural defence (the skin) with a foreign object, risking the entry of pathogens from the healthcare practitioner, the environment or the patient's own resident skin flora. The choice of skin-cleaning agent will depend on local protocol but will commonly be an alcohol-impregnated swab or chlorhexidine solution. It is essential to allow the solution to evaporate fully (at least 30 seconds); once this process has been completed, it is important for the site not to be touched or palpated again (Dougherty 2012). If repalpation is necessary, then the skin-cleansing process must be completed again *to reduce the risk of pathogens entering the patient's bloodstream.*

- If using a safety needle device and holder, these should be assembled following the manufacturer's instructions. If a 'butterfly'-type needle is being used, this should be removed from the sterile packaging and the wings folded upwards and inwards in preparation for use. Asepsis must be maintained. Follow these practices *to prepare the equipment and maintain asepsis.*
- With the tourniquet still in situ and the skin cleansed ready for venepuncture, your non-dominant hand should be used to apply light skin traction below the intended venepuncture site *to stabilize the vein and prevent any movement.*
- Smoothly insert the needle with the bevel facing upwards at an angle of approximately 10–30 degrees (De Verteuil 2011). Advance the needle until it is in the lumen of the vein, taking care not to advance it too far and puncture the back of the vein, as this will cause bleeding, bruising and possible haematoma. Once a 'flashback' of blood is seen in the blood collection equipment chamber or tubing, the needle has entered the vein. If you are using a 'butterfly' device, the wings should be folded back down *to obtain the required blood sample safely.*
- Keeping the equipment as stable as possible, attach the blood collection bottle to the other end of the tubing, or advance the collection bottle into the blood bottle holder. These collection bottles have a vacuum within them that will draw the blood from the vein and fill the bottle *to obtain the required blood sample safely* (Fig. 39.3).
- Once the required blood sample has been obtained, the collection bottle should be disconnected. Where more than one sample of blood is needed, it is important to ensure that the blood bottles are used in the correct order, as cross-contamination of the bottles' reagents can affect the accuracy of results (Dojcinovska 2011). Follow these practices *to ensure that blood samples are correctly obtained and that accurate results are returned.*

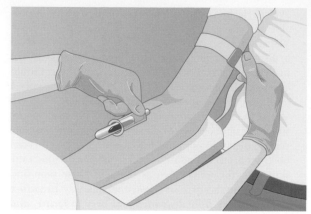

Fig. 39.3 Obtaining the required blood sample.

- Release the tourniquet, withdraw the needle from the patient's arm and apply firm pressure using a gauze swab until any bleeding has stopped, *to prevent bleeding and reduce any bruising.*
- The used needle must be disposed of safely and immediately in a suitable sharps container in line with local policy, *to prevent the risk of needle-stick injury and the risk of transmission of blood-borne infections.*
- After ensuring that the patient does not have any allergies to such dressings, an adhesive plaster can then be applied *to cover the puncture site, keeping it clean and dry.*
- Label all blood bottles meticulously to eliminate any risk of misidentification, which could lead to adverse clinical outcomes, *to ensure that blood results are accurate and results are assigned to the correct patient.*
- When the procedure has been completed, ensure that the patient is left feeling comfortable. Dispose of any contaminated equipment, remove gloves and apron, and dispose of all of them safely in line with local policy. Wash and dry your hands thoroughly *to reduce the risk of cross-infection.*
- Provide the patient (and carer, if present and appropriate) with information in relation to self-care following the procedure (see 'Patient/Carer Education').
- Arrange safe transfer of the blood specimen to the laboratory in a timely fashion in line with local policy.
- Document the procedure, noting any adverse reactions, *to ensure accurate record-keeping in line with your NMC requirements* (Nursing and Midwifery Council 2018b).

PATIENT/CARER EDUCATION: KEY POINTS

Prior to performing the nursing practice, it is important for the nurse to discuss any potential adverse effects or complications. This is part of the process of gaining informed consent (Nursing and Midwifery Council 2018b).

Before certain blood tests are taken, the patient may be required to modify their diet or to fast (e.g. for certain cholesterol investigations or fasting blood glucose levels). If this is the case, this needs to be clearly explained and a rationale provided.

Certain blood tests may require additional information from the patient/carer, e.g. when they last took a particular medication, when they last drank alcohol, or whether or not they may be pregnant or menstruating. This information should be obtained sensitively through effective communication to maintain patient dignity and confidentiality.

Following the venepuncture, the nurse must ensure that the patient is left comfortable. They should be aware of who to contact should they encounter any complications following the procedure, e.g. bleeding, excessive bruising, pain, swelling, or pins and needles/tingling (which may indicate nerve damage).

Patients/carers should be advised that the plaster should be removed 24–48 hours following the venepuncture.

REFERENCES

Ahlin, C., Klang-Söderkvist, B., Johansson, E., et al., 2017. Assessing nursing students' knowledge and skills in performing venepuncture and inserting peripheral venous catheters. Nurse Education in Practice 23, 8–14. Available from: https://doi.org/10.1016/j.nepr.2017.01.003.

De Verteuil, A., 2011. Procedures for Venepuncture and Cannulation. In: Phillips, S., Collins, M., Dougherty, L. (Eds.), Venepuncture and Cannulation. Blackwell, Oxford, pp. 131–174.

Dojcinovska, M., 2011. Selection of equipment. In: Phillips, S., Collins, M., Dougherty, L. (Eds.), Procedures for Venepuncture and Cannulation. Wiley-Blackwell, Oxford.

Dougherty, L., 2008. Obtaining peripheral venous access. Intravenous Therapy in Nursing Practice 225–270.

Dougherty, L., 2012. Venepuncture. In: O'Brien, L. (Ed.), District Nursing Manual of Clinical Procedures. Wiley-Blackwell, Oxford.

Dougherty, L., 2016. Venepuncture using a needle and holder Available from: https://www.clinicalskills.net.

Hobson, P., 2008. Venepuncture and cannulation: theoretical aspects. British Journal of Healthcare Assistants 2 (2), 75–78. Available from: https://doi.org/10.12968/bjha.2008.2.2.28386.

Nursing and Midwifery Council, 2018a. Future Nurse: Standards of Proficiency for Registered Nurses. NMC, London. Available at: https://www.nmc.org.uk/globalassets/sitedocuments/education-standards/future-nurse-proficiencies.pdf.

Nursing and Midwifery Council, 2018b. The Code: Professional Standards of Practice and Behaviour for Nurses, Midwives and Nursing Associates. NMC, London. Available at: https://www.nmc.org.uk/globalassets/sitedocuments/nmc-publications/nmc-code.pdf.

Ritz, T., Meuret, A., Ayala, E., 2010. The psychophysiology of blood-injection-injury phobia: looking beyond the diphasic response paradigm. International Journal of Psychophysiology 78 (1), 50–67. Available from: https://doi.org/10.1016/j.ijpsycho.2010.05.007.

Weinstein, S.M., 2007. Plumer's Principles and Practice of Intravenous Therapy. Lippincott Williams & Wilkins, Philadelphia.

World Health Organization, 2018. Five moments for hand hygiene. Available from: http://www.who.int/gpsc/tools/Five_moments/en.

SELF-ASSESSMENT

1. Which veins of the arm are usually most suitable for venepuncture, and why?
2. Why is it important to ensure that the patient is in a comfortable and well-supported position before undertaking this nursing practice?
3. Why is the consideration of patient skin cleansing important prior to undertaking this nursing practice?
4. What are the potential complications of venepuncture?

Wound Care

There are three parts to this chapter:

1. Wound bed preparation
2. Wound drain care
3. Removal of stitches, clips and staples.

The concluding boxes, 'Patient/Carer Education: Key Points' and 'Self-Assessment', refer to the chapter as a whole.

LEARNING OUTCOMES

By the end of this chapter, you should be able to:
- assess the patient for these three nursing practices
- collect and prepare appropriate equipment
- carry out these nursing practices.

BACKGROUND KNOWLEDGE REQUIRED

- Revision of the physiology of wound healing and the factors that affect wound healing
- Revision of the principles of wound assessment
- Review of existing local policy and national guidelines regarding all three components of this chapter
- Review of the common wound dressings available and their individual properties (in hospitals, available dressings may vary depending on stock held by the pharmacy; in the community setting, a wider selection is usually accessible)

The concept of wound care is vast, with an ever-evolving knowledge base offering direction for best practice. This chapter therefore presents the basic knowledge required for these practices and encourages you to reflect on your own learning needs to develop a relevant knowledge base. References and useful web addresses are provided at the end of this chapter as a starting point for this process.

1. WOUND BED PREPARATION

INDICATIONS AND RATIONALE FOR WOUND BED PREPARATION

Wound bed preparation is a process that assists in optimizing conditions at the wound bed to encourage healing. This process requires the nurse to have a basic knowledge of the physiology of the stages of wound healing, as this will help in understanding the reasons why some wounds fail to heal effectively and/or quickly.

The main aims of wound bed preparation are:

- to *provide a method for continual assessment of the wound bed for tissue type*
- *to monitor and treat any signs or symptoms of critical colonization or clinical infection appropriately*
- *to address any moisture imbalance evident in the wound bed* by either rehydrating sloughy or necrotic tissue, or removing excess volumes of exudate
- *to monitor the edges of the wound for signs and symptoms of effective healing.*

ASSESSMENT

The first step of wound bed preparation should focus on the holistic assessment of the patient, not the wound (Flanagan 2013). Wound assessment tools are of value within this process, as they provide prompting and direction for appropriate care (Brown 2015). The tool chosen should address both local and systemic factors that may have an impact on the ability of the patient to heal effectively (Brown 2015). Examples of local factors that may need to be addressed include pressure area assessments, continence assessments and evidence of trauma. Examples of systemic factors include peripheral vascular disease, immunosuppression and nutritional status. Once these have been identified, action must be taken to rectify any unmet need that might delay effective wound healing, such as:

- use of specialist pressure-reducing or continence equipment
- referral on to relevant members of the multidisciplinary team.

Assessment tools also collect basic information, such as the position and depth of the wound; the cause of the wound, e.g. trauma, surgical incision; how long the wound has been there; and any allergies the patient may have to previously tried dressings. The use of clinically assessed, research-based assessment tools offers not only a direction for care but also a means of objective monitoring that can be used within clinical audit. Pressure ulcers can be graded by means of recognized classification scales, a process that will help in the accurate description of these wounds (Charlton 2014; Chamanga et al. 2015).

A grid map can be used to assess the original size of a wound and consequent changes to size and tissue type on the wound bed. Care should be taken, however, to ensure that consensus is reached within the clinical area in relation to the counting of the squares within the wound bed (Hampton 2015). Photography may be used to record both the size and the tissue type of the wound bed effectively; this should be done in conjunction with local protocols to adhere to legal requirements including the Data Protection Act (DOH 2018). The Joint Commission (2011) has produced standards in relation to the use of photography in patient care. Again, knowledge of local guidelines and protocols should guide practice (Spear 2011).

A Doppler ultrasound can also be used by skilled personnel as part of the holistic assessment of leg ulcers to determine if the ulcer has developed as a result of venous, arterial or mixed aetiology disease, and to assist and guide the management of the leg ulcer (Furlong 2013; Benbow 2014). This is important, as treatment will vary significantly depending on the result of this test. Vascular wounds will require referral to a vascular clinic for further assessment, while venous leg ulcers are appropriate for compression bandaging. Assessment, clinical investigation and application of compression bandaging should be undertaken only by healthcare professionals educated in leg ulcer management, as badly applied bandaging can cause damage to the lower limb (Benbow 2014).

Tissue Type

Appropriate identification of tissue type on the wound bed determines the wound status and directs treatment (Benbow 2016). There are five main types of tissue found in wounds, and a popular way to describe these types objectively is by colour (Benbow 2016).

- black – necrotic
- yellow – sloughy
- green – infected

- red – granulating
- pink – epithelializing.

Infection

Wounds that are taking longer to heal than expected but do not appear clinically infected should be assessed for 'critical colonization'. This means that bacteria in the wound are of a great enough number to compete for existing nutrients and oxygen against healthy cells, but are not of a great enough number to cause a clinically infected wound (Hughes 2016). Signs of critical colonization include delayed healing, wound breakdown and discoloration of the granulation tissue from red to dusky red/purple.

Clinically infected wounds will require further assessment by medical staff to assess if an antibiotic is required. Critically colonized wounds will benefit from the use of dressings that contain broad-spectrum antimicrobial properties, such as silver or iodine (Leaper et al. 2012; Chamanga et al. 2015). It is important to note that these dressings are expensive and require frequent reassessment to ensure their effectiveness. Once healthy tissue is observed in the wound bed, these dressings can be stopped and other dressings can be applied (Hughes 2016).

Moisture

An assessment of the volume, colour and viscosity of any exudate present should be included (Leaper et al. 2012). If there is too little exudate, a scab (eschar) will form, precluding the moist, warm environment required for effective wound healing. High volumes of exudate will have an impact on surrounding tissue, causing maceration and preventing the wound from healing further. Dressings for necrotic (black) or sloughy (yellow) tissue with low volumes of exudate should be chosen to rehydrate the eschar or slough, e.g. hydrogels or hydrocolloids. Wounds with high volumes of exudate require dressings that will absorb the exudates effectively, e.g. foams or hydrofibres.

Wound Edges

As already stated, excess volumes of exudates will have a detrimental effect on surrounding tissue. Assessment should also involve gentle probing of the wound margins to rule out any undermining of tissue. In a healing wound the margins advance across the wound bed, thereby leading to an epithelialized (pink) wound. If this process fails, reassessment is required to identify the cause of this failure.

WOUND CLEANSING

Though it was once a routine procedure, it is important for the nurse to question the need for wound cleansing prior to each individual dressing change. Evidence suggests, however, that cleansing the wound bed can improve the wound environment and accelerate healing. Residual debris on the wound bed can provide an environment that encourages bacterial growth and prevent healing (Wilkins & Unverdorben 2013). Hughes (2016) suggests that wound cleansing may be necessary only under certain circumstances:

- when specifically indicated by the dressing manufacturer, e.g. hydrogels, alginates
- when assistance is needed in visualizing the wound bed, removing debris, non-viable tissue and moderate to severe exudate.

If cleansing is indicated, informed decision-making should direct the choice of fluid chosen. Tap water can be used to irrigate wounds, with no greater incidence of wound infection compared to normal saline (Ljubic 2013); however, risk assessment guidelines should be followed to ensure the quality of the water used (Ljubic 2013). No other fluid, e.g. chlorhexidine or betadine, should be used to cleanse a wound unless required by a specific aseptic technique or requested by a clinical specialist with research to support the request (Wilkins & Unverdorben 2013).

Reference should be made to the use of an aseptic technique, once a routine procedure, within this discussion. A risk assessment will direct the nurse in the appropriate decision as to whether this practice is necessary. For certain procedures, e.g. care of a Hickman line, an aseptic technique is vital to protect the patient from infection. However, in general, chronic wounds, e.g. leg ulcers and pressure ulcers (Hughes 2016), do not require an aseptic technique.

CHOOSING A WOUND DRESSING

Nurses are accountable for administering topical preparations, as they are for the administration of all other medicines, so they must be familiar with the properties and side-effects of any wound care products they are using. Wound products should protect surrounding healthy skin, support autolytic debridement, and absorb exudate to provide optimal wound healing (Dhivya et al. 2015). Up-to-date information on these preparations is available from the *British National Formulary*. Dressings should provide a moist, warm environment for optimum wound healing to occur (Dhivya et al. 2015). They should also:

- be impermeable to bacteria
- be non-toxic and non-allergenic
- be comfortable and conformable for the patient to wear
- protect the wound from further trauma
- require infrequent dressing changes
- be cost-effective
- have a long shelf life
- be available in both hospital and community settings.

In addition to these qualities, it is also important for the dressing to have the necessary physiological and biochemical properties to facilitate wound healing at a cellular level. Tissue viability nurse specialists offer a wealth of knowledge in wound healing and treatment options, and are available in both acute and community settings for support for complex or delayed healing wounds.

Larval therapy also provides an option for the debridement of necrotic or sloughy wounds (Naik & Harding 2017). Available on prescription, the larvae ingest dead tissue without affecting healthy tissue and can also be used when a wound is infected; indeed, research shows that they may be effective in eradicating meticillin-resistant *Staphylococcus aureus* (MRSA) from infected wounds (Naik & Harding 2017).

Due to budgetary constraints, ward-based nurses may have a limited number of dressings available via the pharmacy. Within the community, most District Nurses have undertaken a nationally accredited course to enable them to prescribe from a wide range of wound care products. Nurse prescribers must ensure that they seek current evidence-based practice to ensure that decision-making is grounded in a balance of cost-effectiveness and the proven effectiveness of the dressing. The Nursing and Midwifery Council (2018) also states that nurse prescribers must remain up to date with knowledge and skills to enable them to prescribe competently and safely.

WOUND ASSESSMENT AND NON-ASEPTIC DRESSING CHANGE

> ◎ **EQUIPMENT**
>
> - Drape/towel
> - Wound assessment tool
> - Grid or camera
> - Dressing pack or swabs (only if required)
> - Flat surface
> - Gloves and apron
> - Disposal bag
> - Water or normal saline (only if required)
> - Alcohol-based hand rub
> - Clean scissors (to cut tape or the dressing to fit the wound)
> - Appropriate dressings or securing bandage, if required

For many dressings a dressing pack will not be required. Simple dressings will require removal of the old dressing and application of a new dressing. Since all dressings are packaged within a sterile field, careful removal of these dressings negates the need for any further sterile field to lay them on. In an institutional environment, the number of air-borne pathogenic microorganisms can be reduced by working in a well-ventilated room used solely for procedures involving aseptic technique, or by performing procedures at least 30 minutes after the completion of ward cleaning and bed-making. This may not always be possible in the home setting, where the community nurse has little control over the environment.

There is no need for the nurse to wear a disposable cap or face mask, but verbal communication should be kept to a minimum during the aseptic technique in order to reduce droplet contamination. When a number of aseptic wound dressings are to be performed, a known contaminated and/or infected wound should be treated last to reduce environmental contamination.

GUIDELINES AND RATIONALE FOR THIS NURSING PRACTICE

- Explain the nursing practice to the patient *to gain consent and cooperation.*
- Collect and prepare the equipment required *to ensure that it is available and ready for use.*
- Ensure the patient's privacy *to reduce anxiety.*
- Help the patient into a comfortable position *to create a sense of well-being.*
- Place a drape or towel under the wound if possible, *to protect the bed/chair/floor from potential leakage of exudates and/or from irrigation fluid (if used).*
- Wash your hands and apply gloves and apron *to reduce cross-infection.*
- Remove any existing dressing *to allow a clear assessment of the wound.*
- Use an appropriate wound assessment tool to assess the patient and the wound bed, *to ensure a holistic assessment of the patient.*
- Assess and record the shape of the wound using a measured grid tracing or grid camera *to permit changes to the wound shape to be noted.* If a camera is used, the appropriate paperwork must be completed to ensure both consent and legal ownership of the photos (Hampton 2015).
- Assess wound bed tissue; any evidence of infection; volume of exudates and wound edges exudate, *to assist with the decision-making process to determine the choice of dressing.*
- Assess and document the wound bed tissue type *to provide information regarding the stage of healing.*
- Carry out a pain assessment *to determine the analgesic requirement and the timing of any medication required.*
- Discuss with the patient previous treatments and their effect, allergies and dressing preferences *to increase concordance with the treatment regime.*

- Decide on the most appropriate dressing for the presenting wound (if this is different from the existing dressing, remove and dispose of gloves; collect the new dressing; wash your hands again and apply new gloves) *to ensure effective treatment for the patient.*
- Irrigate the wound with either warm saline or tap water only if indicated, *to ensure that research-based practice is followed.*
- Apply an appropriate dressing.
- Following the initial assessment, evaluate the wound at regular intervals *to monitor the overall progress of the wound.*
- Ensure that the patient is left feeling as comfortable as possible, *to maintain the quality of this nursing practice.*
- Dispose of the equipment safely *to reduce any health hazard.*
- Document the nursing practice appropriately, monitor the after-effects and report any abnormal findings *to provide a written record and assist in the implementation of any action, should an abnormality or adverse reaction to the practice be noted.*
- In undertaking this practice, nurses are accountable for their actions, the quality of care delivered and record-keeping, according to *The Code*, which includes record-keeping (Nursing and Midwifery Council 2018).

Thorough hand-washing **prior** to the dressing must be performed, further hand preparation being carried out **during** the aseptic technique, as stated in the guidelines just described, and when the nurse accidentally contaminates their hands. An alcohol-based hand rub is used for the subsequent hand preparation; it has the benefit that the nurse does not have to leave the patient during the practice.

It is preferable for the skin-cleansing lotion to be supplied as an individual single-use sterile sachet or bottle. Once a bottle has been opened, environmental contamination can occur and so any residual lotion should be discarded. If an aerosol can of irrigating fluid is used, the nurse should ensure that the dispensing nozzle does not become contaminated and therefore act as a source of infection.

ASEPTIC DRESSING CHANGE

⊚ EQUIPMENT

- Dressings trolley, or an appropriate clean surface if in the patient's home
- Sterile dressing pack containing a gallipot or similar container, low-linting swabs, disposable forceps, a drape and a disposal bag
- Normal saline (if wound irrigation is indicated)

EQUIPMENT—cont'd

- Ethyl alcohol 70%
- Sterile 10 mL syringe for irrigating the wound: may not be required, as some solutions are packaged to allow irrigation
- Additional sterile dressing material: usually packed separately
- Sterile disposable gloves
- Hypoallergenic tape
- Clean pair of scissors for cutting the tape
- Clean disposable plastic apron
- Alcohol-based hand preparation lotion
- Appropriate dressings or securing bandage, if required
- Receptacle for soiled disposable items

GUIDELINES AND RATIONALE FOR THIS NURSING PRACTICE

The guidelines for this procedure are similar, whether it takes place within a hospital setting or within a patient's home. The obvious difference is that within the hospital a dressing trolley will be available; within a patient's home there will be vastly differing levels of cleanliness. An experienced community nurse will adhere as closely to an aseptic technique as the environment allows.

- Explain the nursing practice to the patient *to gain informed consent and cooperation* (Nursing and Midwifery Council 2018).
- Use a treatment room for wound dressing *to reduce the incidence of cross-infection*. If one is not available, prepare the environment around the patient's bed appropriately. If in the community, identify an adequate surface.
- Wash your hands *to reduce the risk of cross-infection*.
- If using a dressing trolley, wash thoroughly with detergent and water, and then dry it *to provide a socially clean surface*.
- Disinfect the dressings trolley with 70% ethyl alcohol immediately prior to every dressing undertaken *to reduce the number of microorganisms on the trolley surface*.
- Collect and prepare the equipment, check the packaging for damage such as tears or leakage, and check the expiry dates of all the materials to be used, *to ensure that the equipment has not been contaminated*.
- In the hospital, place all the equipment on the bottom shelf of the trolley, preferably in order of use, *to leave the top shelf free and clean during the practice and to permit easy access to the equipment*.
- Ensure the patient's privacy *to reduce anxiety*.
- Observe the patient throughout this activity, *to note any signs of distress*.

- In the hospital, adjust the position of the bed *to ensure safe working practice and the most comfortable position to carry out this procedure*.
- Help the patient into a comfortable position *to allow the position to be maintained during the practice*.
- Adjust the patient's clothing, exposing the wound area, *to give the nurse easy access to the wound*.
- Wash your hands *to reduce the risk of cross-infection*.
- Apply the plastic disposable apron *to prevent microorganisms adhering to the nurse's uniform*, which could be a source of cross-infection.
- Open the outer packaging of the dressing pack and slip the contents on to the top shelf of the dressings trolley or flat surface, *to allow the inner cover of the dressing pack to come into contact with a clean surface*.
- Loosen the outer dressing covering the patient's wound *to ease removal after commencing the dressing*.
- Wash your hands using bactericidal soap or an alcohol-based hand lotion *to reduce the risk of cross-infection*.
- Open the dressing pack, touching the sterile covering as little as possible *to reduce contamination from the dresser's hands*.
- Open any additional equipment and drop it on to the sterile field. If using a sachet of saline, pour the contents into the gallipot, *to prepare the equipment for use*.
- Wash the hands with alcohol-based lotion.
- Place one hand inside the disposal bag and arrange the contents of the dressing pack, *to reduce the risk of contamination*.
- With the hand still in the bag, remove the soiled dressing from the wound, *to remove contaminated material from the wound site*.
- Turn the bag inside out with soiled dressing inside and, if using a dressing trolley, attach it to the side of the trolley, below the level of the top shelf, *to reduce the risk of contamination*.
- Apply gloves *to prevent contact with body fluids*.
- Drape the wound with the sterile drape.
- Note the condition of the wound and the surrounding skin *to assess and evaluate the healing rate and identify potential problems*.
- If required, irrigate the wound, ensuring that the tip of the syringe or container does not come into contact with skin surface, *to remove debris without localized trauma*.
- Use the gauze swab to dry the surrounding skin, *to aid dressing adherence and prevent maceration of the skin*.
- Apply the appropriate dressing *to create the optimum wound-healing environment*.
- Discard the gloves or forceps, *to remove contaminated material*.
- *To maintain the position of the dressing*, secure it by the chosen method.

- Ensure that the patient is left feeling as comfortable as possible, *to maintain the quality of this nursing practice.*
- Dispose of all equipment safely *to reduce any health hazard.*
- Document this nursing practice appropriately, monitor the after-effects and report any abnormal findings immediately, *to provide a written record and assist in the implementation of any action, should an abnormality or adverse reaction to the practice be noted.*
- In undertaking this practice, nurses are accountable for their actions, the quality of care delivered and record-keeping according to *The Code* (Nursing and Midwifery Council 2018).

2. WOUND DRAIN CARE

INDICATIONS AND RATIONALE FOR WOUND DRAIN CARE

Wound drains are inserted at the time of surgical intervention by the medical practitioner *to prevent fluid collecting at the operation or wound site,* which may retard tissue healing. The extent and site of the surgery will influence the type and number of drains used. Drains may be inserted away from the original incision, to be dressed and to heal independently. This will help *to prevent the transmission of infection between the incision/operation site and the exit site for the wound drain.* Research studies discuss the need for wound drains following certain types of surgery, e.g. total hip arthroplasty, total knee replacement, abdominal surgery. The suggestion is that drains may not decrease the risk of postoperative wound infection or the development of haematomas; indeed, the presence of a wound drain may instead increase the risk of infection (Mujagic et al. 2019). Despite this emerging research, it remains important to have an understanding of the types of wound drain you may come into contact with and the appropriate nursing practice to manage them.

TYPES OF WOUND DRAIN

Hollow Plastic Tube

This is a deep drain with drainage holes at the proximal (drainage site) end, which is usually stitched in position and attached to a closed-circuit drainage bag. Such a drain may be used following major abdominal surgery to drain fluid collections.

Corrugated Rubber Drain

This is a superficial drain that usually drains directly into the dressing. It may be used to drain an incision site.

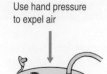

Use hand pressure to expel air

Replace stopper while maintaining pressure to create a vacuum

Fig. 40.1 Wound care: a portable vacuum drain.

T-Tube

A T-tube is a specialized tube inserted into the common bile duct following a cholecystectomy. It allows bile to drain into a closed circuit bag for 6–10 days postoperatively until normal drainage is re-established.

Portable Vacuum Suction Drain

This is a perforated plastic catheter attached to a specialized sterile vacuum suction bag (Fig. 40.1). Two or more may be attached to the same vacuum bag with a Y-connection. This system is used *to prevent the formation of a haematoma, by maintaining gentle suction.* It may be used following joint replacement surgery or surgery to the face or neck area, where fluid may collect rapidly because of the efficient local blood supply.

Soft Fluted Silicone Drain

This may be less painful than a rigid drain, especially if a large-calibre drain is required.

⊚ EQUIPMENT

- As for 'Aseptic Dressing Change' earlier

Additional Equipment as Required
- Sterile gloves: should be used when dressing wound drains to help to maintain asepsis
- Sterile scissors
- Sterile stitch-cutters
- Sterile drainage bag
- Portable wound suction equipment
- Sterile specialized keyhole dressing
- Extra sterile dressing material
- Sterile safety pin
- Sterile wound pads
- Measuring jug
- Sterile specimen container

GUIDELINES AND RATIONALE FOR THIS NURSING PRACTICE

- Explain the nursing practice *to the patient to gain consent and cooperation, and encourage participation in care.*
- Ensure the patient's privacy *to respect their individuality.*
- Help the patient into a comfortable position, depending on the area of the wound drain, *to ensure that the area for dressing is easily accessible and the patient is able to maintain the position with minimum distress.* In some instances, carefully timed, prescribed analgesia may be given *to ensure its maximum effect during wound care.*
- Observe the patient throughout this activity *to monitor any adverse effects.* This continual evaluation ensures that nursing or medical intervention can be altered as necessary.
- Collect and prepare the equipment *to ensure an efficient use of time and resources.*
- Remove the patient's clothes and covers from the area of the wound, ensuring that, with the exception of that area, the patient remains covered, *to expose only the site for wound care and respect the patient's dignity.*
- Perform the dressing for the surgical incision line first if necessary, maintaining asepsis. Dressings will usually be removed from the incision line after 24 hours and the wound may be covered by a plastic spray dressing *to encourage healing by first intention.* After this, only the drainage tube sites need to be dressed *to promote healing and prevent infection.*
- Prepare the sterile field for dressing the drainage tube site as an essential component of the aseptic technique.
- Put on sterile gloves after efficient hand-washing *to prevent any contamination with body fluids.*
- Proceed as for 'Aseptic Dressing Change' earlier until the drainage tube has been exposed.
- Cleanse the skin round the wound drain with normal saline (if required) and then dry surrounding skin *to allow any subsequent dressings to adhere properly.*
- Prepare a 'keyhole' dressing *to allow the dressing to fit snugly round the drain* (Fig. 40.2).
- Shorten the drain as ordered by the medical practitioner (see next section). This will depend on the healing process of the individual wound.
- Apply the keyhole or other dressing as required, *to maintain asepsis and promote healing.*
- Secure the dressing *to prevent its slipping.*
- Change the drainage bag and secure it in such a position *to ensure that gravity will help the fluid to drain away from the wound efficiently.*

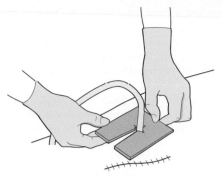

Fig. 40.2 Applying a keyhole dressing.

- Measure the drainage fluid and note its colour, consistency and smell *to monitor the process of healing and to be able to report any adverse condition.*
- Ensure that the patient is left as comfortable as possible *to create an environment that will promote healing.*
- Dispose of the equipment safely *to maintain a safe environment.*
- Document this nursing practice appropriately, monitor the after-effects and report any abnormal findings immediately *to ensure that any nursing or medical intervention can be evaluated and altered as required.*
- In undertaking this practice, nurses are accountable for their actions, the quality of care delivered and record-keeping, according to *The Code* (Nursing and Midwifery Council 2018).

Shortening Wound Drains

Deep wound drains may be shortened, as ordered by the medical practitioner, once or twice during the postoperative period as healing proceeds.

- Expose the drain site, maintaining asepsis and cleansing the skin as above. Sterile gloves should be worn after effective hand-washing *to prevent contamination with body fluids.*
- Remove any stitches holding the drain in position (*see* 'Removal of Stitches, Clips and Staples' later) *to release the drain.*
- Support the skin round the drain site with one hand, using a sterile swab, and gently withdraw the drain as far as ordered by the medical practitioner, e.g. 3–5 cm. Support the surrounding area *to reduce discomfort and prevent damage to healthy tissue.*
- Insert a sterile safety pin through the drain near the entry site *to prevent the drain from falling back into the wound.*
- Cut off the extra length of drain if necessary *to ensure that it lies neatly at the drain site and causes no*

discomfort. Drains attached to drainage bags will not need to be cut.

- Apply one sterile keyhole dressing under the safety pin and another over it, *to help to maintain the drain in position and prevent the safety pin from damaging the skin.*
- Secure the dressing in position *to prevent any drag on the drain or contamination of the wound.*
- Proceed as for the guidelines in the previous section.

Removing Wound Drains

Removal of wound drains will be ordered by the medical practitioner when there is no longer any significant drainage from the wound.

- Expose the drain site.
- The skin should be cleansed only if this is needed, *to ensure that the suture is visible.*
- Gloves should be worn *to prevent contamination with body fluids.*
- Release the vacuum or clamp the tubing *to prevent suction during removal,* which may cause tissue damage or pain.
- Remove any stitches holding the drain in position.
- Support the skin round the drain site with one hand, using a sterile swab, and gently withdraw the drain using either a sterile gloved hand or sterile forceps held in the other hand. Do this *to prevent damage to the surrounding tissues and to help to reduce discomfort, as well as maintaining asepsis.*
- Maintain pressure over the wound after the drain has been removed.
- The tip of the drain should be cut off with sterile scissors and placed in a sterile specimen container, maintaining asepsis, *if it is required for microbiological investigation.*
- Cleanse and dry the wound site again, if necessary.
- Apply and secure an appropriate sterile dressing *to maintain asepsis and promote healing.*
- Proceed as for the guidelines in the previous section.
- Immediately dispatch the labelled specimen to the laboratory, along with the completed form, *to enable investigative procedures to be completed as soon as possible.*

Emptying the Portable Wound Suction Container

The containers should be emptied as soon as they are no longer maintaining a vacuum suction, or every 12 hours as required, *to measure drainage and prevent ascending infection.*

As a wound drain is in direct contact with the underlying tissues, pathogenic microorganisms could gain entry to a wound through the drain site. The maintenance of a closed drainage system and aseptic technique may help to reduce the chance of wound infection.

- Clamp the drainage tubing above the level of the wound drainage container *to prevent backflow.*
- Remove the stopper or bung from the container, maintaining asepsis, *to release the vacuum.*
- Obtain a specimen of drainage fluid *for microbiological investigation if required.*
- Pour the remaining contents into a measuring jug, *avoiding contamination.*
- Wipe the outside of the entry channel with an alcohol solution, e.g. Mediswab, *to remove any drainage fluid that might cause infection.*
- Press the two rigid surfaces of the container together and maintain the pressure until the stopper is firmly in position. Once the pressure is removed, a gentle vacuum suction is created.
- Secure the drainage bag in position as before.
- Document the amount and details of the drainage fluid in the patient's records *to enable accurate monitoring of the healing process and an evaluation of treatment to continue.*
- In undertaking this practice, nurses are accountable for their actions, the quality of care delivered and record-keeping, according to *The Code* (Nursing and Midwifery Council 2018).

3. REMOVAL OF STITCHES, CLIPS AND STAPLES

INDICATIONS AND RATIONALE FOR REMOVAL OF STITCHES, CLIPS AND STAPLES

Following surgery, stitches, clips, staples or tissue glue/Superglue are used *to place the skin edges in apposition and promote rapid healing.* Unless absorbable, these are removed when there is:

- evidence that the wound has healed
- infection in part of the wound.

If the wound is greater than 15 cm in length or if healing is slow, alternate sutures or clips may be removed. The remaining sutures should be removed when clinically indicated.

Wounds that will heal quickly, requiring temporary support, are usually closed with absorbable sutures or glue. Non-absorbable material (staples, non-absorbable sutures) offers longer mechanical support.

Adhesive sutures are sometimes applied to the wound edges when healing is not complete. Some wounds are sutured using a subcuticular method or tissue glue, e.g. Dermabond; since biodegradable material is used, this does not require manual removal. Research studies demonstrate ongoing discussion surrounding the various methods for surgical wound closure (Levi et al. 2016) and the associated benefits and risks of each technique. Local preference will also influence the techniques used within different areas.

During suture, clip or staple removal, care must be taken to prevent the sharp equipment causing accidental injury to the patient.

◎ EQUIPMENT

- Dressing trolley or flat surface
- Sterile dressing pack
- Sterile normal saline: only if required to visualize the incision line
- Sterile stitch-cutter or scissors, clip or staple remover
- Receptacle for soiled disposable items

GUIDELINES AND RATIONALE FOR THIS NURSING PRACTICE

- Explain the procedure to the patient *to gain consent and cooperation.*
- Ensure the patient's privacy *to maintain dignity and a sense of self.*
- Collect the equipment *to help the efficiency of the practice.*

- Observe the patient throughout this activity *to detect any signs of discomfort or distress.*
- Clean the wound with normal saline only if it is necessary *to gain access to the stitches, clips or staples.*
- Examine the wound *to ensure that it is appropriate to remove the sutures or clips.*

Removing Sutures

There are two main types of suture: continuous and individual (Fig. 40.3). The method of removal is similar for both.

Removing Individual Stitches

- Hold the stitch-cutter or scissors in your dominant hand and the dissecting forceps in the other hand *to lift the knot of the stitch gently* (see Fig. 40.3A).
- Cut between the knot and the skin so that no part of the stitch above the skin surface is pulled under the tissues; then gently pull out the cut stitch. This helps *to reduce the risk of introducing infection.*
- Ensure that no piece of the stitch is left in the wound *to prevent the eventual formation of a wound sinus.*

Removing Continuous Stitches

- Hold the stitch-cutter or scissors in your dominant hand and the dissecting forceps in the other hand *to lift gently the knot at one end of the suture line* (see Fig. 40.3B).

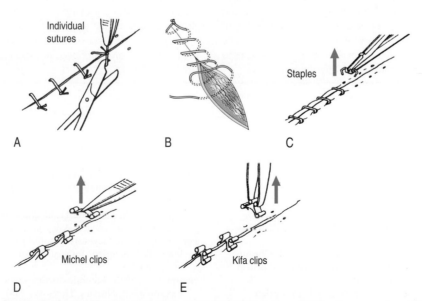

Fig. 40.3 Removal of sutures, clips and staples. (A) Individual suture. (B) Continuous suture. (C) Staples. (D) Michel clips. (E) Kifa clips.

- Cut between the knot and the skin, so that no part of the stitch above the skin surface is pulled under the tissues. This helps *to reduce the risk of introducing infection.*
- Grasp the knot at the other end of the suture line and pull gently away from the wound *to remove the total suture intact.*

Removing Clips or Staples

- Hold the remover in your dominant hand and the dissecting forceps in the other hand when removing clips or staples (*see* Fig. 40.3C–E).
- Steady the clips or staples with the dissecting forceps. Depending on the type of clip or staple, either insert one blade of the remover under the centre of the clip or staple and the other blade over it, then gently squeeze the blades together; alternatively, place one blade of the remover on the outside of each wing on top of the clip

and squeeze the blades together. Depending on the clip or staple type, one or other of these actions should *lift the clip from the skin on either side of the wound.*

Care After Removing all Types of Closure

- Follow local policy for the aftercare of a wound. The wound may be cleaned if necessary and then left exposed, or covered with a dressing if discharge is present.
- Ensure that the patient is left as comfortable as possible.
- Dispose of all equipment safely *to protect others.*
- Document the nursing practice appropriately, monitor the after-effects and report any abnormal findings immediately.
- In undertaking this practice, nurses are accountable for their actions, the quality of care delivered and record-keeping, according to *The Code* (Nursing and Midwifery Council 2018).

🖐 PATIENT/CARER EDUCATION: KEY POINTS

In partnership with the patient and/or carer, ensure that they are competent to carry out any practices required. Information should be given on an appropriate point of contact for any concerns that may arise.

The nurse should discuss the identified factors that may interfere with wound healing for each patient and, where possible, agree on realistic goals for these factors with the patient. The nurse should provide information and education for the patient and/or carer relating to the care of the wound between each dressing change. The community nurse should agree and confirm the place, date and time of the next dressing change with the patient.

At home, the patient or carer may assume some or all of the responsibility for wound care; the nurse therefore has an important role in the education of all concerned.

Some education and guidance may have to be given to allay patients' fears that the wound will open up once the clips or sutures have been removed. Advice and guidance should be given on any lifestyle restrictions. Smoking in particular should be discouraged, as it delays wound healing by causing vasoconstriction and reduced prostaglandin and fibrinogen production (McDaniel & Browning 2014).

REFERENCES

Benbow, M., 2014. An introduction and guide to effective Doppler assessment. British Journal of Community Nursing 19, S21–S26.

Benbow, M., 2016. Best practice in wound assessment. Nursing Standard 30 (29), 40.

Brown, A., 2015. The principles of holistic wound assessment. Nursing Times 111 (46), 14.

Chamanga, E.T., Hughes, M., Hilston, K., et al., 2015. Chronic wound bed preparation using a cleansing solution. British Journal of Nursing 24 (12), S30–S36.

Charlton, S., 2014. Pressure ulcer grading and appropriate equipment selection. British Journal of Nursing 23 (15), S4–S13.

Data Protection Act, 2018. Available at: https://www.legislation.gov.uk/ukpga/2018/12/pdfs/ukpga_20180012_en.pdf.

Dhivya, S., Padma, V.V., Santhini, E., 2015. Wound dressings – a review. Biomedicine / [Publiee Pour L'A.A.I.C.I.G.] 5 (4), 1–5.

Flanagan, M., 2013. Wound Healing and Skin Integrity Principles and Practice. Wiley-Blackwell, Oxford.

Furlong, W., 2013. How often should patients in compression have ABPI recorded? Journal of Community Nursing 27 (5), 60–62, 64–65.

Hampton, S., 2015. Accurate documentation and wound measurement. Nursing Times 111 (48), 16–19.

Hughes, M., 2016. Wound infection: a knowledge deficit that needs addressing. British Journal of Nursing 25 (6), S46.

Joint Commission, 2011. National Patient Safety Goals. https://www.jointcommission.org/standards_information/npsgs.aspx.

Leaper, D.J., Schultz, G., Carville, K., et al., 2012. Extending the TIME concept: what have we learned in the past 10 years? International Wound Journal 9 (2), 1–19.

Levi, K., Ichiryu, K., Kefel, P., et al., 2016. Mechanics of wound closure: emerging Tape-Based wound closure technology vs. Traditional methods. Cureus 8 (10), e827.

Ljubic, A., 2013. Cleansing chronic wounds with tap water or saline: a review. Journal of Community Nursing 27 (1), 19–21.

McDaniel, J.C., Browning, K.K., 2014. Smoking, chronic wound healing, and implications for evidence-based practice. Journal of Wound, Ostomy, and Continence Nursing 41 (5), E1–E2.

Mujagic, E., Zeindler, J., Coslovsky, M., et al., 2019. The association of surgical drains with surgical site infections – A prospective observational study. American Journal of Surgery 217 (1), 17–23.

Naik, G., Harding, K.G., 2017. Maggot debridement therapy: the current perspectives. Chronic Wound Care Management and Research 2017, 121–128.

Nursing and Midwifery Council, 2018. The Code: Professional Standards of Practice and Behaviour for Nurses, Midwives and Nursing Associates. NMC, London. Available at: https://www.nmc.org.uk/globalassets/sitedocuments/nmc-publications/nmc-code.pdf.

Spear, M., 2011. Wound photography: considerations and recommendations. Plastic Surgical Nursing 31 (2), 82.

Wilkins, R.G., Unverdorben, M., 2013. Wound cleaning and wound healing: a concise review. Advances in Skin & Wound Care 26 (4), 160–163.

WEBSITES

https://tvs.org.uk/ Tissue *Viability Society*
www.worldwidewounds.com/ *World Wide Wounds*
https://www.wounds-uk.com/ *Wounds UK*

SELF-ASSESSMENT

1. What is wound bed preparation?
2. List the five types of tissue to be found in wound beds.
3. What properties should you look for when choosing a dressing?
4. How do you decide whether to cleanse a wound or not?
5. Discuss the different types of ways to close a surgical wound.

Page numbers followed by "*f*" indicate figures, "*t*" indicate tables, and "*b*" indicate boxes.